Cancer and Pre-cancer of the Vulva

Edited by

David M Luesley MA, MD, FRCOG
Professor of Gynaecological Oncology, University of
Birmingham, UK

A member of the Hodder Headline Group
LONDON
Co-published in the USA by
Oxford University Press Inc., New York

First published in Great Britain in 2000 by
Arnold, a member of the Hodder Headline Group,
338 Euston Road, London NW1 3BH

http://www.arnoldpublishers.com

Co-published in the United States of America by
Oxford University Press Inc.,
198 Madison Avenue, New York, NY 10016
Oxford is a registered trademark of Oxford University Press

British Library Cataloguing in Publication Data
A catalogue record for this book is available from the British Library

Library of Congress Cataloging-in-Publication Data
A catalog record for this book is available from the Library of Congress

ISBN 0 340 74210 0 (hb)

1 2 3 4 5 6 7 8 9 10

Commissioning Editor: Joanna Koster
Project Editor: Sarah de Souza
Production Editor: Wendy Rooke
Production Controller: Sarah Kett

Typeset in 10/12pt Minion by J&L Composition Ltd, Filey, N. Yorks
Printed and bound in Great Britain by The Bath Press, Bath

What do you think about this book? Or any other Arnold title?
Please send your comments to feedback.arnold@hodder.co.uk

To Gabrielle for her support,
encouragement and understanding.

Contents

Contributors

Barbara L Andersen, PhD
Professor of Psychology, and Obstetrics and Gynecology, Department of Psychology, Ohio State University, 1885 Neil Ave, Columbus, OH 43210, USA

Anca C Ansink, MD PhD
Staff Specialist in Gynecological Oncology, Department of Obstetrics and Gynecology, Academic Medical Center, Meibergdreef 9, 1105 AZ Amsterdam, The Netherlands

Laurence JR Brown, MBBS, FRCPath
Consultant Histopathologist, Department of Histopathology, Leicester Royal Infirmary, Leicester, UK

Christopher P Crum, MD
Division of Women's and Perinatal Pathology, Department of Pathology, Brigham and Women's Hospital and Harvard Medical School, Boston, MA 02115, USA

George C Du Toit, MB, FCOG (SA), ChB, MMed,
Principle Specialist/Lecturer, Head, Unit of Gynaecological Oncology, Department of Obstetrics and Gynaecology, Tygerberg Hospital/University of Stellenbosch, Republic of South Africa

Patricia Eifel, MD
Professor of Radiation Oncology, Department of Radiation Oncology, The University of Texas MD Anderson Cancer Center, Houston, TX 77030, USA

C William Helm, FRCS, MRCOG, FACOG
Director, Division of Gynecologic Oncology, Temple University School of Medicine, 3401 N Broad St, Philadelphia, PA 19140, USA

Jonathan O Herod, MRCOG
Gynaecology Oncology Fellow, Department of Gynaecological Oncology, St Bartholomew's Hospital, Liverpool Women's Hospital, Crown Street, Liverpool L8 7SS, UK

Anuja Jhingran, MD
Assistant Professor of Radiation Oncology, Department of Radiation Oncology, The University of Texas MD Anderson Cancer Center, Houston, TX 77030, USA

Ronald W Jones, FRCS, FRCOG, FRANZCOG
Visiting Gynaecological Oncologist, Gynaecology Service, National Women's Hospital, and Clinical Reader in Gynaecological Oncology, The University of Auckland, PO Box 26090, Epsom, Auckland 3, New Zealand

Marjolein J Kagie, MD, PhD
Consultant Gynaecologist, Department of Obstetrics and Gynaecology, Medical Center Haaglanden, Location Westeinde, PO Box 432, 2501 CK Den Haag, The Netherlands

Frank G Lawton, MD, FRCOG
Consultant Gynaecological Cancer Surgeon, Department of Obstetrics and Gynaecology, King's College Hospital, Denmark Hill, London SE5 8RX, UK

Min-Chieh Lin, MD
Attending Pathologist, Department of Pathology, National Taiwan University Hospital, 7 Chung-Shan South Road, Taipei, Taiwan

Allan B MacLean, MD, FRCOG
Professor of Obstetrics and Gynaecology, University Department of Obstetrics and Gynaecology, Royal Free and University College Medical School, Rowland Hill Street, Hampstead, London NW3 2PF, UK

John B Murdoch, MD, MRCOG
Consultant Gynaecologist and Gynaecological Oncologist, Department of Gynaecology, St Michael's Hospital, United Bristol Healthcare Trust, Bristol BS2 8EG, UK

Álvaro Piazzetta Pinto, MD
Assistant Professor of Pathology, Constultant in Gynecological Pathology, Department of Pathology, Hospital de Clínicas, Universidade Federal do Paramá, Rua General Carneiro, 181, CEP 80069-900, Curitiba, Paraná, Brazil

Terence P Rollason, MB, ChB, FRCPath
Consultant Gynaecological Pathologist and Senior Clinical Lecturer in Pathology, Department of Pathology, Birmingham Women's Hospital, Edgbaston, Birmingham, UK

John H Shepherd, FRCS, FRCOG, FACOG
Consultant Gynaecological Surgeon and Oncologist, Department of Gynaecological Oncology, Directorate of Women's and Children's Health, King George Vth Block, St Bartholomew's Hospital, West Smithfield, London EC1A 7BE, UK

Mark E Sherman, MD
Associate Professor of Pathology, and Gynecology and
Obstetrics, and Visiting Scientist, National Cancer Institute,
Bethesda, Department of Pathology, Johns Hopkins
Medical Institutions, Ross 659, 720 Rutland Avenue,
Baltimore, MD 21205, USA

Frederick H Sillman, MD
Associate Professor, Gynaecology and Reproductive
Biology, Harvard Medical School; Attending, Brigham and
Women's and Massachusetts General Hospitals (partners),
Boston, MA 02115, USA

Susan R Sturgeon, DrPH
Epidemiologist, Division of Cancer Epidemiology and
Genetics, National Cancer Institute, 6120 Executive Blvd,
EPS-MSC 7334, Rockville, Bethesda, MD 20852, USA

Jacobus van der Velden, MD, PhD
Staff Specialist in Gynecological Oncology, Department of
Obstetrics and Gynecology, Academic Medical Center,
Meibergdreef 9, 1105 AZ Amsterdam, The Netherlands

Preface

Pre-malignant and malignant vulval diseases are uncommon. This fact may well have contributed to the relative neglect of the subject in standard texts. Although ovarian and cervical cancer in particular have held centre stage for many years, vulvar cancer has remained very much in the wings with at most a 'walk-on' role comprising one or two chapters in 'multisite' texts. This book attempts to remedy this situation by placing vulvar cancer 'centre stage'. Apart from previous omissions, there are other important reasons for providing a sharper focus on this particular problem.

Over the last 20 years there has been a considerable change in the approaches to management of vulval cancer. One must admit that this has been both gradual and based on just observational data, with few robust randomized clinical trials. One must also accept that, in the case of uncommon conditions, this is likely to be the case and, for this reason, those providing material for this book were asked specifically to synthesize and critically appraise what evidence was available. These data are far from ideal for generating change; nevertheless, it clearly demonstrates that change can take place and care can be improved by careful analyses of the available evidence. The driving-force for change has almost certainly been the need to minimize morbidity, both physical and psychological. The gradual realization of these objectives without the sacrifice of survival is encouraging, and these important lessons might now be applied to other gynaecological cancers. A final point is the increasing use of multimodality treatment. This has allowed a much more critical approach to the individual woman with cancer and has been facilitated considerably by significant moves towards team-working in gynaecological cancer.

In this book, we have tried to capture the feel of this change and the team approach. All of the major areas of care have been covered in some detail and, where doubt and confusion exists, this has been highlighted by posing arguments for and against, backed up by whatever data might be available. Those chapters dealing with pre-neoplastic conditions perhaps best exemplify this. The pathology, molecular basis and clinical perspectives have been approached, both comprehensively and critically, by acknowledged experts in their fields.

One might conclude by suggesting that a text devoted to a rare condition is unlikely to impact on a reading public already overwhelmed by a variety of information sources. I believe nothing could be further from the truth, as I also believe that, in precisely these areas, there is a need to bring together all of the information in a format that will provide sound and robust factual knowledge combined with the most contemporary thinking on the subject.

I am very much indebted to those who have provided chapters for this book, especially for following a fairly tight editorial brief. All of the contributors exceeded my expectations and made the editing process less daunting than I had originally thought it would be. I know they, like myself, can feel that this text fills an important niche in oncology as a whole and in gynaecological oncology in particular.

David M Luesley

Epidemiology: VIN and vulvar cancer

SR STURGEON, ME SHERMAN

This chapter summarizes our current knowledge regarding the epidemiology of vulvar intraepithelial neoplasia (VIN) and vulvar cancer, with an emphasis on recent research into the possible aetiological diversity of different histopathological types of vulvar cancer. Attention is focused on the emerging hypothesis that human papillomavirus (HPV) is related to most VINs and some vulvar cancers, but a proportion of invasive tumours is entirely unrelated. Other points of discussion include the potential role of cigarette smoking, other sexually transmitted viruses, diabetes, obesity and immunosuppression.

HISTOPATHOLOGY

The histopathology of vulvar cancer is reviewed in detail elsewhere in this volume (Chapters 2 and 3). Approximately 80 per cent of invasive vulvar cancers are squamous cell tumours; the remaining histological types include basal cell carcinoma, Paget's disease, adenocarcinomas, malignant melanoma, sarcoma and other rare neoplasms.[1] More recently, three histological subtypes of invasive squamous vulvar cancer have been described morphologically: (1) keratinizing squamous carcinoma (KSC); (2) basaloid carcinoma (BC); and (3) warty squamous carcinoma (WC). As these last two subtypes have been related to HPV, pathological and epidemiological studies have often combined them into one group (basaloid warty carcinoma or BWC).[2] Various small studies have found that between 50 per cent and 85 per cent of invasive vulvar cancers are KSC and that 15–50 per cent are BWC.[3–9] The proportion containing oncogenic types of HPV DNA appears to vary across these histological subtypes. HPV DNA has been detected in 4–39 per cent of KSCs using methods based on the polymerase chain reaction (PCR).[3,5,7–9] A higher proportion of BWC, between 50 per cent and 86 per cent, have been reported to be HPV DNA positive using PCR methodology.[3,5,7–9] Among women with invasive vulvar carcinoma, several studies suggest that women with HPV-positive tumours are younger than those with HPV-DNA-negative tumours.[2] It has also been reported that VIN 3 and BWC are more likely to be adjacent to cervical cancer and other lower genital tract tumours than KSC.[10]

Pathological data suggest that VIN 3 represents the precursor of BWC but not of KSC.[2] Between 50 per cent and 90 per cent of VIN 3 lesions have been found, in various studies, to contain HPV DNA.[10–15] In contrast to the variable proportion of HPV-DNA-positive vulvar cancers, HPV DNA is found in nearly all cervical intraepithelial neoplasia (CIN) lesions and invasive cervical cancers.[16] As in cervical cancer, HPV 16 is the most frequent type associated with vulvar cancer, but HPV 18, -31 and -45 play a much larger role in the cervix than in the vulva.[16]

Clinicopathological studies indicate that KSC may be more common than BWC, and that HPV is associated mainly with BWC and its precursor lesion, VIN 3. Investigation of a large, population-based series of VIN 3 and vulvar cancer is an essential next step in evaluating the relationship between histopathological types of vulvar cancer and HPV infection.

INCIDENCE AND MORTALITY

Invasive vulvar cancer is rare, with incidence rates rarely exceeding 2 per 100 000 women in different parts of the world. Variations between countries in the incidence of invasive vulvar cancer are generally unremarkable, with the possible exception that elevated rates have been reported from Portugal and parts of Brazil.[17] In the USA, the age-adjusted incidence rates of invasive vulvar cancer for 1990–94 among whites and blacks were 1.8 and 1.5, respectively.[18] As a point of reference, the age-adjusted incidence rates of invasive cervical cancer for 1990–94 among whites and blacks were 7.7 and 12.2, respectively.[18] Age-specific incidence rates of vulvar cancer and cervical cancer also vary dramatically. The incidence of squamous carcinoma of the cervix increases rapidly between the ages of 20 and 40 and then plateaus, whereas the incidence of vulvar cancer is low at younger ages and rises sharply only after the age of 50.[2]

Sturgeon and colleagues[1] examined the US incidence trends for VIN 3 and invasive squamous vulvar cancer between the period 1973–77 and 1985–87.

Invasive vulvar cancer rates among white women were remarkably stable during this period, with annual age-adjusted rates of 1.3 per 100 000 and 1.2 per 100 000 in 1973–77 and 1985–87, respectively. Consistent with clinical observations that vulvar cancer is a disease of older women, almost 80 per cent of the invasive squamous cases were diagnosed among women aged 55 years and older.

In contrast to the pattern for invasive cancer, the incidence of VIN 3 nearly doubled from 1.1 to 2.1 per 100 000 among white women during this same period, surpassing the rate for invasive squamous cell cancer. The largest proportional increase occurred among women younger than 35 years, for whom the rate almost tripled. The peak rate of VIN 3 shifted over this time period from women aged 35–54 years to those aged 35 years or younger.

Changes in sexual behaviour in the USA over the last several decades have translated into increases in the prevalence of HPV infection. Thus, changes in sexual behaviour may explain the increase in VIN 3 over time. Increasing detection and reporting, related partly to a better appreciation of the link between HPV and lower genital tract neoplasia of multiple sites, could also explain some of the rise. The discordant incidence trends for VIN 3 and invasive vulvar carcinoma are consistent with the hypothesis that almost all cases of VIN 3 are aetiologically linked to HPV, whereas significant numbers of invasive carcinomas are related to other factors. Alternatively, it is possible that the cohort of women affected by changes in sexual behaviour or other putative factors is not yet old enough to develop invasive vulvar cancer, or that early diagnosis and treatment of VIN 3 has blunted the anticipated increase in invasive vulvar cancer.

The age-adjusted mortality of vulvar cancer among both blacks and whites for 1990–94 was 0.3 per 100 000 women in the USA.[18] The mortality rate from this cancer declined by about 17.8 per cent between 1973 and 1994. The 5-year relative survival rate for vulvar cancer is approximately 75 per cent.

METHODOLOGICAL CONSIDERATIONS IN EVALUATING EPIDEMIOLOGICAL DATA

As a result of the rarity of vulvar cancer, only a few, relatively small, case–control studies have been performed.[19–23] Moreover, the validity of these studies has been limited by several methodological problems. Interview participation rates for vulvar cancer cases were between 60 per cent and 74 per cent in several investigations[19,23] and participation rates were even lower for the serological component of these studies.[9,24] Furthermore, one study did not investigate the potential aetiological role of sexually transmitted diseases[20] and two other investigations ascertained a history of sexually transmitted viruses by interview only.[21,22]

Many large epidemiological studies of cervical cancer and its precursor have used cytological samples collected in special buffers or frozen tissue for HPV-DNA testing. Epidemiological studies of vulvar cancer, by contrast, have relied on the detection of serum levels of antibodies to assess HPV exposure in cases and controls, a technique that is believed to be less sensitive and specific than detection of cellular HPV DNA. HPV-DNA testing in epidemiological studies of vulvar cancer has largely been carried out on formalin-fixed, paraffin-embedded tumour tissue, which is a technique that is historically less sensitive than testing fresh specimens.

As epidemiological studies of vulvar cancers have been limited by their small numbers and incomplete evaluation of HPV infection, investigators may have been unable to control adequately for potential confounding factors. Another limitation of published studies is that only one small study investigated the possibility that histologically distinct forms of squamous carcinoma may be aetiologically distinct.[13] The failure to analyse risk factors for different histological types of vulvar cancer separately may have led to an underestimation of the relevant risk factors for specific tumour types. Thus, the risk factors that have emerged from these studies (see below) remain to be confirmed in larger studies involving detailed histological information and epidemiological risk factor assessment.

BEHAVIOURAL CORRELATES OF SEXUALLY TRANSMITTED INFECTIONS

Several epidemiological studies have examined vulvar cancer risk and correlates of sexually transmitted infections, including number of sexual partners and age at first intercourse. Mabuchi and colleagues,[21] in a US case–control study consisting of 149 vulvar cancers of unspecified type, and a similar number of hospitalized controls, found no increased risk among women who had one or more sexual partners compared with women who had no partners. However, the effect on risk of increasing number of sexual partners was not

evaluated. In an Italian case–control study involving 73 invasive cases and 572 hospitalized controls,[22] no association was observed between number of sexual partners and vulvar cancer (relative risk or RR = 1.2, 95 per cent confidence interval or 95%CI = 0.4–4.1, for three or more partners versus one or no partners).

In two other larger case–control studies conducted in the USA, a positive association was observed between number of sexual partners and vulvar cancer.[19,23] A study of 209 vulvar cancer cases (96 VIN 3, 113 invasive) and 348 community controls reported that multiple sexual partners was a more convincing risk factor for VIN 3 than invasive vulvar cancer. For example, the RR associated with five to nine partners compared with no to one partner was 5.1 (95%CI = 1.7–14.8) for VIN 3 and 1.5 (95%CI = 0.6–3.9) for invasive cancer. Adjustment in these analyses was made for age, number of sexual partners, smoking, previous abnormal Papanicolaou smear and a history of genital warts. In a subsequent analysis involving a small subset of the subjects from this same study (48 cases of SC, 21 cases of BWC, 54 VIN 3 cases and 87 matched controls),[13] the age-adjusted RRs associated with two or more sexual partners were 2.2 (95%CI = 0.7–7.4) for KSC and 2.9 (95%CI = 1.0–8.4) for VIN 3. By contrast, the age-adjusted RR for BWC was 8.1 (95%CI = 1.7–37.9).

In another US case–control study of 180 VIN 3 cases, 53 invasive cases and 459 population-based controls,[23] women with 15 or more sexual partners had RRs of approximately sixfold and eightfold for invasive carcinoma and VIN 3, respectively. Adjustment in these analyses was made for age, education and age at first intercourse. In several studies,[19,23] early age at intercourse has not been related to vulvar cancer risk, after adjustment for number of sexual partners.

GENITAL WARTS

In an analysis of cancer registry data from Washington State between 1974 and 1981, it was noted that 16.6 per cent of women with squamous vulvar cancer had coexisting condyloma, compared with none of the women with non-squamous vulvar cancer.[25] These data, along with clinical observations that women with vulvar squamous tumours may have one or more condylomata,[26–30] led to the suggestion that genital warts are involved in the development of vulvar cancer.

In two subsequent case–control studies,[19,23] a self-reported history of genital warts was associated with substantially increased risks of vulvar cancer. One study reported RRs of 15.8 (95%CI = 8.4–29.8) for VIN 3 and 17.3 (95%CI = 6.3–47.2) for invasive disease.[23] In these analyses, adjustment was made for age, smoking, number of sexual partners and education. Comparable RRs in the study by Brinton and colleagues were 18.5 (95%CI = 5.5–62.5) and 14.6 (95%CI = 1.7–125.6).[19] Adjustment was made in this study for age, cigarette smoking, number of sexual partners and a previous abnormal Papanicolaou smear. In a reanalysis involving a subset of cases from this study,[13] a self-reported history of genital warts was reported by 21 per cent of the VIN 3 cases, 25 per cent of the BWC cases and none of the KSC cases. This observation supports the hypothesis that KSC is less clearly linked to a sexually transmitted agent such as HPV than BWC.

The interpretation of these data is puzzling because genital warts are usually caused by HPV 6 and HPV 11, HPV types that are not generally believed to be oncogenic.[31] Although the association between vulvar cancer risk and genital warts has been observed even for warts occurring 10 or more years before the diagnosis of vulvar cancer,[19,23] it is possible that some genital warts are an exophytic preinvasive phase of BWC. Other possible explanations are that women diagnosed with condyloma may tend to have infections with multiple HPV types or that a history of condyloma serves as a marker of poor host response.[19]

HUMAN PAPILLOMAVIRUS

Human papillomavirus is now known to be the major causal factor involved in the development of cervical cancer. As vulvar and cervical cancer often occur synchronously or asynchronously in the same patient,[32–36] it is often proposed that these two tumours share a common aetiology. Two epidemiological studies have examined the association between presence of serum antibodies to HPV 16 virus-like particles and risk of vulvar cancer.[9,24] In one study,[24] a much stronger association between HPV 16 seropositivity and disease was observed for VIN 3 (RR = 13.4; 95%CI = 3.9–46.5) than for invasive disease (RR = 2.9; 95%CI = 0.9–8.7). Adjustments in these analyses were made for herpes simplex virus (HSV), Chlamydia trachomatis, age, number of sexual partners, education, cigarette smok-ing and oral contraceptive use. Further analyses suggested that the association was stronger for BWC (RR = 3.8; 95%CI = 0.8–18.9) than for KSC (RR = 1.6; 95%CI = 0.4–7.4), but age was the only adjustment factor considered in these analyses.

In contrast, Madeleine and colleagues[9] reported that HPV 16 seropositivity was associated with similarly elevated risks for VIN 3 (RR = 3.6; 95%CI = 2.6–4.8) and invasive disease (RR = 2.8; 95%CI = 1.7–4.7). Adjustment was made in this study for age, education, smoking and body mass index (BMI). Furthermore, HPV 16 seropositivity was also associated with HPV-DNA-positive (RR = 4.5; 95%CI = 3.0–6.8) and -negative tumours (RR = 2.9; 95%CI = 1.6–5.0). The authors speculated that those seropositive case subjects whose tumours are HPV negative could be revealing a response to HPV infection that is no longer necessary to maintain the tumour, an infection that is unrelated to tumour development or methodological problems in the PCR or serological assays.

Human papillomavirus infection almost certainly plays a role in the aetiology of vulvar cancer, the molecular basis of which is explored further in Chapter 4. On present epidemiological evidence, it is unclear whether there is a subgroup of vulvar cancers that are non-HPV related.

OTHER SEXUALLY TRANSMITTED INFECTIOUS AGENTS

Although some studies have found associations between cervical cancer risk and serological markers of sexually transmitted infections, such as HSV 2 and Chlamydia trachomatis infections, it is difficult to rule out the possibility of confounding by HPV status.[37] Few epidemiological data are available to address the question of the role of specific infectious agents other than HPV in the development of vulvar cancer. In one case–control study,[24] HSV 2 seropositivity was associated with an increase in vulvar cancer risk, after adjustment for HPV 16 serology, Chlamydia trachomatis, cigarette smoking and oral contraceptive use (RR = 3.2; 95%CI = 1.0–10.0). In another study,[9] HSV 2 seropositivity was weakly associated with VIN 3 (RR = 1.9; 95%CI = 1.4–2.6) and invasive vulvar cancer (RR = 1.5; 95%CI = 0.9–2.6) after adjustment for age, HPV 16 serology, smoking and BMI.

Sherman and colleagues[23] found a modest association between a self-reported history of an infection with *Trichomonas vaginalis* and risk of VIN 3 (RR = 1.5), but an inverse association with invasive disease, after adjustment for age, number of partners, smoking, education, a history of genital warts and gonorrhoea. In the study by Hildesheim and colleagues,[24] *Chlamydia trachomatis* seroprevalence was associated with a 1.5-fold increase in vulvar cancer risk, decreasing to 1.4 (95%CI = 0.8–2.8), after adjustment for HPV 16 and other confounding factors. The interpretation of this finding is not clear because *Chlamydia* does not infect vulvar tissue. It is therefore likely that the modest association between *Chlamydia* and vulvar cancer risk represents confounding by HPV or other sexually transmitted infections.

There is some anecdotal evidence that syphilis is associated with vulvar cancer, especially in areas with high prevalence rates of this condition.[38,39] Several epidemiological studies have reported that cases are more likely than controls to have a self-reported history of syphilis or gonorrhoea,[21,23] but it is difficult to interpret these studies because of the rarity of these conditions and the potential for confounding by HPV status.

In summary, studies demonstrate inconsistent associations between sexually transmitted diseases other than HPV and vulvar cancer. It is unclear whether the associations observed between sexually transmitted diseases and vulvar cancer reflect incomplete control for HPV infection, a role for other sexually transmitted diseases as cofactors for progression of HPV infection to cancer or a separate aetiological role for some infectious diseases.

CIGARETTE SMOKING

Studies of cervical cancer have usually observed RRs of about 2 among cigarette smokers, but questions remain about whether these associations reflect confounding by HPV infection.[37] In the few studies that have examined the effects of smoking, controlling for HPV, no residual effect of smoking was observed.[40,41] A number of investigations that have not accounted for HPV status also reported a positive association between cigarette smoking, especially current use, and vulvar cancer.[19–21,42] Relative risks associated with current smoking in these studies have ranged from 1.5 to 4.8. Most of these studies reported a stronger association between cigarette smoking and VIN 3 compared with invasive disease.[19,20,42]

The relationship between cigarette smoking and vulvar cancer has been investigated in only two studies that included information on HPV infection. In an analysis of a subset of data from the original study by Hildesheim and colleagues,[24] the RR associated with early age at initiation of smoking remained elevated (RR = 1.7; 95%CI = 0.7–3.8), after adjustment for age, HPV 16 antibody serology, HSV, *Chlamydia trachomatis*, number of sexual partners, education and oral contraceptive use. In a reanalysis involving a larger study population than in the original investigation by Madeleine and colleagues,[9] current smoking was associated with VIN 3 (RR = 6.4; 95%CI = 4.4–9.3) and invasive disease (RR = 3.0; 95%CI = 1.7–5.3), after adjustment for age, education and HPV 16 antibody serology. Among current smokers, intensity and number of years smoked further increased the risk of disease.

It has been proposed that the immunosuppressive effects of cigarette smoke could enhance the persistence of HPV infection and, in turn, increase the risk of HPV-related tumours.[43] Some indirect support for this hypothesis is derived from the observation that cigarette smoking seems to be more strongly linked with VIN 3 as opposed to invasive vulvar cancers. Furthermore, two studies have reported that the effect of HPV antibody seropositivity on vulvar cancer risk is greater among cigarette smokers than among non-smokers.[9,24] As an interesting corollary, several studies have found a substantial degree of effect modification between genital warts and smoking.[19,23] For example, compared with non-smokers with no genital warts, smokers with genital warts had a 51-fold greater risk of developing vulvar cancer, after adjustment for age, number of sexual partners, cigarette smoking and a history of an abnormal Papanicolaou smear.[9]

Data on the role of cigarette smoking in non-HPV-related vulvar cancers are limited and conflicting. Trimble and colleagues[13] reported that ever smoking was associated with age-adjusted RRs of 4.9 (95%CI = 1.7–14.3) and 12.3 (95%CI = 1.5–101) for VIN 3 and BWC, respectively. By contrast, the age-adjusted RR for KSC, the histological type presumed to be unrelated to HPV, was 0.26 (95%CI = 0.1–0.8). Madeleine and colleagues[9] found that cigarette smoking was somewhat more strongly associated with HPV-DNA-positive than with HPV-DNA-negative tumours, but it still appeared to be an important risk factor for both tumour types, suggesting that cigarette smoking may play a role in HPV-related and non-HPV-related tumours.

OBESITY

Several case–control studies have examined the relationship between obesity and vulvar cancer risk. In a study restricted to invasive vulvar cancer, an age-adjusted RR of 2.3 (95%CI = 1.1–4.5) was observed among women with a body mass index (BMI, kg/m^2) of 30 or more compared with women with one of less than 25.[22] In another study,[44] an elevated risk of invasive disease (RR = 2.9; 95%CI = 1.5–5.8) but not VIN 3 (RR = 1.0; 95%CI = 0.7–1.5) was observed among women in the highest versus those in the lowest category of BMI. These analyses were adjusted for age, number of sexual partners, smoking, education and history of genital warts. Newcomb and colleagues[20] also found no association between weight at age 30 and risk of VIN 3 but heavier women, after adjustment for height, had a slightly higher risk of invasive cancer. Brinton and colleagues[19] reported that obesity was unrelated to risk of vulvar cancer (RR = 1.2 for BMI ≥ 25 versus < 21). A lack of association between weight at age 20 and 40 and vulvar cancer risk was also reported in another case–control study.[21] Risk estimates from the last two studies relate to a mixture of VIN 3 and invasive vulvar cancer cases. Overall, the data suggest, but do not conclusively demonstrate, that obesity may be a risk factor for invasive carcinoma but not for VIN 3. This pattern of findings has the potential to reveal an aetiological clue for non-HPV-related vulvar cancers. It is possible that chronic vulvar dermatitis involving the genital skinfolds of overweight women may be important. Other possible factors that may be involved include hyperinsulinaemia or insulin-like growth factors, which have been related to breast cancer in some studies.[45]

REPRODUCTIVE FACTORS

Although multiparity has been linked with cervical cancer risk,[40,41] there is little evidence that various reproductive factors are involved in the aetiology of vulvar cancer. In one study, multiparity was associated with an increased risk mainly of VIN 3,[20] but this finding was not replicated in another study.[44] Other studies have reported either an inverse association[21] or no association between parity and vulvar cancer.[19,22,23,44] Other reproductive variables, including age at first live birth, age at menarche and age at menopause, have also not been convincingly linked with vulvar cancer risk.[19–22,44]

EXOGENOUS HORMONES

Some experimental evidence suggests that hormones may enhance viral wart infections[46] and mediate the malignant transformation of HPV-infected cells.[47] There is some evidence that prolonged use of oral contraceptives may increase the risk of cervical cancer.[37] Newcomb and colleagues[20] reported a fourfold increase in risk associated with ever-use of oral contraceptives for VIN 3. These analyses were adjusted only for age, education and obesity. Sherman and colleagues[44] reported a slight increase in risk of VIN 3 associated with 5 or more years of oral contraceptive use (RR = 1.3), but an inverse association with invasive disease. These analyses were adjusted for age, number of sexual partners, smoking, education and a history of genital warts. Brinton and colleagues[19] also found a slight increase in risk of vulvar cancer with increasing years of use, rising to 1.3 among women who used oral contraceptives for 10 or more years. These analyses were adjusted for age, number of sexual partners, previous abnormal Papanicolaou smear, history of genital warts and current cigarette smoking. Menopausal oestrogens, with or without concomitant progestins, have not been associated with vulvar cancer risk, but few studies included women with extensive usage.[19,20]

MEDICAL HISTORY

Women with VIN 3 and invasive vulvar cancer are substantially more likely to have a history of anogenital tumours than women in the general population.[48] A number of other disorders have been linked with vulvar cancer clinically, but most of these associations have not been confirmed in epidemiological investigations. The association most deserving of additional attention is a possible link between diabetes and vulvar cancer risk. O'Mara and colleagues[49] reported a positive association between diabetes mellitus and a combined category of cancers of the vulva and vagina, after adjustment for age and obesity. The greatest risk was observed among women diagnosed with diabetes before the age of 29 years. In the case–control study by Newcomb and colleagues,[20] a history of diabetes was associated with an almost eightfold increase of invasive vulvar cancer, after controlling for age, education and obesity. By contrast, a history of diabetes was unrelated to risk of VIN 3. A history of diabetes was associated with a non-significant 1.3-fold increase in risk in the study by Brinton and colleagues.[19] This analysis was adjusted for age, education, number of sexual partners, oral contraceptive use and a prior abnormal Papanicolaou smear. In a study conducted in Israel, Voliovitch and colleagues[50] reported that the frequency of vulvar cancer patients with a history of diabetes was higher than in the general Jewish population of the same age range. Although Mabuchi and colleagues[21] observed no association between a history of diabetes and vulvar cancer risk, a limitation of this study is the use of hospitalized controls. Further exploration is needed on the possible role of chronic candidiasis with inflammation and the potential role of different types of diabetes in risk.

Most epidemiological studies have not found associations with hypertension,[19,21] gallbladder disease[19] or thyroid disease.[19,20] Newcomb and colleagues[20] reported a small non-significant association between hypertension and invasive disease but no association with VIN 3. In a retrospective cohort study of 3000 patients who had undergone cosmetic augmentation mammoplasty,[51] five vulvar cancers were observed where only one was expected. This finding may reflect various characteristics of the population compared with the general population, including number of sexual partners and cigarette smoking.

PERSONAL HYGIENE

At present there is no evidence that poor personal hygiene plays a role in the development of vulvar cancer. It has been reported that vulvar cancer is uncommon among orthodox Moslem women who wash after the acts of micturition and elimination.[52] However, the case–control study by Brinton and colleagues showed no relationship between risk and various hygiene factors, including number of times bathed per week, use of vaginal douches, use of vaginal deodorants and tampon use.[19]

DIET

Decreased consumption of fruit and vegetables has been linked with increased risk of various epithelial tumours, including cancer of the cervix.[53] Two studies have examined the relationship between dietary factors and risk of vulvar cancer. In the study by Sturgeon and colleagues,[54] the risk decreased with increasing consumption of dark yellow–orange vegetables, but the risk was unrelated to intake of dark-green vegetables, citrus fruits, legumes, and vitamins A and C and folate. Risk increased modestly with decreased intake of dark yellow–orange vegetables. Analyses were adjusted for age, cigarette smoking and number of sexual partners. Parazzini and colleagues[55] also found that the risk of invasive vulvar cancer was inversely related to green vegetable and carrot consumption, after adjustment for age, education and BMI.

Coffee drinkers were at increased risk of vulvar cancer in one study.[19] In another study,[54] however, the effect of coffee was modest and there were irregular changes in risk with increased frequency of coffee intake, after adjustment for age, cigarette smoking and number of sexual partners. Parazzini and colleagues[55] also found no association between coffee and vulvar cancer risk, after adjustment for age, education and BMI. Neither alcohol nor intake of specific types of alcoholic beverages has been shown to be associated with vulvar cancer risk.[54,55]

OCCUPATIONAL HISTORY AND CHEMICAL EXPOSURES

An increased risk of vulvar cancer has been found among maids and servants in private households and women employed in laundry, cleaning and other garment services.[21] It is possible, however, that these associations reflect confounding by sexual behaviour. There are also several case reports linking vulvar cancer to oil-saturated waste in cotton-mill workers[56] and to arsenic compounds on a tobacco farm.[57] Hennekens and colleagues[58] reported that the risk of developing vaginal/vulvar cancer was elevated among nurses in the USA who used permanent hair dyes, but adjustment was made only for age and cigarette smoking.

IMMUNOSUPPRESSION

Consistent with the presumption that immune impairment is involved in the acquisition or maintenance of HPV infection, numerous case–control and cohort studies have suggested a higher incidence of

CIN among transplant recipients than in the general population.[31] Data for vulvar cancer are much more sparse, but two cohort studies of organ transplant recipients have reported surprisingly high risks of vulvar cancer (observed to expected ratio or O:E = 56) or vulvar and vaginal cancer combined (O:E = 31).[59,60] By contrast, only four- to ninefold increases in cervical cancer risk were observed in these two studies. In another study, women with systemic lupus erythematosus, an autoimmune disease of unknown aetiology, were more likely to develop vulvar/vaginal cancer.[61] There are also various reports in the literature of VIN and invasive vulvar cancer among HIV-infected individuals, but the potential for confounding by sexual behaviour precludes any causal association with immune impairment.[62,63]

As HPV infection is very common in sexually active populations and major immunosuppressive states have been linked to increased risk of vulvar cancer, it is likely that host immune response to HPV is an important predictor of the risk of development of vulvar cancer. The importance of the host immune response has been demonstrated in several recent studies of cervical cancer.[64,65]

IONIZING RADIATION

Several studies have been performed to determine whether there is an increased risk of developing a second cancer in the genital area after pelvic irradiation. In two large multinational studies, each involving more than 150 000 cervical cancer patients, there was no evidence that radiotherapy increased the risk of vulvar cancer.[66,67] A subsequent study by Kleinerman and colleagues,[68] involving approximately 86 000 patients with cervical cancer, also found that vulvar cancer risk was similarly increased in irradiated (O:E = 4.4) and non-irradiated women (O:E = 3.5). However, the observation that risk tended to increase with increasing years since radiotherapy led the authors to speculate that radiotherapy may play a role in the development of vulvar cancer.

SCREENING

In several studies,[19,22] a history of prior Papanicolaou smears has been associated with a decreased risk of invasive vulvar cancer. As women participating in Pap smear programmes are likely to undergo physical pelvic examinations, it is possible that the protective effect is the result of the detection and treatment of cancer precursors.

SECOND PRIMARIES

Women with vulvar cancer have been shown to be at elevated risk of developing second primaries related to cigarette smoking, including cancers of the lung, oesophagus, buccal cavity and pharynx, and nasal cavity and larynx. Sturgeon and colleagues[69] reported that women with VIN 3 were 2.8 times more likely to develop smoking-related cancers than women in the general population. Women with invasive vulvar carcinoma had a 1.6-fold increased risk of developing smoking-related tumours. These data are consistent with epidemiological studies that suggest that cigarette smoking may be involved in vulvar cancer, particularly VIN 3.

Women with VIN 3 and invasive vulvar cancer have been found to be at increased risk of cancers of the cervix, vagina and anus.[69] This observation is consistent with the role of HPV infection in the development of several anogenital tumours. Sturgeon and colleagues[69] also found that women with VIN 3 and invasive vulvar cancer were also at increased risk of developing non-Hodgkin's lymphoma. As the women in whom non-Hodgkin's disease developed were elderly in this study, it seems unlikely that they were infected with HIV.

EPIDEMIOLOGICAL CORRELATES OF *p53* GENE MUTATION AND EXPRESSION

Most clinicopathological studies have demonstrated that *p53* abnormalities are uncommon in VIN. Kagie and colleagues[70] reported that *p53* was immunohistochemically detectable in 13–18 per cent of VIN lesions of varying grade associated with carcinomas compared with 13 per cent of tissues removed from normal women. Similarly, Kohlberger and colleagues[71] did not detect *p53* with immunohistochemistry in 28 VIN lesions not associated with carcinoma. HPV DNA was detected in 92.8 per cent of these cases. Kurvinen and colleagues[72] also did not identify *p53* mutations in exons 5 to 9 among eight cases of VIN or vulvar cancer tested with a single-strand conformation polymorphism analysis and DNA sequencing. In contrast, Milde-Langosch and colleagues[8] identified *p53* mutations and/or abnormal expression in VIN associated with carcinomas harbouring *p53* mutations. In summary, most data suggest that *p53* mutations are not related to VIN, a lesion that is linked to HPV infection.

Analysis of invasive carcinomas has also demonstrated that *p53* abnormalities are uncommon in HPV-related carcinomas. Lee and colleagues[73] detected a *p53* mutation in only 1 of 12 HPV-associated carcinomas, compared with four (44.4 per cent) of nine tumours that tested negative for HPV. One tumour contained HPV DNA and showed a *p53* mutation. Milde-Langosch and colleagues[8] reported that 52.5 per cent of vulvar carcinomas were associated with a *p53* mutation, compared with 7.8 per cent of cervical cancers. In this study, HPV was detected in 80.4 per cent of cervical cancers and only 27.5 per cent of vulvar cancers; however, *p53* mutations were not detected more commonly in HPV-negative as opposed to HPV-positive vulvar tumours. The authors noted that *p53* immunohistochemistry results and gene mutation analyses were not closely correlated. In contrast, Pilotti and colleagues[74] reported that HPV-related carcinomas contained wild-type *p53* as assessed with immunohistochemistry and molecular techniques, whereas 75 per cent of HPV-negative tumours showed *p53* mutations or expression.

In summary, data from several studies indicate that HPV-related VIN and cancers usually contain wild-type *p53*, whereas lesions unrelated to HPV are associated with *p53* abnormalities in a variable, but relatively small, percentage of cases. These data suggest two different aetiologies of vulvar carcinoma that share a common endpoint: inactivation of *p53* function. In HPV-related tumours, this is most probably accomplished through binding to HPV-E6 protein, with degradation via a ubiquitin-dependent pathway. In tumours unrelated to HPV, mutation leading to loss of *p53* function seems to be frequently involved. The molecular basis for vulvar oncogenesis is explored in more detail in Chapter 4.

Recently, Storey and colleagues[75] reported that a polymorphism in codon 72 of the *p53* gene renders the protein product more susceptible to degradation by the HPV oncogene E6, and confers an increased risk of cervical cancer compared with other *p53* alleles. If confirmed in large epidemiological studies of cervical cancer, this finding would suggest that the risk of HPV-related vulvar cancer might also involve a genetic component.

SQUAMOUS HYPERPLASIA

Kim and colleagues[76] studied the clonality of four invasive carcinomas associated with *p53* mutations and multiple adjacent areas of normal epithelium and squamous hyperplasia. The authors found that all three informative cancers were monoclonal with the assay used, whereas the adjacent normal and hyperplastic tissues were polyclonal and did not contain detectable *p53* mutations. The authors concluded that either *p53* mutation is a late event in vulvar carcinogenesis or squamous hyperplasia is not a precursor of these tumours. In contrast, Lin and colleagues[77] demonstrated that loss of heterozygosity was detectable in both squamous hyperplasia and atypical squamous hyperplasia (differentiated VIN), and that the pattern in the latter overlapped with an associated invasive carcinoma. Another study from the same laboratory[78] demonstrated monoclonality in six of eight evaluable hyperplasias, one of which was associated with lichen sclerosus. These authors suggested that hyperplasias deserve consideration as possible cancer precursors.

The relationship between lichen sclerosus and vulvar carcinoma has been a subject of controversy, but most studies suggest that the neoplastic potential of lichen sclerosus is minimal. The relationship between lichen sclerosus and other 'benign' maturation disorders and possible carcinogenesis is explored in detail in Chapter 6.

In summary, VIN is the likely precursor of HPV-related vulvar cancers, but the precursor(s) of vulvar carcinomas that are unrelated to HPV is unknown. Data concerning the neoplastic potential of atypical squamous hyperplasia are sparse and not derived from population-based studies. The association between lichen sclerosus and carcinoma is tenuous. Furthermore, the diagnostic reproducibility of non-neoplastic vulvar disease has not been established.

FUTURE DIRECTIONS

Human papillomavirus is a major risk factor for vulvar cancer but there is compelling evidence that some forms of vulvar cancer are non-HPV related. Pathologists have proposed a dualistic model of carcinogenesis based on histopathological classifications of vulvar cancer. In this model, BWCs are HPV-related tumours that arise from VIN 3. As in the cervix, it is postulated that the E6 and E7 HPV oncoproteins contribute to the development of these tumours by degrading the key cell cycle regulatory proteins p53 and retinoblastoma gene product. By contrast, KSCs are hypothesized to be unrelated to HPV. In these non-HPV-related tumours, *p53* mutation may play a role. Using large population-based studies, further research will be required to confirm this hypothesis. It is acknowledged that the rarity of vulvar cancer, and methodological difficulties related to the measurement of exposure to HPV infection, complicate the epidemiological study of this tumour. Additional research should also consider the possible role of cigarette smoking, other sexually transmitted infections, diabetes, obesity, exogenous hormones and immune response.

ACKNOWLEDGEMENTS

The authors gratefully acknowledge the thoughtful review of this chapter by Dr Robert J Kurman.

REFERENCES

1 Sturgeon SR, Brinton LA, Devesa SS, Kurman RJ. In situ and invasive vulvar cancer incidence trends (1973 to 1987). *Am J Obstet Gynecol* 1992; **166:** 1482–5.

2 Kurman RJ, Trimble CL, Shah KV. Human papillomavirus and the pathogenesis of vulvar carcinoma. *Curr Opin Obstet Gynecol* 1992; **4:** 582–5.

3 Monk BJ, Burger RA, Lin F, Parham G, Vasilev SA, Wilczynski SP. Prognostic significance of human papillomavirus DNA in vulvar carcinoma. *Obstet Gynecol* 1995; **85:** 709–15.

4 Kurman RJ, Toki T, Shiffman MH. Basaloid and warty carcinomas of the vulva. *Am J Surg Pathol* 1993; **17:** 133–45.

5 Hording U, Junge J, Daugaard S, Lundvall F, Poulsen H, Bock JE. Vulvar squamous cell carcinoma and papillomaviruses: indications for two different etiologies. *Gynecol Oncol* 1994; **52:** 241–6.

6 Trimble CL, Hildesheim A, Brinton LA, Shah KV, Kurman RJ. Heterogeneous etiology of squamous carcinoma of the vulva. *Obstet Gynecol* 1996; **87:** 59–64.

7 Toki T, Kurman RJ, Park JS, Kessis T, Daniel RW, Shah K. Probable nonpapillomavirus etiology of squamous cell carcinoma of the vulva in older women: A clinicopathologic study using in situ hybridization

and polymerase chain reaction. *Int J Gynecol Pathol* 1991; **10:** 107–25.

8 Milde-Langosch K, Albrecht K, Joram S, Schlechte H, Giessing M, Loning T. Presence and persistence of HPV infection and p53 mutation in cancer of the cervix uteri and vulva. *Int J Cancer* 1995; **63:** 639–45.

9 Madeleine MM, Daling JR, Carter JJ et al. Cofactors with human papillomavirus in a population-based study of vulvar cancer. *J Natl Cancer Inst* 1997; **89:** 1516–23.

10 Hording U, Daugaard S, Iversen AKN, Knudsen J, Bock JE, Norrild B. Human papillomavirus type 16 in vulvar carcinoma, vulvar intraepithelial neoplasia and associated cervical neoplasia. *Gynecol Oncol* 1991; **42:** 22–6.

11 Jones RW, Park JS, McLean MR, Shah KV. Human papillomavirus in women with vulvar intraepithelial neoplasia III. *J Reprod Med* 1990; **35:** 1124–6.

12 Park JS, Jones RW, McLean MR et al. Possible etiologic heterogenity of vulvar intraepithelial neoplasia. *Cancer* 1991; **67:** 1599–607.

13 Kagie MJ, Kenter GG, Zomerdijk-Nooijen Y, Hermans J, Schauring E, Timmers PJ, Trimbos JB, Fleuren GJ. Human papillomavirus infection in squamous cell carcinoma of the vulva, in various synchronous epithelial changes and in normal vulvar skin. *Gynecol Oncol* 1997; **67:** 178–83.

14 Junge J, Poulson H, Horn T, Hording U, Lundvall F. Prognosis of vulvar dysplasia and carcinoma in situ with special reference to histology and types of human papillomavirus (HPV). *AMPIS* 1997; **105:** 963–71.

15 Hording U, Daugaard S, Junge J, Ludvall F. Vulvar intraepithelial neoplasia III: a viral disease of undetermined progressive potential. *Gynecol Oncol* 1996; **56:** 276–9.

16 Bosch FX, Manos MM, Munoz N et al. Prevalence of human papillomavirus in cervical cancer: A worldwide perspective. *J Natl Cancer Inst* 1995; **87:** 796–802.

17 Parkin DM, Muir CS, Whelan SL, Gao YT, Ferlay J, Powell J (eds). *Cancer incidence in five continents*, Vol VI. *IARC Scientific Publications No. 120*, Lyon, IARC: 1992.

18 Ries LAG, Kosary CL, Hankey BF, Miller BA, Harras A, Edwards BK (eds). *SEER Cancer Statistics Review, 1973–1994*. NIH Pub. No. 97–2789. Bethesda, MD: National Cancer Institute, 1997.

19 Brinton LA, Nasca PC, Mallin K, Baptiste MS, Wilbanks GD, Richart RM. Case–control study of cancer of the vulva. *Obstet Gynecol* 1990; **75:** 859–66.

20 Newcomb PA, Weiss NS, Daling JR. Incidence of vulvar carcinoma in relation to menstrual, reproductive and medical factors. *J Natl Cancer Inst* 1984; **73**: 391–6.

21 Mabuchi K, Bross DS, Kessler II. Epidemiology of cancer of the vulva. A case–control study. *Cancer* 1985; **55**: 1843–8.

22 Parazzini F, La Veccia C, Garsia S et al. Determinants of invasive vulvar cancer risk: An Italian case–control study. *Gynecol Oncol* 1993; **48**: 50–5.

23 Sherman KJ, Daling JR, Chu J, Weiss NS, Ashley RL, Corey L. Genital warts, other sexually transmitted diseases, and vulvar cancer. *Epidemiology* 1991; **2**: 257–62.

24 Hildesheim A, Cheng-Long H, Brinton LA, Kurman RJ, Schiller JT. Human papillomavirus Type 16 and risk of preinvasive and invasive vulvar cancer: Results from a seroepidemiological case–control study. *Obstet Gynecol* 1997; **90**: 748–54.

25 Daling JR, Chu J, Weiss NS, Emel L, Tamini HK. The association of condylomata acuminata and squamous carcinoma of the vulva. *Br J Cancer* 1984; **50**: 533–5.

26 Buscema J, Woodruff JD, Parmley T et al. Carcinoma in situ of the vulva. *Obstet Gynecol* 1980; **55**: 225–30.

27 Friedrich EG Jr, Wilkinson EJ, Fu YS. Carcinoma in situ of the vulva. A continuing challenge. *Am J Obstet Gynecol* 1980; **136**: 830–43.

28 Rastkar G, Okagaki T, Twiggs LB, Clark BA. Early invasive and in situ warty carcinoma of the vulva: clinical, histologic, and electron microscopic study with particular reference to viral association. *Am J Obstet Gynecol* 1982; **143**: 814–20.

29 Kovi J, Tillman L, Lee SM. Malignant transformation of condyloma acuminatum. *Am J Clin Pathol* 1974; **61**: 702–10.

30 Woodruff JD, Julian C, Puray T, Mernut S, Katayama P. The contemporary challenge of carcinoma in situ of the vulva. *Am J Obset Gynecol* 1973; **115**: 677–86.

31 IARC. *Monographs on the evaluation of the carcinogenic risks to humans*, Vol 64. *Human papillomaviruses*. Lyon: IARC, 1995.

32 Figge DC, Gaudenz R. Invasive carcinoma of the vulva. *Am J Obstet Gynecol* 1974; **19**: 382–95.

33 Franklin EW, Rutledge FD. Epidemiology of epidermoid carcinoma of the vulva. *Obstet Gynecol* 1972; **39**: 165–72.

34 Japaze H, Garcia-Bunuel R, Woodruff JD. Primary vulvar neoplasia. A review of in situ and invasive carcinoma, 1935–1972. *Obstet Gynecol* 1977; **49**: 404–11.

35 Jimerson GK, Merrill JA. Multicentric squamous malignancy involving both cervix and vulva. *Cancer* 1970; **26**: 150–5.

36 Rose PG, Herterick EE, Boutselis JG, Moesberger M, Sachs L. Multiple primary neoplasms. *Am J Obstet Gynecol* 1987; **157**: 261–7.

37 Schiffman MH, Brinton LA, Devesa SS, Fraumeni JF Jr. Cervical cancer. In: Schottenfeld D, Fraumeni JF Jr (eds). *Cancer epidemiology and prevention*. New York: Oxford University Press, 1996: 1090–1116.

38 Sengupta BS. Carcinoma of the vulva in Jamaican women. *Acta Obstet Gynecol Scand* 1981; **60**: 537–44.

39 Hay DM, Cole FM. Primary invasive carcinoma of the vulva in Jamaica. *Obstet Gynaecol Br Commonwealth* 1969; **76**: 821–30.

40 Bosch FX, Munoz N, de Sanjose S et al. Risk factors for cervical cancer in Columbia and Spain. *Int J Cancer* 1992; **52**: 750–8.

41 Eluf-Neto J, Booth M, Munoz N, Bosch FX, Meijer CJLM, Walboomers JMM. Human papillomavirus and invasive cervical cancer in Brazil. *Br J Cancer* 1994; **69**: 114–19.

42 Daling JR, Sherman KJ, Hislop TG et al. Cigarette smoking and the risk of anogenital cancer. *Am J Epidemiol* 1992; **135**: 180–9.

43 Barton SE, Maddox PH, Jenkins D, Edwards R, Cuzick J, Singer A. Effect of cigarette smoking on cervical epithelial immunity: a mechanism for neoplastic change? *Lancet* 1988; **ii**: 652–4.

44 Sherman KJ, Daling JR, McKnight B, Chu J. Hormonal factors in vulvar cancer: A case–control study. *J Reprod Med* 1994; **39**: 857–61.

45 Kaaks R. Nutrition, hormones and breast cancer: Is insulin the missing link? *Cancer Causes Control* 1996; **62**: 403–6.

46 Crum CP, Burkett BJ. Papillomavirus and vulvovaginal neoplasia. *J Reprod Med* 1989; **34**: 566–71.

47 Weiss NS, Hill DA. Postmenopausal estrogens and progestogens and incidence of gynecologic cancer. *Maturitas* 1996; **23**: 235–9.

48 Sherman KJ, Daling JR, Chu J, McKnight B, Weiss NS. Multiple primary tumours in women with vulvar neoplasms: a case–control study. *Br J Cancer* 1988; **57**: 423–7.

49 O'Mara BA, Byers T, Schoenfeld E. Diabetes mellitus and cancer risk: A multisite case–control study. *J Chronic Dis* 1985; **38**: 435–41.

50 Voliovitch V, Menczer J, Modan M, Modan B. Clinical features of Jewish Israeli patients with squamous cell carcinoma of the vulva. *Isr J Med Sci* 1984; **20**: 421–5.

51 Deapen DM, Brody GS. Augmentation mammaplasty

and breast cancer: a 5-year update of the Los Angeles study. *Plas Reconstr Surg* 1992; **89:** 660–4.

52 Barber H. *Manual of gynecologic oncology.* Philadelphia: JP Lippincott Co., 1980.

53 Potischman N, Brinton LA. Nutrition and cervical neoplasia. *Cancer Causes Control* 1996; **7:** 113–26.

54 Sturgeon SR, Ziegler RG, Brinton LA, Nasca PC, Mallin K, Gridley G. Diet and the risk of vulvar cancer. *Ann Epidemiol* 1991; **1:** 427–37.

55 Parazzini F, Moroni S, Negri E, LaVecchia C, Pino DD, Cavalleri E. Selected food intake and risk of vulvar cancer. *Cancer* 1995; **76:** 2291–6.

56 Gerrard EA. Epithelioma vulvae as an occupational disease among cotton operatives. *Trans North Engl Obstet Gynaecol* 1932: 65.

57 Way S. Carcinoma of the vulva. *Am J Obstet Gynecol* 1960; **79:** 692–7.

58 Hennekens CH, Rosner B, Belanger C, Speizer FE, Bain CJ, Peto R. Use of permanent hair dyes and cancer among registered nurses. *Lancet* 1976; **i:** 1390–3.

59 Fairley CK, Sheil AGR, McNeil JJ et al. The risk of anogenital malignancies in dialysis and transplant patients. *Clin Nephrol* 1994; **41:** 101–5.

60 Birkeland SA, Storm HH, Lamm LU L et al. Cancer risk after renal transplantation in Nordic countries, 1964–1986. *Int J Cancer* 1995; **60:** 183–9.

61 Mellemkjaer L, Anderson V, Linet MS, Gridley G, Hoover R, Olsen JH. Non-Hodgkin's lymphoma and other cancers among a cohort of patients with systemic lupus erythematosis. *Arthritis Rheum* 1997; **40:** 761–8.

62 Wright TC, Koulos JP, Liu P, Sun XW. Invasive vulvar carcinoma in two women infected with human immunodeficiency virus. *Gynecol Oncol* 1996; **60:** 500–3.

63 Korn AP, Abercrombie PD, Foster A. Vulvar intraepithelial neoplasia in women infected with human imunodeficiency virus–1. *Gynecol Oncol* 1996; **61:** 384–6.

64 Tsuki T, Hildesheim A, Schiffman MH. Interleukin 2 production in vitro by peripheral lymphocytes in response to human papillomavirus-derived peptides: correlation with cervical pathology. *Cancer Res* 1996; **56:** 3967–74.

65 Clerici M, Merola M, Ferrario E. Cytokine production patterns in cervical intraepithelial neoplasia: Association with human papillomavirus infection. *J Natl Cancer Inst* 1997; **89:** 245–50.

66 Boice JD, Day NE, Andersen A et al. Second cancers following radiation treatment for cervical cancer. An international collaboration among cancer registries. *J Natl Cancer Inst* 1985; **74:** 955–75.

67 Boice JD, Engholm G, Kleinerman RA et al. Radiation dose and second cancer risk in patients treated for cancer of the cervix. *Radiat Res* 1988; **116:** 3–55.

68 Kleinerman RA, Boice JD, Storm HH et al. Second primary cancer after treatment for cervical cancer. *Cancer* 1995; **76:** 442–52.

69 Sturgeon SR, Curtis RE, Johnson K, Ries L, Brinton LA. Second primary cancers after vulvar and vaginal cancers. *Am J Obstet Gynecol* 1996; **174:** 929–33.

70 Kagie MJ, Kenter GG, Tollenaar RAEM, Herman J, Trimbos JB, Fleuren GJ. p53 protein overexpression, a frequent observation in squamous cell carcinoma of the vulva and in various synchronous vulvar epithelia, has no value as a prognostic parameter. *Int J Gynecol Pathol* 1997; **16:** 124–30.

71 Kohlberger PD, Kirnbauer R, Bancher D et al. Absence of p53 protein overexpression in precancerous lesions of the vulva. *Cancer* 1998; **82:** 323–7.

72 Kurvinen K, Tervahauta A, Syrjanen, Chang F, Syrjanen K. The state of the p53 gene in human papillomavirus (HPV)-positive and HPV-negative genital precancer lesions and carcinomas as determined by single-strand conformation polymorphism analysis and sequencing. *Anticancer Res* 1994; **14:** 177–82.

73 Lee YY, Wilczynski SP, Chumakov A, Chih D, Koeffler HP. Carcinoma of the vulva: HPV and p53. *Oncogene* 1994; **9:** 1655–9.

74 Pilotti S, Donghi R, D'Amato L et al. Papillomavirus, p53 alteration and primary carcinoma of the vulva. *Eur J Cancer* 1993; **29A:** 924–5.

75 Storey A, Thomas M, Kalita A et al. Role of p53 polymorphism in the development of human papillomavirus-associated cancer. *Nature* 1998; **393:** 229–34.

76 Kim Y, Thomas NF, Kessis TD, Wilkinson EJ, Hedrick L, Cho KR. p53 mutations and clonality in vulvar carcinomas and squamous hyperplasias: Evidence suggesting that squamous hyperplasias do not serve as direct precursors of human papillomavirus-negative vulvar carcinomas. *Human Pathol* 1996; **27:** 389–95.

77 Lin M, Mutter GL, Trivijisilp P, Boynton KA, Sun D, Crum CP. Patterns of allelic loss (LOS) in vulvar squamous carcinomas and adjacent noninvasive epithelia. *Am J Pathol* 1998; **152:** 1313–18.

78 Tate JE, Mutter GL, Boynton KA, Crum CP. Monoclonal origin of vulvar intraepithelial neoplasia and some vulvar hyperplasias. *Am J Pathol* 1997; **150:** 315–22.

2

Pathology of preinvasive lesions of the vulva

VULVA: ANATOMY AND LOCAL ENVIRONMENT

The vulva is a uniquely moist and usually occluded environment. This has an impact on the appearance of any vulvar skin condition. Clinically, keratotic areas tend to be white and often soggy, masking flaky exfoliation, whereas ulcerated or partially denuded foci remain moist and red without the development of a dry crust. These white and red patches have been recognized clinically in a constellation of obsolete terms that includes leukoplakia, neurodermatitis, atrophic vulvitis and kraurosis vulvae. Furthermore, the close apposition of skinfolds, particularly in overweight subjects, causes occlusion and friction leading to a degree of maceration. Supervening infection further changes the environment and clinical appearance.[1]

The vestibule and inner aspects of the labia minora are covered by skin-like mucous membrane, richly endowed with sebaceous glands. The outer aspects of the labia minora and labia majora are covered by skin. As both dermatologists and gynaecologists are involved in treating this area, the spread of interest across clinical disciplines has lead to a variety of terms for what are essentially the same conditions. Hence the dermatologists' lichen simplex chronicus shares many of the features of squamous hyperplasia, and probably

represents one end of the spectrum of changes in this condition.

The scope of vulval preinvasive disease includes:

- vulvar intraepithelial neoplasia (VIN):
  - warty VIN
  - basaloid VIN
  - squamous VIN
- extramammary Paget's disease
- in situ melanoma.

Other conditions in which a premalignant role is less well defined include:

- lichen sclerosus
- squamous hyperplasia
- lichen planus.

VULVAR INTRAEPITHELIAL NEOPLASIA

The concept of an intraepithelial precursor of vulvar squamous carcinoma, carcinoma in situ, although recognized for some time, was infrequently diagnosed before the second half of the twentieth century.[2] The term 'vulvar intraepithelial neoplasia' (VIN) was proposed in the early 1980s[3] to incorporate the full spectrum of grades of dysplasia, including carcinoma in situ, erythroplasia of Queyrat, hyperplastic dystrophy with atypia, bowenoid papulosis and Bowen's disease. The classification of VIN supported by the International Society for the Study of Vulvar Disease (ISSVD), the International Society of Gynaecological Pathology (ISGYP) and the World Health Organization (WHO) also includes Paget's disease and intraepithelial melanoma. However, it is common practice to use VIN to refer to squamous lesions and to use specific titles to identify the other two types. Only squamous VIN will be covered in this section.

Recent studies have shown that all grades of VIN are becoming more common.[2,4] The disease appears to be arising in a younger age group, mirroring the increase in the number of cases of squamous carcinoma of the vulva in young women[5–7] but not all studies show this trend.[8] The mean age of VIN has reduced from the sixth decade in 1960–70 to around 35 years in the mid-1990s.[6,9] The epidemiology of this condition and its invasive counterpart is discussed in greater detail in Chapter 1.

The initial descriptions detailed minor degrees of atypia limited to the basal one-third of the epithelium (VIN 1), more noticeable changes involving the basal two-thirds (VIN 2) and full-thickness dysplasia (VIN 3). However, this is a misleading, but unfortunately enduring, concept[9,6] that is actually refuted by the illustrations that were used to support it.[10] In all grades of VIN there are abnormal cells throughout the full

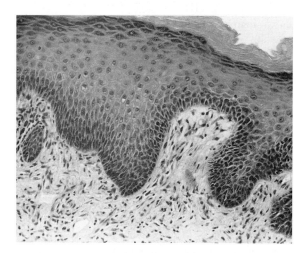

Figure 2.1 *Basaloid VIN 1 showing parabasal cells and mitoses limited to the lower third of the epithelial height. Note that all epithelial cells, including the surface layer, have significantly enlarged nuclei with prominent nucleoli. The surface is moderately keratinized.*

epithelial thickness: it is the degree of abnormality that grades the severity of the intraepithelial neoplasia (Fig. 2.1). A moment's consideration of the role of exfoliative cytology at this site[10] and in the cervix would show that, as cytological examination involves removal of largely surface cells, these must be abnormal in all grades for cytology to detect any change. If this were not the case, then cytology could detect only high-grade disease. It must follow that, even in low-grade intraepithelial neoplasia, VIN 1, cells at all levels of the epithelium are abnormal. Surface cells with enlarged hyperchromatic nuclei are clearly depicted through all grades of VIN in the original illustrations.[10]

Patients complain of pruritus, burning or pain depending on the location of the lesion. Vulvar swelling, discoloration, pigmented areas or discharge may be noted. On examination, affected areas may be red, white, warty or ulcerated, and there may be multiple symptoms and signs. VIN may be detected incidentally during cervical screening and colposcopy may reveal diffuse reddening or acetowhite areas. One-third of cases may exhibit multifocal involvement.[4,6,8,11] VIN may involve any part of the vulva, but most commonly affects the central areas, including the inner aspects of the labia minora, vestibule and introitus.[12] The posterior non-hair-bearing area, especially the fourchette, is commonly involved. The epithelium may be atrophic but is usually thickened up to 1.9 mm.[12] In about a third to a half of cases, VIN may extend along the pilosebaceous units of both the hair-bearing skin and the mucous membrane. Where the appendages are involved, VIN does not usually reach the deepest parts. The depth of VIN in appendages is 2.03–3.4 mm (hair-bearing) and 1.07 mm (non-hairy), measured from the bottom of the keratin/parakeratin layer, and up to 4.6 mm from the epithelial surface[12–14] (Fig. 2.2). The more recent studies, in which orientation of the sample and measurement have been meticulously controlled, have recommended that any laser ablation of VIN need not be deeper than 3 mm to avoid unnecessary damage to skin appendages and subcutaneous tissue.[12,14]

Current classifications of VIN distinguish basaloid and warty (bowenoid) forms. Common to all these forms is the presence of abnormal maturation and mitotic activity above the germinative layer of the epithelium. The lesions are graded 1–3 by:[15]

- the extent to which undifferentiated basaloid or parabasal cells extend through the height of the epithelium;
- the height at which abnormal mitoses, often tripo-

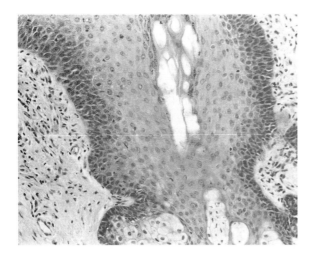

Figure 2.2 *Basaloid VIN 1 involving a sebeceous gland ostium. Although parabasal cells and mitoses are limited to the basal third of the epithelium, cells throughout the whole epithelial thickness are abnormal.*

lar, quadripolar, V shaped, irregularly grouped or dispersed, appear in the epithelium;

- the degree of nuclear enlargement of the cells;
- the degree of nuclear abnormalities such as pleomorphism, hyperchromasia, granular or irregularly dispersed chromatin, and variable numbers of nucleoli;
- the degree of nuclear abnormalities in the surface cells.

In VIN 1, mitoses and basaloid cells are limited to the basal third, in VIN 2 to the lower two-thirds and in VIN 3 they appear in the upper third. Abnormal cells occupy the full epithelial thickness in all grades, but the increasing nuclear:cytoplasmic ratio of the surface cells mirrors the other changes with increasing grade.

A third type, differentiated VIN, is not graded because it shows only basal or parabasal atypia and mitotic activity. It shares many of the morphological features of well-differentiated squamous carcinoma, but does not show any stromal invasion in biopsies.[16,17]

Basaloid VIN

There is no attempt at cellular differentiation in this form. The cells do not keratinize and maturation is abnormal, with basal cells present above the basal layer of the epithelium to varying degrees. Multinucleated and dyskeratotic cells are rare, but most of the cells display nuclear pleomorphism and hyperchromasia. The chromatin is granular with an abnormal pattern

and multiple nucleoli. The surface is usually not keratinized but may be covered by a thin keratotic or parakeratotic layer, and the surface contour is usually flat with no papillae (Figs 2.3 and 2.4).

Warty or bowenoid VIN

Maturation and differentiation may be variably accompanied by koilocytosis of differing degrees. Multinucleated and dyskeratotic cells are common and there may be marked nuclear pleomorphism. Papillomatosis is often present associated with a surface layer of keratin or parakeratin of variable thickness (Fig. 2.5).

Areas of basaloid and warty VIN may coexist in the same vulva and are often intimately admixed.[18] In one series of 60 cases of all types of VIN, microscopic changes characteristic of human papillomavirus (HPV) infection were seen in 50 per cent.[11] Koilocytosis is a basic diagnostic feature of HPV infection, but, because of the frequency with which it is seen in VIN, it cannot be used to distinguish between neoplastic and non-neoplastic lesions.[15]

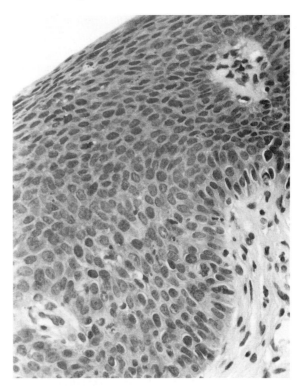

Figure 2.3 *Basaloid VIN 2. Some differentiation of the superficial third of the epithelium is seen, although the surface layer cells are still abnormal with hyperchromatic, enlarged nuclei.*

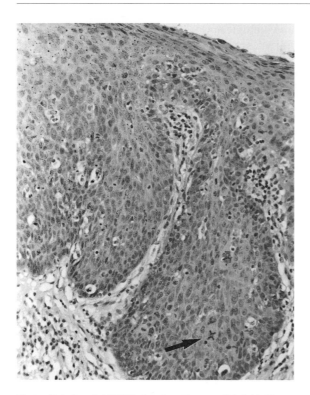

Figure 2.4 *Basaloid VIN 3. Less than the superficial third is showing signs of differentiation. Many of the surface cells are grossly enlarged and hyperchromatic with abnormal cells occupying most of the epithelial thickness. Note the abnormal tri- and quadripolar mitsoses (arrow).*

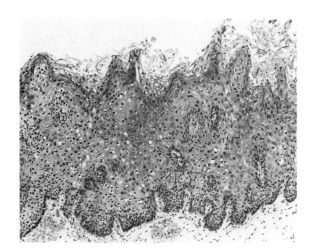

Figure 2.5 *Warty VIN 2. There is marked papillomatosis with numerous koilocytes displaying cleared cytoplasm. Parabasal cells are limited to less than the basal third of the epithelium, but there are abnormal mitoses in the middle third. Note the hyperchromasia and enlargement of the surface cells.*

Differentiated VIN

A characteristic feature of this type of VIN is small squamous pearls or 'eddies' in the basal layers, often within a sharply pointed epithelial downgrowth. The nuclear changes associated with neoplasia may be quite subtle. Single-cell dyskeratosis, basaloid cells and mitoses are usually limited to the basal or parabasal layers and consequently a grading system 1–3 is not used. This type of VIN is usually unifocal, seen in the vicinity of a well-differentiated squamous carcinoma, but occasionally may be multifocal and found at some distance from the tumour.[19] Consequently, as there is a high possibility of nearby invasion, multiple levels must be examined. Indeed, there is agreement with some authors that differentiated VIN cannot easily be separated from squamous carcinoma and may be a biological part of that lesion[2,20] (Fig. 2.6).

Aneuploidy has been used to separate VIN from benign epithelium but, morphologically, it can often be difficult to distinguish VIN 1 from inflammatory or warty changes.[15,21] Not surprisingly there is considerable intra- and interobserver variation in the diagnosis of low-grade lesions. In one study, where two observers re-examined a series of 'mild dysplasias', the diagnosis of VIN 1 could be confirmed only in 19 per cent of cases.[22] This may explain why many studies deal only with VIN 3 [4,23,24] and why there is some doubt over the premalignant role of those dermatoses, such as lichen sclerosus and squamous hyperplasia, that may be confused with VIN 1. Accordingly, VIN 3 is the

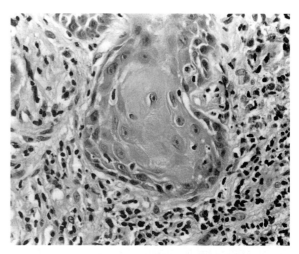

Figure 2.6 *Differentiated VIN. A squamous pearl within an epithelial downgrowth. The basement membrane appears to be intact.*

most commonly reported subtype accounting for 65–90 per cent of cases in most large series, with grades 2 and 1 accounting for the remainder more or less equally.[4,8,25]

Although morphologically similar to cervical intraepithelial neoplasia (CIN), there does not appear to be the same age-related progression through the grades in all types of VIN. Most cases have behaved in an indolent fashion (see below) and did not progress to squamous carcinoma, yet, in one series, seven of eight untreated cases of VIN 3 resulted in invasion over a period of 3 years.[7] No morphological or clinical characteristics indicate whether VIN will progress to invasion.[26] Patients with HPV-associated VIN are younger than those with VIN, seen together with non-neoplastic epithelial disorders (NNEDs) in the absence of HPV. Viral-linked VIN shows a tendency to a more severe grade with advancing age, but this trend is not seen in VIN without HPV.[6]

Overexpression of the mutated tumour suppressor oncogene *p53* has been used as a marker of tumour progression in various sites, but in vulvar carcinoma there is no apparent relationship between *p53* and survival, tumour grade or vascular space invasion.[27,28] One study showed *p53* overexpression in one of five cases of basaloid VIN 3 and two of eleven cases of warty VIN 3,[29] whereas another showed *p53* overexpression in 16 of 33 cases of VIN 3.[27] However, two other studies did not show this feature.[28,30] These discrepancies may reflect the fact that *p53* seems to be overexpressed only in lesions adjacent to carcinoma in the vulva and may reflect a local tumour effect, or further emphasizes the heterogeneity of this range of lesions. It may be that not all cases of VIN express *p53* as an early event in carcinogenesis.

Angiogenesis is believed to be an essential stage in tumour growth and the development of invasion, as the appearance of a supplying vessel system is followed by a phase of rapid tumour growth. Preliminary work shows that vascular endothelial growth factor (VEGF) is more often expressed in VIN 3 than in VIN 1 or VIN 2, but in the three invasive vulvar tumours studied there was no increase in VEGF expression. The variability of VEGF expression may reflect differing malignant potential, but it must be recognized that very few cases have been studied.[31,32]

As with CIN, the proliferation markers Ki67 and proliferating cell nuclear antigen (PCNA) are expressed above the basal layers in high-grade VIN and may be used to identify intraepithelial neoplasia. Most dyskaryotic cells react with Ki67 and a smaller proportion with PCNA, and the distribution of reacting cells appears to be correlated to the degree of atypia. Although few cases have been studied, reactions to Ki67 in formalin-fixed material have been promoted as a diagnostic tool for VIN.[33]

Vulvar squamous carcinoma is a heterogeneous condition in which two main types and modes of pathogenesis are postulated. In younger women, basaloid or warty carcinomas seem to arise in the context of HPV infection against a background of basaloid or warty VIN. HPV 16 is the genotype seen in up to 90 per cent of VIN 3, but HPV 33, HPV 11 and HPV 6 may also be found.[18,23,26,30,34,35] Differentiated VIN is not associated with HPV infection in most cases[20] but HPV serology will not distinguish between warty and basaloid types.[25] Older women develop keratinizing, often well-differentiated, squamous carcinoma with no morphological features of viral infection in the epithelium, showing a variety of NNEDs or differentiated VIN.[5,20]

It was generally believed that VIN has a low malignant potential in the absence of immunosuppression,[2,36–38] but in many of those cases the outcome was modified by treatment.[39–40] Only a minor proportion, approximately 5–10 per cent, of treated VIN 3 will progress to squamous carcinoma, although up to 16 per cent will have superficially (depth< 1 mm, diameter < 2 cm) invasive squamous carcinoma at the time of presentation.[4,8,18] These figures may be an underestimate as long-term follow-up is lacking in several studies, despite the fact that progression, up to 18 years later, is well recognized.[8,7] There seems to be little risk of squamous carcinoma arising in areas of VIN 1 and VIN 2.[8,21]

Multifocal disease

Multiple areas of VIN constituting multifocal disease are seen in 32–35 per cent of cases of VIN 3, but usually only in those cases linked to HPV infection.[5,6,41] Around 40 per cent of patients have had at least one abnormal cervical smear: 19–37 per cent metachronous cervical neoplasia, 6 per cent vaginal intraepithelial (VaIN) and 4 per cent anal intraepithelial neoplasia (AIN).[4–6,8] The lower incidence of vaginal neoplasia militates against direct spread and supports the concept of widespread change. In most cases, the same genotype of HPV will be found in VIN, CIN and VaIN occurring in the same patient.[41] This 'field response' was proposed to be the result of a common carcinogen as long ago as 1961 and accords well with extensive HPV infection.[42] Multifocal disease associated with HPV is more often seen in patients aged under 35, will recur more often and is more likely to progress to invasion;[24,41] in fact when widespread disease is present VaIN 3 may recur in a surgically constructed neovagina.[43] Extensive vulvovaginal condylomatas and multifocal VIN are seen as a result of immunosuppression in HIV infection and in transplant recipients.[36]

Changes associated with HPV

Up to 85 per cent of cases of VIN may be associated with features of HPV infection.[5,8] In the absence of atypia or intraepithelial neoplasia, HPV presents a characteristic appearance. Infection by the papillomavirus is indicated by koilocytosis, in which the cytoplasm around the nucleus is cleared and the nuclei are hyperchromatic and angulated.[9,15] Occasional multinucleated cells, single-cell dyskeratosis, hyperkeratosis and papillomatosis are all commonly seen. Mitotic figures may be present above the germinative layer, but abnormal forms are diagnostic of intraepithelial neoplasia. The common wart, condyloma acuminatum, will usually show all of these features, but flat areas, without papillae, can often be difficult to distinguish from low-grade intraepithelial neoplasia.[8,15] In VIN, koilocytes are usually seen only in the upper epithelial layers, hence their presence in the basal or parabasal layers is a useful indicator of a condyloma.[15]

PAGET'S DISEASE OF THE VULVA

Vulvar Paget's disease is an intraepithelial lesion displaying adenocarcinomatous differentiation that generally affects women aged over 60. It presents a similar clinical appearance to Paget's disease of the breast, displaying red, moist or scaly eczematous patches on all parts of the vulva, but mainly on the labia majora. Typically, the lesions are itchy and well defined.

Histologically, large, vacuolated or pale cells lie singly, and form nests or sheets along the basal vulvar epithelium. The abnormal cells have the morphological characteristics of adenocarcinoma cells with large vesicular nuclei and occasional signet ring forms. Mitoses may be numerous and the nuclei typically contain large nucleoli. As the disease evolves, the basal groups enlarge and single cells permeate the upper

epithelial layers where they may exfoliate to be detected by cytology. Most of the abnormal cells are separated from the basement membrane by a flattened layer of epithelial keratinocytes. This does not occur in melanoma in situ where melanoma cells abut the basement membrane.[45] In contrast to Paget's disease of the breast, the cells of vulvar Paget's disease may form tubules within the epithelium. Paget cells often extend down around the ducts of apocrine and eccrine ducts and involve sebaceous glands.[44–47]

The major histological differential diagnoses are intraepithelial melanoma and, to a lesser extent, bowenoid VIN, but a panel of histochemical and immunohistochemical reactions can readily differentiate the conditions (Table 2.1). Paget cells react for short chain cytokeratins (CAM 5.2),[48] neutral and acidic mucins (periodic acid–Schiff [PAS] with diastase and Alcian blue at pH 2.5) and carcinoembryonic antigen (CEA), whereas melanoma cells in the epidermis are positive for HMB45 and S100 antigens.[49,50] A recent paper advocates CK7 (present in eccrine and apocrine glands) for the identification of Paget cells in rare mucin- and CEA-negative cases (probably associated with an underlying transitional cell tumour).[51] The pale vacuolated cells in bowenoid VIN that may cause confusion are negative for all of the above, but react for long-chain cytokeratins.[52] Paget's disease reacts with a monoclonal antibody, B72.3, that binds to tumour-associated glycoprotein-72 found in a wide variety of adenocarcinomas and mature glandular tissues,[53] and is a useful discriminator from melanoma (Fig. 2.7).

The immunohistochemical reactions may be focal, with Paget's cells reacting differently to the underlying

Table 2.1 *Differentiation of Paget cells, intraepithelial melanoma and bowenoid VIN*

Stain/ antigen	Paget's disease	Melanoma	Bowenoid VIN
PAS	+ve	−ve	−ve
Alcian blue	+ve	−ve	−ve
EMA	+ve	−ve	−ve
Colloidal iron	+ve	−ve	−ve
CAM 5.2	+ve	−ve	−ve
B72.3	+ve	−ve	−ve
CEA	+ve	−ve	−ve
CK1	−ve	−ve	+ve
S100	−ve	+ve	−ve
HMB45	−ve	+ve	−ve

PAS, periodic acid–Schiff; EMA, epithelial membrane antigen; CEA, carcinoembryonic antigen.

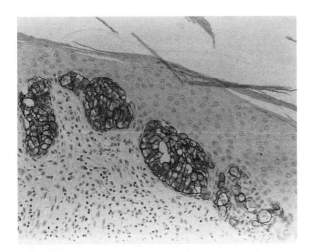

Figure 2.7 *Paget's disease of the vulva. Immunohisto-chemical reacion with short-chain cytokeratins (CAM 5.2) to highlight groups of malignant cells showing adenocarcinomatous differentiation along the basement membrane.*

adenocarcinoma.[53] Punch biopsies may be confusing as the reactions for mucin may also be discontinuous.[51] Occasional Paget cells in dark-skinned individuals may contain small amounts of melanin, but heavy melanin deposits invariably indicate melanoma.

A vast literature has addressed the histogenesis of extramammary Paget's disease resulting in three main theories: origin from apocrine sweat glands, an underlying adenocarcinoma or pluripotential epithelial cells.

APOCRINE GLANDS

A predilection for those sites rich in apocrine glands, such as the genitals, axillae, eyelids (Moll's glands) and external auditory canals (ceruminous glands), with positivity for adenocarcinoma antigens,[53] apocrine epithelial antigen, and gross cystic fluid antigen, accords with the suggestion that Paget cells are derived from apocrine gland ducts.[43,50,52,54,55] Electron microscopy has supported both eccrine and apocrine glandular differentiation with clear intracytoplasmic vacuoles and occasional cell surface specialization such as microvilli and intracytoplasmic lumina. Epidermal cell features such as cytokeratin filaments and hemidesmosomes are not present.[50,56,57]

UNDERLYING ADENOCARCINOMA

Unlike Paget's disease of the breast, extramammary Paget's disease is not associated with an underlying carcinoma in most cases. A carcinoma of an associated apocrine gland is found in 21 per cent of patients[58,46] with about 24–38 per cent[53] associated with a malignancy of underlying skin adnexae, Bartholin's glands, large bowel or bladder. In these cases, Paget cells are believed to grow from the underlying tumour to involve the overlying or adjacent epithelium. Around 25 per cent of cases of vulvar Paget's disease may invade and a further 20 per cent will be associated with distant invasive adenocarcinomas.[59,60]

PLURIPOTENTIAL EPITHELIAL CELLS

Paget's disease also occurs in areas that do not support apocrine glands, lending weight to the more widely accepted theory that the lesion represents malignant recapitulation of apocrine differentiation from pluripotential epidermal stem cells.[58,46] Eccrine glands develop from the epidermis by a process of downgrowth, indicating that there is a potential for glandular development. Clear cell papulosis is a benign counterpart arising in the epidermis, which has been suggested as a possible precursor; this illustrates that the final differentiation might not reflect the cell of origin.[61]

However, as vulvar Paget's disease may be seen with a variety of carcinomas and show variable patterns of immunohistochemistry, it is probably a heterogeneous condition with several different histogenetic mechanisms that lead to a common clinical and microscopic appearance.[53]

The prognosis of vulvar Paget's disease depends on whether there is dermal invasion or an associated underlying or distant adenocarcinoma. Flow cytometry has shown that aneuploidy is more likely to be associated with invasion of the dermis, adenocarcinoma in situ of underlying sweat glands, lymphatic invasion or frank underlying adenocarcinoma.[62]

Excision of an intraepidermal lesion should effect a cure, but recurrences may even be seen in grafted skin[63] or a myocutaneous flap[64] after incomplete removal. Intraoperative frozen sections have been deemed necessary to assess the margins, but painstaking sampling and interpretation must be undertaken to avoid a significant error rate, and may not offer any information other than clinical observation.[65,66] Consequently, frozen sections are not recommended unless an associated invasive lesion is suspected.

Non-neoplastic epithelial disorders

The most recent classifications of these conditions and their development are presented in Chapter 6.

LICHEN SCLEROSUS

Clinical features

The earliest lesions are small white papules with a central depression marking the site of a skin appendage ostium, but these are rarely seen on the vulva except at the margins of larger involved areas.[67] The papules merge to form large white or pale pink waxy plaques, which lend a wrinkled, atrophic appearance to the skin. These 'cigarette paper', crinkly changes have been used to justify the clinical suffix 'et atrophicus', but it has been known for many years that epidermal cell turnover is actually increased by up to sixfold in lichen sclerosus.[68]

Small superficial dermal blood vessels eventually become telangiectatic, and may be damaged by rubbing, causing purpura and larger areas of bruising. This is particularly relevant in children where lichen sclerosus must not be confused with the effects of abuse.[69,70] Bullae and areas of depigmentation are common. Eventually, marked scarring and atrophy lead to loss of the normal vulvar contour. The labia minora are absorbed and the clitoris becomes buried by fusion across the prepuce and the labia majora. The introitus becomes progressively narrowed until there is a small anteriorly placed opening that may cause dyspareunia. Any areas of lichenified epithelium are brittle and may split, leaving painful fissures.[67] Although quite characteristic, the changes can be confused with cicatricial pemphigoid.[71]

Histology

The most characteristic aspect of the histology is hyalinization and homogenization of the superficial dermal collagen (Fig. 2.8). Special stains show loss of elastic fibres in these areas. A loss of integrity of the dermis leads to bullae and separation of the epithelium. Small telangiectatic blood vessels are poorly supported by the altered dermal collagen and are associated with extravasated red blood cells (Fig. 2.9). The skin appendages are atrophic or absent, as a result of the effects of dermal fibrosis and occlusion of the

ostia. The epidermis may appear thin or irregularly acanthotic, with attenuated, sharply pointed rete ridges extending into the dermis. Marked hyperkeratosis is caused by rubbing as a result of pruritus, but pronounced acanthosis is classified as superimposed squamous hyperplasia and probably forms part of the spectrum of changes of lichen simplex chronicus.[72]

Lymphocytes and smaller populations of plasma cells form collections predominantly in the upper dermis. Pigmented dermal macrophages contain melanin

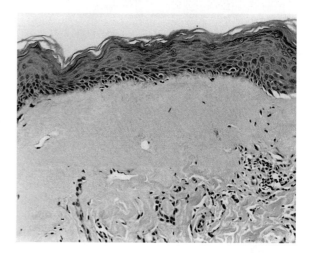

Figure 2.8 *Lichen sclerosus displaying mild epithelial thinning and a prominent zone of hyalinized collagen in the superficial stroma. The epithelium is slightly keratinized and there is a sparse chronic inflammatory cell exudate in the deeper stroma.*

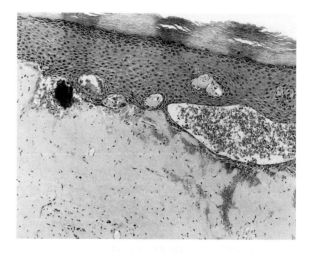

Figure 2.9 *Heavily keratinized lichen sclerosus showing a blood-filled subepithelial bulla. Extravasated red blood cells are also present in the dermis.*

released from the damaged epidermis. In the early stages, lymphocytes permeate the lower epithelial layers where there is associated oedema and vacuolar degeneration. These changes are difficult to distinguish from lichen planus.

Aetiology

Several pieces of work have suggested multiple aetiological factors involved in lichen sclerosus. Local effects seem to be important: the site-specific conditions of the vulva are such that normal skin transplanted to the vulva will develop lichen sclerosus, and affected skin moved to the thigh reverts to normal.[73] Friction and moisture appear to play a role because lichen sclerosus may be seen under pendulous breasts in obese subjects.

Notwithstanding the dangers of confusing the intradermal haemorrhage of lichen sclerosus with sexual abuse, a recent paper has shown an association with abuse in approximately 25 per cent in a series of childhood cases. The authors recognize the causative effect of physical local trauma.[74]

There appears to be a familial incidence with a relationship to HLA types A29 and B44.[75] There is also a strong relationship to autoimmune disease.[76] In one study of 350 women, 42 per cent had significantly raised autoantibodies, 21.5 per cent had an autoimmune disease and 21 per cent had a first-degree relative with an autoimmune disorder.[70]

Levels of serum testosterone, androstenedione and dihydrotestosterone are decreased in lichen sclerosus. Abnormal 5α-reductase (the enzyme that converts testosterone to the active form, dihydrotestosterone) activity is believed to underlie the restitution of normal testosterone and dihydrotestosterone levels after topical testosterone therapy.[77]

The spirochaete, *Borrelia burgdorferi*, has been proposed as a pathogenic organism because of the similarities between lichen sclerosus and acrodermatitis chronica atrophicans (one type of borreliosis). However, recent work has confused the issue by only detecting the bacterial DNA in a few small studies from Germany and Japan, but not in larger series from the USA and Spain.[78] The concept that the same disorder has separate aetiologies in different countries does not seem to be tenable.

Natural history

There has been much debate concerning the possible premalignant role of lichen sclerosus compounded by the wide variation in the reporting of lichen sclerosus adjacent to squamous carcinoma (9–76 per cent of cases).[19,33,79–81] This may be the result of under-reporting of lichen sclerosus in routine practice,[82,83] but when the type of carcinoma is considered there does appear to be a stronger link with well-differentiated tumours in older women.[19,20,79,80] Lichen sclerosus is also more frequently associated with differentiated VIN (50–77 %) than with undifferentiated VIN (0–19%)[6,19,20,81] and it has been suggested that lichen sclerosus acts independently of undifferentiated VIN 3 in the development of squamous carcinoma.[19] However, it is difficult to derive any information about the premalignant risk of the condition because all these studies take a series of malignancies as their starting point. Furthermore, secondary inflammatory changes around an invasive lesion may mask or mimic lichen sclerosus, possibly also contributing to the variability in reported incidence.[19]

The pattern of the proliferation markers Ki67 and PCNA in lichen sclerosus has no similarities with that in premalignant conditions. In most cases, lichen sclerosus displays the same basal pattern of reactivity with these reagents as normal vulvar epithelium: in VIN, Ki67 and PCNA react with suprabasal cells.[33,84] The MIB 1 index (a reaction for Ki67 in fixed tissues) shows that in the cell cycle in vulvar lichen sclerosus the proportion of cells is lower than in normal vulvar epithelium, but higher than in normal non-genital skin,[85] despite overexpression of *p53*.[28] This may reflect the response of *p53* under these conditions to limit DNA damage by blocking the cell cycle, but could also represent an initial premalignant step.[28,86] A proportion of lichen sclerosus cases has been shown to be monoclonal using DNA-based technology, demonstrating that a clonal expansion might be the first premalignant stage.[87]

The immunohistochemical reactions against a number of cytoplasmic keratins can separate normal and hyperplastic vulvar epithelium from VIN, but cannot reliably distinguish lichen sclerosus from VIN.[29]

SQUAMOUS HYPERPLASIA

Squamous hyperplasia is often considered together with lichen sclerosus, and hence the true incidence is not known. The lesions are found around foci of invasive squamous carcinoma in around 31 per cent of cases[23,82,83] and associated with 69–95 per cent of VIN (30–61 per cent VIN 3).[6,83] Clonal expansion has been shown in a series of cases, and the lesions occasionally contain HPV 16 DNA.[23,26,87] Overexpression of *p53* has been seen in examples adjacent to squamous cell carcinoma.[29] Consequently, treatment and long-term follow-up have been advocated in every case, especially if accompanied by lichen sclerosus.[80]

Clinical appearance

Clinically, squamous hyperplasia presents as a raised white patch or less well-defined area. The colour depends on the degree of keratinization with less heavily keratinized areas showing a dull dusky-red appearance. Depigmentation results from pigmentary incontinence secondary to inflammation, and the inability of rapidly proliferating keratinocytes to produce melanin. Maceration may cause soggy white patches. Intense pruritus leads to excoriation, redness and swelling. The continued rubbing causes lichenification, accentuating the normal rhomboidal pattern of skin markings. The epithelium is rendered stiff and brittle by the keratin layer, leading to splitting and fissuring. Any part of the vulva may be affected and the changes can extend on to the inner thighs. Unlike lichen sclerosus, atrophy does not occur and there is no loss of vulvar contour. The vagina is not involved and there is no tendency to introital narrowing.[1,88]

Histology

Microscopically, squamous hyperplasia is characterized by irregular epithelial growth, resulting in a thick layer of stratified squamous epithelium surmounted by a variably thickened keratotic or partially parakeratotic layer. The rete ridges may not be unduly prominent, but are more usually irregularly lengthened resulting in pointed or club-shaped profiles. The superficial dermis usually contains a sparse-to-moderate exudate of chronic inflammatory cells, and dermal capillaries may be numerous (Fig. 2.10). It is claimed that the absence of dermal inflammation and vertically streaked collagen will distinguish squamous hyperplasia from lichen simplex chronicus[88] but most now recognize squamous hyperplasia and lichen simplex chronicus as part of the same spectrum of disease. Furthermore, one review of 114 non-neoplastic vulvar

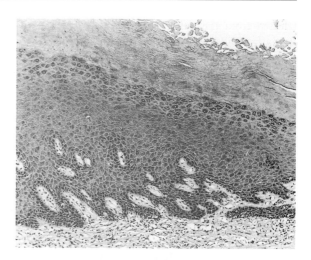

Figure 2.10 *Squamous hyperplasia exhibiting marked hyperkeratosis and irregular epithelial acanthosis*

biopsies suggests that squamous hyperplasia does not exist separately from other non-erosive dermatoses such as lichen simplex chronicus, psoriaform dermatitis, dermatophytosis and spongiotic dermatitis.[89]

The changes of squamous hyperplasia may be superimposed on lichen sclerosus or any other dermatosis, altering the appearance considerably. In particular, care must be taken to avoid confusion with differentiated VIN by paying particular attention to detecting any dysplasia or abnormal mitotic activity in the basal layers.

Combined lichen sclerosus and squamous hyperplasia – mixed NNEDs

Squamous hyperplasia and lichen sclerosus may coexist separately in different parts of the same vulva or may be superimposed (formerly called mixed dystrophy), in which case there is a danger of overlooking the lichen sclerosus component. In one study, all but two cases (96 per cent) of lichen sclerosus were associated with squamous hyperplasia.[19] It is important for the histological report to detail separately the presence of squamous hyperplasia and lichen sclerosus, so that the likely behaviour may be gauged and appropriate management commenced. When the lesions are separate, they involve their sites of election, with squamous hyperplasia tending to involve the outer vulva and lichen sclerosus affecting the labia minora, vestibule and introitus.

Histologically, where squamous hyperplasia is superimposed on lichen sclerosus the characteristic hyalinized dermal collagen layer supports a markedly thickened and heavily keratinized, stratified squamous epithelium. These changes most probably represent reaction to long-term irritation and rubbing.

Mixed lesions of lichen sclerosus and squamous hyperplasia have been detected around areas of VIN in 12–77 per cent of cases[6,19] and it has been suggested that mixed NNEDs have a higher risk of progression to invasive malignancy than each separate condition.[1,90]

Coexistence of squamous hyperplasia and VIN

Any example of VIN may be superimposed on hyperplastic areas and VIN may become thickened and hyperkeratinized as a result of rubbing. These lesions where abnormalities of maturation, mitotic activity and nuclear morphology are seen with marked epithelial thickening and hyper- or parakeratosis were formerly termed 'atypical hyperplasia' or 'dystrophy with atypia'. These terms are no longer included in the recommended classification because they do not allow grading of the neoplastic lesion. Any neoplastic changes should always be reported separately from hyperplasia.

Lichen planus

Lichen planus is a common dermatological condition that frequently involves mucous membranes, but rarely involves the vulva (two cases in a series of 114 NNEDs).[89] The importance of this condition lies in the possible premalignant potential and confusion with other, particularly ulcerating, vulvar disorders.

Lichen planus may involve the skin of the external vulva or the mucous membrane of the vestibule, introitus or vagina. Patients tend to complain of burning pain or rawness when there is vestibular or vaginal involvement and pruritus with disease of the external vulva. Erosive disease is more common on glabrous skin and there may be desquamation in the vagina. The lesions appear as characteristic, flat-topped, shiny white or violaceous papules on the skin. On mucous membranes, lichen planus presents as a fine grey or white reticulate pattern of lines (Wickham's striae), similar to that seen on the gingivobuccal mucosa, or as shiny, red, eroded, painful areas. Vaginal disease tends to form well-defined ulcerated areas that support a scanty inflammatory exudate, involving the upper vaginal fornices and extending on to the cervix. This has been defined previously as a desquamative inflammatory vaginitis. Chronic disease may lead to loss of the labia minora and vaginal adhesions between the walls of the vagina.[91,92] The differential diagnosis of erosive disease includes Behçet's disease, lupus erythematosus and other blistering dermatoses, but these rarely involve the vagina. Fusion of the labia and loss of gross vulvar morphology may cause confusion with lichen sclerosus, but this does not involve the vagina or mouth.

Histology of a non-eroded area on hair-bearing or glabrous skin will show the following: hyper- or parakeratosis; irregular, often saw-toothed acanthosis; and a characteristic band-like infiltrate of chronic inflammatory cells, predominantly lymphocytes with a few plasma cells, which is closely applied to the undersurface of the epithelium. Lymphocytes permeate the basal epithelium where there is associated epithelial oedema and vacuolar degeneration of the basal layer. Apoptotic cells about 10 µm in diameter are often seen in the basal epithelium in inflamed areas where they have been called Civatte bodies (Fig. 2.11). In eroded areas, the histology may be entirely non-specific but may show the more typical changes of lichen planus around the margins.

Erosive oral lichen planus has been known to have an increased risk of malignancy for some time[93] and recently some evidence has appeared of a probable increased risk in the vulva.[94,95] These workers have advised that long-standing vulvar lichen planus should be kept under review.

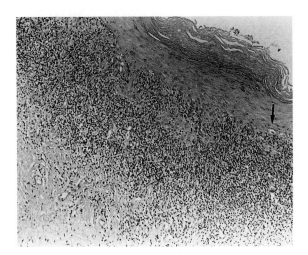

Figure 2.11 *Lichen planus. A dense band of chronic inflammatory cells occupies the upper stromal layers and permeates the basal epithelium. Note the Civatte body (arrow).*

PREINVASIVE MELANOMA

Abnormalities of pigmentation are common in the vulva and it is vitally important to be able to distinguish changes caused by pigmentation from melanocytic proliferations.

The range of melanocytic lesions of the vulva includes:

- melanosis
- lentigines
- junctional, compound and intradermal naevi
- atypical/dysplastic naevi
- melanoma in situ
- malignant melanoma.

Malignant melanoma is rare, but the incidence appears to be increasing, accounting for 2–10 per cent of vulval malignancies.[96,97] The tumour often presents at an advanced stage, highlighting the importance of early diagnosis by recognition of preinvasive disease.[98]

The range of melanocytic lesions in the vulva seems to be the same as elsewhere in the body, although the relative proportion of lentigines, and junctional, compound and intradermal naevi, suggests a preponderance of junctional and compound types.[99] The histopathology of these lesions is essentially the same as on skin and mucous membranes elsewhere, and consequently attention is directed towards those conditions that pose specific problems in the vulva.

Melanosis is used to refer to patches of abnormal vulvar coloration caused by increased basal epithelial pigmentation, accompanied by slight, if any, melanocytic proliferation. Genital lentigines have a similar clinical appearance to melanosis, but they also feature varying degrees of melanocytic proliferation along the basal epithelial layer (lentiginous proliferation). Cytological atypia is not a feature and there is no malignant potential in either of these two conditions.[100,101]

Melanomas may develop from pre-existing normal skin but it is said that the risk of developing melanoma depends on the number of naevi on the body, familial factors (as in the dysplastic naevus syndrome) and exposure to sunlight. It is true that ultraviolet radiation has been cited as a major aetiological factor, but this is inappropriate in this site and no environmental risk factors for vulvar melanoma have been identified.

It is well recognized that acquired and congenital naevi can undergo malignant change, but there have been no studies on this phenomenon at this site. Junctional proliferation is required for growth and, consequently, any naevus showing junctional activity is theoretically capable of malignant transformation. The claim that naevi on the vulva have a greater malignant potential than elsewhere has not been supported by epidemiological analysis.[99]

The premalignant melanocytic lesions are represented by:

- atypical/dysplastic naevi
- intraepidermal melanoma.

There has been much debate on the premalignant role of dysplastic melanocytic naevi.[102] The histological features suggest melanocytic proliferation by the irregular grouping of angulated, hyperchromatic or enlarged melanocytes in variably sized groups along the dermoepidermal junction. Melanocytes appear singly, spread in lentiginous fashion or in groups. Nests of cells may be fused and occur on the shoulders, in addition to the tips of the rete ridges. There is often lamellar dermal fibrosis accompanied by many fine dermal capillaries forming telangiectasias. Atypical naevi have been described in the vulva[103] but classic dysplastic naevi are rare.[104]

It is well recognized that there are increased numbers of atypical naevi in those families in which a high risk of melanoma is inherited as an autosomal dominant (the dysplastic naevus syndrome), but many contend that the risk posed by sporadic dysplastic or atypical naevi is low.[102] There have been no reports on the progression of dysplastic naevi in the vulva.[99]

In melanoma in situ, melanocytic proliferation is confined to the epithelium. An initial radial growth phase can be recognized by a lentiginous proliferation of atypical melanocytes along the dermoepidermal junction. Cellular atypia is recognized by nuclear enlargement, prominent nucleoli, occasionally cleared cytoplasm, variation in nuclear size and variable nuclear staining. Upward invasion results in single cells or groups of atypical melanocytes becoming scattered throughout the epidermis or epithelium of the mucous membrane.[105] Groups of naevus cells may be eliminated through the epidermis in the centre of some benign lesions, but upward migration by atypical cells, particularly towards the margins of the lesion, is a major feature of malignant change. This pattern of intraepithelial invasion is also often seen around the margins of invasive malignant melanomas. The presence of large, atypical, often vacuolated cells arranged in groups or scattered throughout the epithelium can be morphologically similar to Paget's disease (hence the term 'pagetoid spread'). However, melanoma in situ of the vulva can be distinguished from Paget's disease by histochemistry, immunohistochemistry and electron microscopy as detailed earlier in this chapter. Other possible sources of confusion are the cleared cells of koilocytes and normal glycogenated epithelial cells, the 'cellules claires'. Attention to the pattern of cellular distribution and nuclear morphology will prevent diagnostic confusion. Atypical or dysplastic naevi differ from melanoma in situ by their symmetry and the absence of transepidermal permeation.[106]

Invasion of the dermis by mitotically active melanocytes as single cells or groups of cells marks the distinction of in situ from invasive melanoma. It can be difficult to separate true invasion from intraepithelial nests at the tips of epithelial downgrowths. Multiple levels may need to be examined and it may be necessary to stain the basement membrane and highlight dermal melanoma cells with immunohistochemistry for MHB45 and S100 antigens.

HANDLING VULVAL BIOPSIES

Diagnostic material from gynaecologists, genitourinary physicians and dermatologists will be sent as punch or ellipse biopsies. Simple and radical vulvectomies will not be considered here. Laser vaporization will not, of course, generate material for histology and should not be used before a diagnosis has been established.[8] In many cases, it will not be necessary for a pathologist to handle the specimen and it will be more efficient for technical staff to follow protocols for dealing with the tissue. Samples should usually be trimmed fixed but may be cut fresh, partially fixed or after heat-assisted fixation to speed processing. A plane ground skin-graft or dermatome blade will be needed to trim fresh tissue accurately. Intraoperative frozen sections may be required to assess margins in Paget's disease, but are rarely needed for routine biopsies when rapid processing of small samples can deliver a diagnosis in 4–6 hours.[107] The surgeon must identify the surface to orientate the specimen and to avoid tangential cutting in trimming, embedding and section cutting. A vertically orientated section through the surface is essential to distinguish invasion from the irregular epithelial thickening often seen in squamous hyperplasia and VIN.

Punch biopsies

The surface should be identified, the punch orientated and the specimen bisected through the surface. This will provide a rectangular profile to aid the technical staff at the embedding stage. A minimum of three standard step sections should be cut.

Ellipses

The clinician should be aware that a narrow ellipse could twist and be difficult to orientate. The minimum sized biopsy of at least 2 mm across the transverse axis will be embedded as received and sectioned at three step levels; larger biopsies are cut at right angles to the shortest axis. All tissue received must be examined to detect any areas of intraepithelial neoplasia or foci of invasion.

Reporting vulval biopsies

The gross description will give the number, shape, dimensions, colour and surface characteristics of all submitted tissue.

The histological report must detail neoplastic and non-neoplastic processes including HPV-related changes. All grades of intraepithelial neoplasia, not only the worst area, should be documented. All reports of neoplasia must specify the presence or absence of invasion with an indication of whether vascular space permeation is seen. The depth and lateral extent of invasion must be accompanied by the number of blocks in which invasion is present to give an indication of the tumour volume. Most samples will be biopsies of part of a larger lesion, but a mention of incomplete excision must indicate which margins are involved.

REFERENCES

1 Lawrence DW. Non-neoplastic epithelial disorders of the vulva (vulvar dystrophies): historical and current perspectives. *Pathol Annu* 1993; **28**: 23–51.

2 Woodruff JD. Carcinoma in situ of the vulva. *Clin Obstet Gynecol* 1991; **34**: 669–77.

3 Crum CP. Vulvar intraepithelial neoplasia: the concept and its application. *Hum Pathol* 1980; **13**: 187–9.

4 Shafi MI, Luesley DM, Byrne P et al. Vulval

intraepithelial neoplasia – management and outcome. *Br J Obstet Gynaecol* 1989; **96**: 1339–44.

5 Jones RW, Baranyai J, Stables S. Trends in squamous cell carcinoma of the vulva: the influence of vulvar intraepithelial neoplasia. *Obstet Gynecol* 1997; **90**: 448–52.

6 Italian Study Group on Vulvar Disease. Clinicopathologic analysis of 370 cases of vulvar intraepithelial neoplasia. *J Reprod Med* 1996; **41**: 665–70.

7 Jones RW, Rowan DM. Vulvar intraepithelial neoplasia III: a clinical study of the outcome in 113 cases with relation to the later development of invasive vulvar carcinoma. *Obstet Gynecol* 1994; **84**: 741–54.

8 Herod JJO, Shafi MI, Rollason TP et al. Vulvar intraepithelial neoplasia: longterm follow up of treated and untreated women. *Br J Obstet Gynaecol* 1996; **103**: 446–52.

9 Lininger RA, Tavassoli FA. The pathology of vulvar neoplasia. *Curr Opin Obstet Gynaecol* 1996; **8**: 63–8.

10 Buckley CH, Butler EB, Fox H. Vulvar intraepithelial neoplasia and microinvasive carcinoma of the vulva. *J Clin Pathol* 1984; **37**: 1201–11.

11 Barbero M, Micheletti L, Preti M et al. Vulvar intraepithelial neoplasia. A clinicopathologic study of 60 cases. *J Reprod Med* 1990; **35**: 1023–8.

12 Benedet JL, Wilson PS, Matisic J. Epidermal thickness and skin appendage involvement in vulvar intraepithelial neoplasia. *J Reprod Med* 1991; **36**: 608–12.

13 Mene A, Buckley CH. Involvement of the vulval skin appendages by intraepithelial neoplasia. *Br J Obstet Gynaecol* 1985; **92**: 634–8.

14 Shatz P, Bergeron C, Wilkinson EJ et al. Vulvar intraepithelial neoplasia and skin appendage involvement. *Obstet Gynecol* 1989; **74**: 769–74.

15 Crum CP, Fu YS, Levine RU et al. Intraepithelial squamous lesions of the vulva: biologic and histologic criteria for the distinction of condylomas from vulvar intraepithelial neoplasia. *Am J Obstet Gynecol* 1982; **144**: 77–83.

16 Ridley C. The aetiology of vulval neoplasia. *Br J Obstet Gynaecol* 1994; **101**: 655–7.

17 Report of the ISSVD terminology committee. Proceedings of the 8th World Congress, Stockholm, Sweden. *J Reprod Med* 1986; **31**: 973–83.

18 Hording U, Junge J, Poulsen H, Lundvall F. Vulvar intraepithelial neoplasia III: a viral disease of undetermined progressive potential. *Gynecol Oncol* 1995; **56**: 276–9.

19 Vilmer C, Cavelier-Balloy B, Nogues C et al. Analysis of alterations adjacent to invasive vulvar carcinoma and their relationship with the associated carcinoma: a study of 67 cases. *Eur J Gynaecol Oncol* 1998; **19**: 25–31.

20 Haefner HK, Tate JE, McLachlin CM et al. Vulvar intraepithelial neoplasia: age, morphological phenotype, papillomavirus DNA, and coexisting invasive carcinoma. *Hum Pathol* 1995; **26**: 147–54.

21 Evans AS, Monaghan JM, Anderson MC. A nuclear deoxyribonucleic acid analysis of normal and abnormal vulvar epithelium. *Obstet Gynecol* 1987; **69**: 790–3.

22 Micheletti L, Barbero M, Preti M et al. Vulvar intraepithelial neoplasia of low grade: a challenging diagnosis. *Eur J Gynaecol Oncol* 1994; **15**: 70–4.

23 Trimble CL, Hildesheim A, Brinton LA et al. Heterogeneous etiology of squamous carcinoma of the vulva. *Obstet Gynecol* 1996; **87**: 59–64.

24 Jones RW, McLean MR. Carcinoma in situ of the vulva: a review of 31 treated and 5 untreated cases. *Obstet Gynecol* 1986; **68**: 499–503.

25 van Beurden M, ten Kate FJ, Smits HL et al. Multifocal vulvar intraepithelial neoplasia grade III and multicentric lower genital tract neoplasia is associated with transcriptionally active human papillomavirus. *Cancer* 1995; **75**: 2879–84.

26 Kagie MJ, Kenter GG, Zomerdijk-Nooijen Y et al. Human papillomavirus infection in squamous cell carcinoma of the vulva, in various synchronous epithelial changes and in normal vulvar skin. *Gynecol Oncol* 1997; **67**: 178–83.

27 McConnell DT, Miller ID, Parkin DE, Murray GI. p53 protein expression in a population-based series of primary vulval squamous cell carcinoma and immediate adjacent field change. *Gynecol Oncol* 1997; **67**: 248–54.

28 Kohlberger PD, Kirnbauer R, Bancher D et al. Absence of p53 protein overexpression in precancerous lesions of the vulva. *Cancer* 1998; **82**: 323–7.

29 Kajie MJ, Kenter GG, Tollenar RAEM et al. p53 protein overexpression, a frequent observation in squamous cell carcinoma and in various synchronous vulvar epithelia, has no value as a prognostic parameter. *Int J Gynecol Pathol* 1997; **16**: 124–31.

30 Pilotti S, D'Amato L, Della Torre G et al. Papillomavirus, p53 alteration and primary carcinoma of the vulva. *Diagn Mol Pathol* 1995; **4**: 239–48.

31 Bancher-Todesca D, Obermair A, Bilgi S et al. Angiogenesis in vulvar intraepithelial neoplasia. *Gynaecol Oncol* 1997; **64**: 496–500.

32 Doldi N, Origoni M, Bassan F et al. Vascular endothelial growth factor. Expression in human vulvar neoplastic and non-neoplastic tissues. *J Reprod Med*

1996; **41**: 844–8.

33 Van Hoeven KH, Kovatich AJ. Immunohistochemical staining for proliferating cell nuclear antigen, BCL2 and Ki-67 in vulvar tissues. *Int J Gynecol Pathol* 1996; **15**: 1–16.

34 Hording U, Daugaard S, Iversen AK et al. Human papillomavirus type 16 in vulvar carcinoma, vulvar intraepithelial neoplasia, and associated cervical neoplasia. *Gynecol Oncol* 1991; **42**: 22–6.

35 Park JS, Jones RW, McLean MR et al. Possible etiologic heterogeneity of vulvar intraepithelial neoplasia. *Cancer* 1991; **67**: 1599–607.

36 Chiasson MA, Ellerbrock TV, Bush TJ et al. Increased prevalence of vulvovaginal condyloma and vulvar intraepithelial neoplasia in women infected with the human immunodeficiency virus. *Obstet Gynecol* 1997; **89**: 690–4.

37 Narayan H, Cullimore J, Brown L, Byrne P. Vulvar intraepithelial neoplasia. *Contemp Rev Obstet Gynecol* 1993; **5**: 43–8.

38 Petry KU, Kochel H, Bode U et al. Human papillomavirus is associated with the frequent detection of warty and basaloid high grade neoplasia of the vulva and cervical neoplasia among immunocompromised women. *Gynecol Oncol* 1996; **60**: 30–4.

39 Buscema J. Woodruff JD, Parmley TH, Genadry R. Carcinoma in situ of the vulva. *Obstet Gynecol* 1980; **55**: 225–30.

40 Ragnarsson B, Raabe N, Willems J, Pettersson F. Carcinoma in situ of the vulva. Long term prognosis. *Acta Oncol* 1987; **26**: 227–80.

41 van Beurden M, ten Kate FWJ, Tjong-A-Hung SP, de Craen AJM. Human papillomavirus in multicentric vulvar intraepithelial neoplasia. *Int J Gynecol Pathol* 1998; **17**: 12–16.

42 Bornstein J, Kaufman RH, Adam E, Adler-Storthz K. Multicentric intraepithelial neoplasia involving the vulva. Clinical features and association with human papillomavirus and herpes simplex virus. *Cancer* 1988; **62**: 1601–4.

43 Lathrop JC, Ree HJ, McDuff HC. Intraepithelial neoplasia of the neovagina. *Obstet Gynecol* 1985; **65**: 91s–4s.

44 Pinkus H, Mehregan AH. *A guide to dermatopathology*, 3rd edn. New York: Appleton-Century-Crofts, 1981: 471–5.

45 Elder D, Elenitsas R, Jaworsky C, Johnston B. *Histopathology of the skin lever*, 8th edn. Philadelphia: Lippincott-Raven, 1997: 734–8.

46 Jones RE, Austin C, Ackerman AB. Extramammary Paget's disease. *Am J Dermatopathol* 1979; **9**: 101–32.

47 Murrell TW, McMullan JB. Extramammary Paget's disease. *Arch Dermatol* 1962; **85**: 600–13.

48 Helm KF, Goellner JR, Peters MS. Immunohistochemical stains in extramammary Paget's disease. *Am J Dermatopathol* 1992; **14**: 402–7.

49 Bacchi CE, Goldfogel GA, Greer BE, Gown AM. Paget's disease and melanoma of the vulva. Use of a panel of monoclonal antibodies to identify cell type and to microscopically define adequacy of surgical margins. *Gynecol Oncol* 1992; **46**: 216–21.

50 Ordonez NG, Awalt H, MacKay B. Mammary and extramammary Paget's disease. An immunohistochemical and ultrastructural study. *Cancer* 1987; **59**: 1173–83.

51 Battles OE, Page DL, Johnson JE. Cytokeratins, CEA, and mucin histochemistry in the diagnosis and characterisation of extramammary Paget's disease. *Am J Clin Pathol* 1997; **108**: 6–12.

52 Kariemi AL, Forsman L, Wahlstrom T. Expression of differentiation antigens in mammary and extramammary Paget's disease. *Br J Dermatol* 1985; **100**: 203–10.

53 Olson DJ, Fujimura M, Swanson P, Okagaki T. Immunohistochemical features of Paget's disease with and without adenocarcinoma. *Int J Gynecol Oncol* 1991; **10**: 285–95.

54 Merot Y, Mazoujian G, Pinkus G. Extramammary Paget's disease of perianal and perineal regions. Evidence of apocrine derivation. *Arch Dermatol* 1985; **121**: 750–2.

55 Jones RR, Spaul J, Gusterson B. The histogenesis of mammary and extramammary Paget's disease. *Histopathology* 1989; **14**: 409–16.

56 Demopolous RI. Fine structure of the extramammary Paget's cell. *Cancer* 1971; **27**: 1202–1.

57 Roth LM, Lee SM, Ehrlich CE. Paget's disease of the vulva: a histogenentic study of five cases including ultrastructural observations and review of the literature. *Am J Surg Pathol* 1977; **1**: 193–206.

58 Hart, WR, Millman JB. Progression of intraepithelial Paget's disease to invasive carcinoma. *Cancer* 1977; **40**: 2333–7.

59 Cappuccini F, Tewari K, Rogers LW, DiSaia PJ. Extramammary Paget's disease of the vulva: metastases to the bone marrow in the absence of an underlying adenocarcinoma. *Gynecol Oncol* 1997; **66**: 146–50.

60 Feuer GA, Shevchuk M, Calanog A. Vulvar Paget's disease: the need to exclude an invasive lesion. *Gynecol Oncol* 1990; **38**: 81–9.

61 Kuo TT, Chan HL, Hsueh S. Clear cell papulosis of the skin. A new entity with histogenetic implications for cutaneous Paget's disease. *Am J Surg Pathol* 1987; **11**: 827–34.

62 Cotton J, Kotylo PK, Michael H, Roth LM, Sutton GP. Flow cytometric DNA analysis of extramammary Paget's disease of the vulva. *Int J Gynecol Oncol* 1995; **14**: 324–30.

63 DiSaia PJ, Dorion GE, Cappuccini F, Carpenter PM. A report of two cases of recurrent Paget's disease of the vulva in a split-thickness graft and its possible pathogenesis-labelled 'retrodissemination'. *Gynecol Oncol* 1995; **57**: 109–12.

64 Yoshitatsu S, Hosokawa K, Nishimoto S, Yoshikawa K. A case of Paget's disease of the vulva recurring in a musculocutaneous flap. *J Dermatology* 1997; **24**: 471–4.

65 Stacey D, Burrell MO, Franklin EW. Extramammary Paget's disease of the vulva and anus: use of intraoperative frozen section margins. *Am J Obstet Gynecol* 1986; **155**: 519–23.

66 Fishman DA, Chambers SK, Schwartz PE, Kohorn EI, Chambers JT. Extramammary Paget's disease of the vulva. *Gynecol Oncol* 1995; **56**: 266–70.

67 Ridley CM. (1992) Lichen sclerosus. *Dermatol Clin* **10**: 309–23.

68 Woodruff JD et al Metabolic activity in normal and abnormal vulvar epithelia. An assessment by the use of tritiated nucleic acid precursors. *Am J Obstet Gynecol* 1965; **91**: 809–16.

69 Berth-Jones J, Graham-Brown RAC, Burns DA. Lichen sclerosus et atrophicus – a review of 15 cases in young girls. *Clin Exp Dermatol* 1991; **16**: 14–17.

70 Meyrick Thomas RH, Ridley CM, McGibbon DH, Black MM. Lichen sclerosus et atrophicus – a study of 350 women. *Br J Dermatol* 1988; **118**: 41–6.

71 Marren P, Walkden V, Malon E, Wojnarowska F. Vulval cicatricial pemphigoid may mimic lichen sclerosus. *Br J Dermatol* 1996; **134**: 522–4.

72 Meffert JJ, Davis BM, Grimwood RE. Lichen sclerosus. *J Am Acad Dermatol* 1995; **32**: 393–416.

73 Di Paolo GR, Rueda-Leverone NG, Belardi MG. Lichen sclerosus of the vulva recurrent after myocutanerous graft. A case report. *J Reprod Med* 1982; **27**: 666–8.

74 Warrington SA, de San Lazaro C. Lichen sclerosus and sexual abuse. *Arch Dis Child* 1996; **75**: 512–16.

75 Purcell KG, Spencer LU, Simpson PM et al. HLA antigens in lichen sclerosus et atrophicus. *Arch Dermatol* 1990; **126**: 1043–5.

76 Harrington CI, Dunsmore IR. An investigation into the incidence of autoimmune disorders in patients with lichen sclerosus et atrophicus. *Br J Dermatol* 1981; **104**: 563–6.

77 Freidrich EG, Kalra PS. Serum levels of sex hormones in vulvar lichen sclerosus and the effect of topical testosterone. *N Engl J Med* 1984; **310**: 488–91.

78 Alonso-Llamazares J, Persing DH, Anda P, Gibson LE, Rutledge BJ, Iglesias L. No evidence for *Borrelia burgdorferi* in lesions of morphea and lichen sclerosus et atrophicus in Spain. A prospective study and literature review. *Acta Derm Venereol* 1997; **77**: 299–304.

79 Costa S, Syrjanen S, Vendra C et al. Human papillomavirus infections in vulvar precancerous lesions and cancer. *J Reprod Med* 1995; **40**: 291–8.

80 Gomez Rueda N, Garcia A, Vighi S et al. Epithelial alterations adjacent to invasive squamous carcinoma of the vulva. *J Reprod Med* 1994; **39**: 526–30.

81 Leibowitch M, Neill S, Pelisse M, Moyal-Baracco M. The epithelial changes associated with squamous cell carcinoma of the vulva: a review of the clinical, histological and viral findings in 78 women. *Br J Obstet Gynaecol* 1990; **97**: 1135–9.

82 Zaki I, Dalziel KL, Solomonsz FA, Stevens A. The under-reporting of skin disease in association with squamous cell carcinoma of the vulva. *Clin Exp Dermatol* 1996; **21**: 334–7.

83 Carli P, Cattaneo A, De Magnis A, Biggeri A, Taddei G, Giannotti B. Squamous carcinoma arising in vulval lichen sclerosus: a cohort study. *Eur J Cancer Prev* 1995; **4**: 491–5.

84 Scurry J, Beshay V, Cohen C, Allen D. Ki67 expression in patients with and without associated squamous cell carcinoma. *Histopathology* 1998; **32**: 399–404.

85 Tan SH, Derrick E, McKee PH et al. Altered p53 expression and epidermal cell proliferation is seen in vulval lichen sclerosus. *J Cutan Pathol* 1994; **21**: 316–23.

86 Ansink AC, Krul MR, De Weger RA et al. Human papillomavirus, lichen sclerosus and squamous cell carcinoma of the vulva: detection and prognostic significance. *Obstet Gynecol* 1994; **52**: 180–4.

87 Tate JE, Mutter JL, Boynton KA, Crum CP. Monoclonal origin of vulvar intraepithelial neoplasia and some vulvar hyperplasias. *Am J Pathol* 1997; **150**: 315–22.

88 Wells M, Fox H. *Haines and Taylor. Obstetrical and gynaecological pathology.* London: Churchill Livingstone, 1997: 68–74.

89 O'Keefe RJ, Surry JP, Dennerstein G, Sfameni S, Brenan J. Audit of 114 non-neoplastic vulvar biopsies. *Br J Obstet Gynaecol* 1995; **102**: 780–6.

90 Rodke G, Friedrich EG, Wilkinson EJ. Malignant

potential of mixed vulval dystrophy (lichen sclerosus associated with squamous cell hyperplasia). *J Reprod Med* 1988; **33**: 545–50.

91 Mann MS, Kaufman RH. Erosive lichen planus of the vulva. *Clin Obstet Gynecol* 1991; **34**: 605–13.

92 Edwards L. Vulvar lichen planus. *Arch Dermatol* 1989; **125**: 1677–80.

93 Silverman S, Gorsky M, Lozada-Nur F. A prospective follow-up study of 570 patients with oral lichen planus: persistence, remission and malignant association. *Oral Surg Oral Med Oral Pathol* 1985; **60**: 30–4.

94 Frank JM, Young AW. Squamous cell carcinoma in situ arising within lichen planus of the vulva. *Dermatol Surg* 1995; **21**: 890–4.

95 Dwyer CM, Kerr RE, Millan DW. Squamous carcinoma following lichen planus of the vulva. *Clin Exp Dermatol* 1995; **20**: 171–2.

96 Bradgate MG, Rollason TP, McConkey CC, Powell J. Malignant melanoma of the vulva: a clinicopathological study of 50 women. *Br J Obstet Gynaecol* 1990; **97**: 124–33.

97 Raber G, Mempel V, Jacksch C et al. Malignant melanoma of the vulva. *Cancer* 1996; **78**: 2353–8.

98 Fitzpatrick TB, Rhodes AR, Sober AJ. Prevention of melanoma by recognition of its precursors. *N Engl J Med* 1985; **312**: 115–16.

99 Rollason TP. Malignant melanoma and related lesions. In: Lowe D, Fox H (eds). *Advances in gynaecological pathology.* London: Chuchill Livingstone,

1992: 119–43.

100 Sison-Torre EQ, Ackerman AB. Melanosis of the vulva. *Am J Dermatopathol* 1985; **7**(suppl): 51–60.

101 Barnhill RL, Albert LS, Shama SK et al. Genital lentiginosis: A clinical and histopathologic study. *J Am Acad Dermatol* 1990; **22**: 453–60.

102 Ackerman AB. What naevus is dysplastic, a syndrome and the commonest precursor of malignant melanoma? A riddle and an answer. *Histopathology* 1988; **13**: 241–56.

103 Freidman RJ, Ackerman AB. Difficulties in the histological diagnosis of melanocytic nevi on the vulvae of premenopausal women. In: Ackerman AB (ed). *Pathology of malignant melanoma.* New York: Masson 1981: 119–27.

104 Christensen WN, Freidman KJ, Woodruff JD, Hood AF. Histological characteristics of vulvar nevocellular nevi. *J Cutan Pathol* 1987; **14**: 87–91.

105 Clark WH, Elder DE, Guerry D et al. A study of tumour progression: the precursor lesions of superficial spreading and nodular melanoma. *Hum Pathol* 1984; **15**: 1147–65.

106 Seywright MM, Doherty VR, MacKie RM. Proposed alternative terminology and subclassification of so called 'dysplastic naevi'. *J Clin Pathol* 1986; **39**: 189–94.

107 Brown LJR, Carvell S, Cullen R et al. Re-engineering histopathology to provide a dramatic improvement in the turnaround time. *J Pathol* 1997; **181**: 21a.

3

Pathology of invasive vulvar lesions

TP ROLLASON

TUMOURS OF, OR PRIMARILY INVOLVING, SURFACE EPITHELIUM

Superficially invasive squamous cancer

No generally accepted definition of vulvar 'microinvasive' carcinoma exists, but an excellent review of the problem has been presented by Wilkinson.[1]

The present International Federation of Gynaecologists and Obstetricians (FIGO) classification of stage 1 disease confines itself overall to limiting the lateral extent of the tumour to 2 cm for inclusion in this category but, in early invasive tumours, depth rather than surface diameter has more importance; this has been recognized in the 1994 modification of the FIGO staging system by the inclusion of a stage Ia subgroup (Fig. 3.1). It is difficult to determine from published studies what criteria should be used to include early invasive vulvar carcinomas in any putative microinvasive category. Some studies have shown no metastases to groin nodes with tumours up to a depth of 5 mm;[2] others suggest that a significant number (up to 30 per cent in some series) will have metastasized at this depth.[3–5] Even at a maximum depth of invasion of 3 mm, metastases have been reported in several series at varying rates,[4–6] and tumour volume studies have supported the tendency to spread at smaller size when

compared with cervical carcinomas.[7] Comparison between studies is also hampered by the variable methods of measurement used. Dvoretsky and colleagues[8] suggest that total tumour thickness may be more useful and reproducible than depth of invasion, and Pickel and Haas[7] have indicated that a tumour volume of 300 mm^3 or less may be best to define this group. In the light of the above problems, it has been proposed that the term 'microinvasive' be entirely avoided in vulvar carcinoma and only the new FIGO stage Ia disease used, consisting of tumours showing depth of invasion of less than 1 mm, where risk of metastasis appears negligible; there have been only two cases in the literature known to have metastasized at this depth.[9] 'Superficially invasive' is the only other accepted term for this group.

Depth of invasion should be measured from the epidermal–stromal junction of the most superficial adjacent dermal papilla to the deepest point of the tumour.[10]

As with cervical disease, it is desirable that the presence or absence of vessel invasion be specifically noted in histological reports,[4] but the evidence that this or the tumour growth pattern (diffuse or spray type in contrast to confluent[5,11,12]) is useful in predicting outcome in stage Ia tumours is not convincing[8] and, in view of the rarity of metastases in this group, it is unlikely to be shown to be convincing in the future.

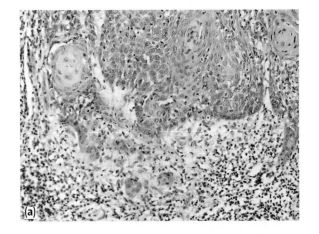

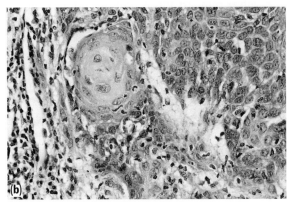

Figure 3.1 *Vulvar epithelium showing VIN with small foci of superficially invasive squamous carcinoma (stage Ia disease). (a) Low and (b) higher power views.*

We suggest avoidance of the term 'confluent' in vulvar tumours generally because it is open to misinterpretation and, as Zaino[13] points out, has been used in different senses by different authors. Tumour differentiation has not been convincingly demonstrated to correlate with prognosis although some dispute this.[14] What is indisputable is that there is no adequate method of grading such small squamous carcinomas.

Invasive squamous carcinoma and its variants

Approximately 90 per cent of all invasive tumours of the vulva are squamous[15] but the tumour at this site makes up only 3–8 per cent of genital tract malignancy.[15,16] Generally, it is a disease of women aged over 50[16] although the incidence in younger women does appear to be increasing.[15,17]

It would appear that present evidence points to two separate groups of vulvar carcinomas: those in younger women associated with human papillomavirus (HPV) infection (in particular types 16 and 18) and pre-existing 'classic' vulvar intraepithelial neoplasia (VIN), and those in older women without the HPV and classic VIN connection but associated, in a proportion of cases, with the 'differentiated' variant of VIN or epithelial hyperplasia.[18–21] There is also evidence suggesting that prognosis for HPV-negative tumours may be worse than that for HPV-positive ones.[22]

'Typical' squamous carcinoma

On gross examination, these tumours are often ulcerated masses, although polypoid and diffuse plaque-like lesions are also not uncommon. No clear predilection for a particular site on the vulva is seen; most involve the labia[23] with the clitoris being the second most common site. In one major series, a tendency for the anterior half of the vulva to be more commonly involved than the posterior half was seen.[24] Approximately 10 per cent are multifocal. The tumours that follow granulomatous vulvar disease tend to be widespread and polypoid.[25] Most of the factors associated with the development of squamous carcinoma in older studies, e.g. obesity, diabetes and low socioeconomic status, are probably not independently important,[26,27] and the putative role of syphilis and other non-HPV-related, sexually transmitted diseases is now also unclear.

Spread of squamous carcinoma is by direct extension and lymphatic invasion, with bloodstream spread occurring only rarely and late in the disease. At the time of presentation, 25–30 per cent of cases have nodal metastases.

Most tumours are histologically well- or moderately well-differentiated being composed of infiltrating tongues of eosinophilic cells showing keratinization, often with 'pearl' formation (Fig. 3.2). Surgical staging by the FIGO method provides the most accurate prognostic information. Histological grading of tumour differentiation has not been universally shown to be prognostically helpful,[5] although some series have claimed good correlation.[28–30] To attempt to address difficulties in reproducibility with older grading methods, a newer grading method based on the percentage of undifferentiated cells has been recommended, but this has not been widely adopted to date.[14] A 'spray' or

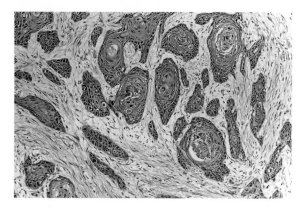

Figure 3.2 *Vulvectomy specimen. There is typical, infiltrating, well-differentiated, keratinizing squamous cell carcinoma present.*

diffuse pattern of invasion appears to confer a poorer prognosis but no clear advantage is evident in grading nuclear:cytoplasmic ratio, desmoplastic reaction, mitotic rate, etc. One recent study showed considerable prognostic value in using a combination of tumour size, nuclear hyperchromasia and site.[31] The presence of vascular invasion appears to be an important guide to the likelihood of lymph-node metastasis.[5,28,29,32] Metastases are usually to groin nodes, which are almost invariably involved before more distant node groups.

To date, there are few studies on ploidy and proliferation index, etc. in vulvar squamous carcinoma and no clear evidence of their prognostic utility is available.[33–35] Morphometry is not of proven value.[31]

Histological variants of invasive squamous carcinoma

VERRUCOUS CARCINOMA

When strict histological criteria are applied these are relatively rare tumours with less than 50 vulvar cases in the English language literature.[36–38] Macroscopically they are usually fungating, cauliflower-like masses, similar to large condylomata. It has been suggested that 50 per cent are associated with 'classic' condylomata acuminata and HPV DNA has been demonstrated in these tumours, particularly HPV type 6, but they are nevertheless predominantly tumours of postmenopausal women with a peak incidence in the 50s and 60s.[38] The vulvar tumours are most often found on the labia majora and are typically malodorous.

Histologically, verrucous carcinoma has a papillary

pattern with virtually no cellular atypia. The epithelium is markedly thickened with florid hyper- and parakeratosis. Deep keratin-filled tunnels are seen, but clearly defined invasion is difficult to demonstrate (Fig. 3.3) and the tumour has a pushing margin. Groin lymph nodes are commonly enlarged as a result of infection, but metastases have not been described in well-documented cases and extragenital tumours of this type also very rarely metastasize.[39] Because of the bland histological appearance, it is imperative that any biopsy is of adequate size and depth. It has been said in the past that irradiation of verrucous carcinomas led to alteration to a more aggressive tumour type, with rapid progression and possibly metastasis, but for non-vulvar tumours this is probably not true and in the case of the vulva the position is unclear. Some have suggested that radiotherapy may have a role in very large tumours not amenable to surgical removal, but support from the larger series in the literature is lacking.[37,38] After wide and complete local excision the prognosis is excellent.

It seems almost certain that this tumour is the same condition as the giant condyloma acuminatum of Bushke and Lowenstein, although some have disputed this;[40] they are said to be inseparable on clinical appearances. Verrucous carcinoma should not be confused with so-called 'warty' carcinoma (see later), where the coexistence of very well-differentiated squamous cell carcinoma and HPV effect produces an exophytic tumour with coexistent koilocytosis but clear stromal invasion.[10,41] Such tumours have a prognosis that is possibly somewhat better than 'classic' keratinizing squamous cell carcinoma, but not as favourable as verrucous carcinoma.

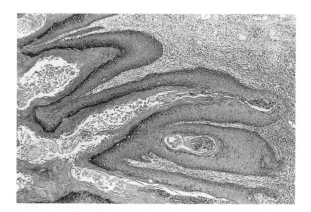

Figure 3.3 *Simple vulvectomy specimen: verrucous carcinoma. The typical keratin-filled tunnels and coarse papillary pattern of a verrucous carcinoma are evident.*

When diagnosing very well-differentiated and verrucous carcinomas of the vulva, the possibility of pseudoepitheliomatous hyperplasia should always be borne in mind because this mimics such tumours, on occasion very closely. It is seen in association with many skin conditions (Fig. 3.4) but, in particular, may be seen on the vulva with lichen sclerosus complicated by florid epithelial hyperplasia, and in association with chronic infective conditions including Crohn's disease. Rarely, it may be encountered above benign granular cell tumours (Fig. 3.5).[42] An adequate, deep biopsy is usually necessary for differential diagnosis.

BASALOID SQUAMOUS CELL CARCINOMA

This type tends to occur in relatively young women (mean age in the mid-50s), has a higher incidence in blacks than in whites and is usually associated with

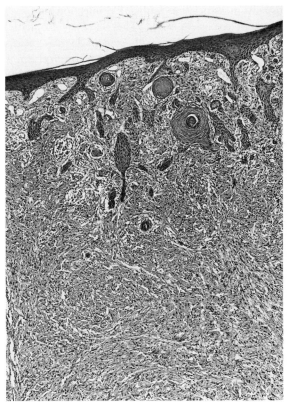

Figure 3.5 *A further example of pseudoepitheliomatous hyperplasia. There is a benign granular cell tumour in the dermis. Such tumours regularly cause changes in the overlying epithelium, mimicking squamous carcinoma.*

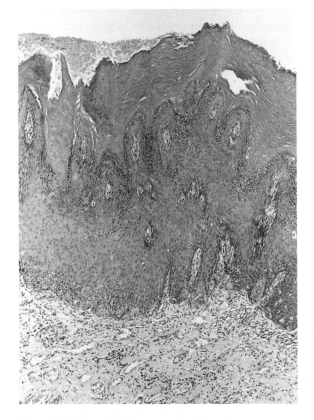

Figure 3.4 *The epithelium shows florid papillary overgrowth (pseudoepitheliomatous hyperplasia), in this case related to Paget's disease of the vulva. The pale Paget cell aggregates can just be discerned at this magnification at the bases of the epithelial rete pegs. (Reproduced from* CPD Bulletin – Cellular Pathology, *vol. 1, 1998, pp 19–25, with the permission of Rila Publications, London.)*

adjacent VIN. They also appear to have a particularly high incidence of coexistent HPV infection, especially HPV 16 and HPV 33,[43] and of synchronous or metachronous cervical intraepithelial neoplasia (CIN) and invasive squamous cell carcinoma of the cervix and vagina, i.e. they are a particular type of squamous cell carcinoma seen in association with 'lower female genital tract neoplasia syndrome'.[10,44] The prognosis is as yet unclear but multifactorial analysis suggests that it is similar to 'classic' keratinizing squamous cell carcinoma. Basaloid squamous carcinoma can be confused histologically with basal cell carcinoma and other small cell tumours because they are composed of a relatively uniform population of small ovoid cells with a high nuclear:cytoplasmic ratio (Fig. 3.6).

WARTY SQUAMOUS CELL CARCINOMA

This tumour probably accounts for about 5–10 per cent of vulvar squamous carcinomas and, as for the basaloid variant, occurs in relatively young women usually in association with HPV infection and evidence of coexistent VIN.[44] They have an exophytic, condylomatous outline with evident hyperkeratosis and parakeratosis (Fig. 3.7). Nuclear pleomorphism is variable in extent but may be prominent in some examples with evidence of multinucleate cells; unlike verrucous carcinoma, invasion is easily recognized at the extending margins. Koilocytes are usually present in the adjacent epithelium and in the more superficial tumour cells. Outcome in comparison to 'usual' squamous carcinoma is as yet unclear, but the tumour may carry some survival advantage, with prognosis lying between the 'usual' squamous carcinoma and verrucous carcinoma.

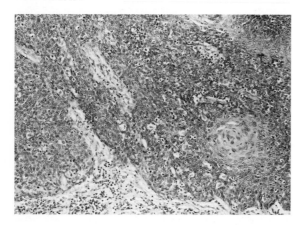

Figure 3.6 *This squamous carcinoma is of basaloid type and is composed predominantly of small, dark cells, forming occasional, paler, whorled, squamous aggregates. Keratinization was seen in the tumour but only very focally. (Reproduced from* CPD Bulletin – Cellular Pathology, *vol. 1, 1998, pp 19–25, with the permission of Rila Publications, London.)*

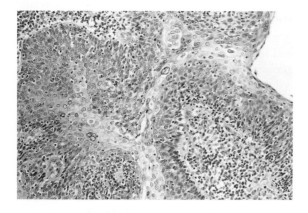

Figure 3.7 *A warty carcinoma of the vulva showing perinuclear cellular vacuoles and multinucleation. Hyperkeratosis was evident elsewhere in the tumour. Haematoxylin and eosin (H&E) stain. (Reproduced from* CPD Bulletin – Cellular Pathology, *vol. 1, 1998, pp 19–25, with the permission of Rila Publications, London.)*

SPINDLE CELL SQUAMOUS CARCINOMA

This tumour is composed histologically of pleomorphic spindle cells in a collagenous stroma. It may be very difficult to differentiate histologically from sarcoma, but immunocytochemistry may be very helpful in this regard because spindle cell carcinoma shows generalized cytokeratin marker positivity in tumour cells. It is a rare tumour with too few acceptable cases in the literature[45] to assess relative prognosis.

ADENOID (ACANTHOLYTIC) SQUAMOUS CARCINOMA

This variant may be seen as an element in an otherwise typical squamous carcinoma or in 'pure' form; essentially it consists of two elements: keratinizing squamous cells and acinar structures with dyskeratotic acantholytic cells in the centre.[46,47] Epithelial mucin is not present. The prognosis relative to squamous carcinoma generally is not known.[47] This tumour should be differentiated from adenoid cystic carcinoma which is a distinct entity (see below).

LYMPHOEPITHELIOMA-LIKE CARCINOMA

These tumours are very rare on the vulva and have usually been seen in elderly people. They show large cells of epithelial origin, with a dense lymphoid infiltrate similar to the pattern evident at the more common sites of occurrence such as the pharynx. Outcome is not clear but probably similar to that for keratinizing squamous carcinoma.

Basal cell carcinoma

Basal cell carcinomas usually occur on the light-exposed skin of elderly people and, although rare on the vulva, are probably also under-reported. They present as long-standing pruritus, soreness or a nodule, polyp, ulcer or area of altered pigmentation,[48,49,50] often on the anterior vulva, and make up between 2 per cent and 5 per cent of vulvar carcinomas.[50,51] Some authors suggest that they are rarely larger than 3 cm in diameter at presentation,[51,52] but others have found a wider size range with evidence of much larger tumours.[53] Multicentricity is common and there is said to be a strong association with malignancy at other sites.[51] Irradiation appears to be a predisposing cause in a small number of cases. As at other sites, local invasion without metastasis is characteristic, although exceptions are recorded in several series.[49,50,53,54]

The vulvar tumour is histologically identical to tumours elsewhere, being composed of small, dark, 'undifferentiated', basal-type cells with a variable architectural pattern (Figs 3.8 and 3.9). The infiltrative growth pattern seems to be the most common and the morphoea-like pattern is rare.[50] An adenoid variant that shows trabecular or gland-like structures in a dense stroma has been described.[55] Basisquamous variants are also well described but opinions vary on whether they represent true basal cell, squamous cell

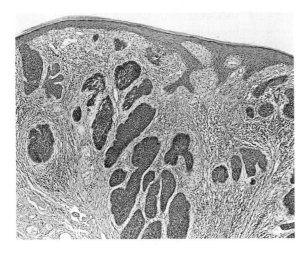

Figure 3.8 *Vulvar biopsy: basal cell carcinoma. Low-power photomicrograph showing a common pattern of basal cell carcinoma with irregular cords of dark cells infiltrating the dermis.*

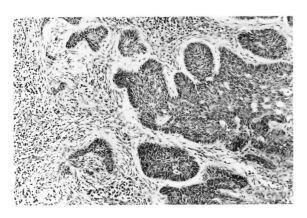

Figure 3.9 *Vulvar biopsy: higher power view of the undifferentiated small dark cells of a basal cell carcinoma.*

or intermediate neoplasms. The great majority probably behave as basal cell carcinomas. In cases where this apparent variant has metastasized, only the squamous component has usually been seen at the metastatic site, suggesting that such cases were in reality squamous cell carcinomas.

Paget's disease of the vulva

This disease has generally been considered to be rare, making up approximately 2 per cent of all vulvar malignancy,[56] it differs from that of the breast in that only about a fifth of cases have a demonstrable underlying adenocarcinoma of the sweat glands, etc.[57] Some cases, as many as 40 per cent in one series,[57] are associated with extragenital cancer (especially breast), other genitourinary tumours or squamous cell carcinomas, but Paget's disease is not considered to be metastatic. In those cases with no underlying vulval adenocarcinoma, it is still unclear whether the primary site of origin is in the ducts, surface mucosa or at different sites in different cases, although the likely cell of origin in all cases is a multipotent cell derived from the epithelial germinal layer. Those cases involving the perineal area have a high incidence of rectal adenocarcinoma.

Macroscopically, the disease appears as a scaly, red area anywhere on the vulvar or perianal surface, usually in middle-aged or elderly women. Histologically, characteristic, large, pale Paget cells, showing a distinct preference for the basal layers, are seen in the epithelium. These cells are often vacuolated and contain epithelial mucin. Cell clusters are typically seen at least focally and acini may be evident (Figs 3.10 and 3.11). Immunohistochemistry has, to date, not been helpful in determining from superficial biopsies whether an underlying invasive tumour was present.[58] The Paget cells often extend into adnexal structures.

Prognosis of Paget's disease is excellent if the disease is confined to the epithelium, though recurrences are common. With dermal invasion or an underlying adnexal carcinoma, prognosis worsens considerably[57,59] and metastases to regional nodes etc. occur. The literature is conflicting about whether frozen section examination of the resection margins during surgery is of value, and even about whether resection margin involvement in permanent sections from the complete specimen predicts recurrence.[60–62] Paget's disease is covered in greater detail in Chapter 2.

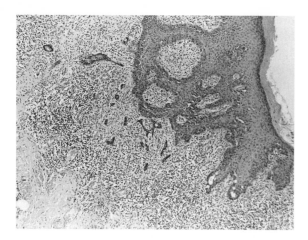

Figure 3.10 *Paget's disease of the vulva. At low power the cell clusters at the base of the epithelium are evident, but the important feature is the presence of dermal invasion by small irregular acini and trabeculae. (Reproduced from* CPD Bulletin – Cellular Pathology, *vol. 1, 1998, pp 19–25, with the permission of Rila Publications, London.)*

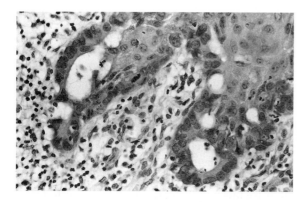

Figure 3.11 *Paget's disease of the vulva. At higher magnification the acinus formation at the base of the surface epithelium is clearly evident. (Reproduced from* CPD Bulletin – Cellular Pathology, *vol. 1, 1998, pp 19–25, with the permission of Rila Publications, London.)*

Malignant melanoma

Approximately 5 per cent of malignant melanomas in white females are said to occur on the vulva making up between 2 per cent and 10 per cent of vulvar malignancies.[63–65] These figures do not appear to have altered with the recent considerable increase generally in the incidence of malignant melanoma.[66] In a survey of the British West Midlands, Bradgate and colleagues[67] found only 50 cases over a 25-year period in an area with a population of 5 million. In this survey,

the tumour accounted for 2.2 per cent of all melanomas in women and 3.6 per cent of all vulvar malignancies.

Malignant melanoma at this site is said to be a disease of postmenopausal women. The mean age in our own series[67] was 63 years (range 22–93). Approximately one-third occur in women aged under 50. Impingement on or localization to mucosal surfaces is seen in more than 60 per cent of cases, manifest in some series as a preference for involvement of the clitoral area and labia minora.[64,68] Macroscopically, they may be pigmented or non-pigmented, nodular, flat or ulcerated. On the skin generally, melanoma may be divided into four main types: superficial spreading (pagetoid), nodular, acral lentiginous and lentigo maligna. It has been suggested that some anogenital and vulval melanomas may constitute a further group (termed mucosal lentigina), having considerable similarities to acral lentiginous tumours and showing a similar mixture of epithelioid and lentiginous features, but with the addition of multinucleation in tumour cells, which is rarely seen at other sites.[69,70] The differentiation of benign naevi from melanomas on the vulva may be particularly difficult because pleomorphic atypical naevi may occur, and Clark and colleagues[71] have described 'atypical melanocytic naevi of genital type' as a definable subgroup that shows a non-specific but diagnostically important stromal reaction. Such atypical naevi appear to show a predilection for the labia minora and clitoral area in contrast to dysplastic naevi, which in this area tend to involve the labia majora. The rarer variants of melanoma such as desmoplastic and neurotropic types are also described on the vulva.[72,73]

In the great majority of cases, lentigo maligna melanoma occurs on light-exposed skin. The relative proportions of the other types described vary greatly in different series,[74] probably as a result of differences in definition of type. In our own series, more than 50 per cent were of invasive superficial spreading type.

Histologically, superficial spreading melanoma shows a 'radial' or in situ growth phase with nests of atypical melanocytes at all levels of the epidermis before the development of invasive foci. Acral and mucosal lentiginous and lentigo maligna types also show a well-developed radial phase of different morphology (Figs 3.12 and 3.13). Nodular malignant melanoma manifests a 'vertical' (invasive) growth pattern from very early in the disease, with the intraepithelial component absent or slight (extending no more than three rete ridges from

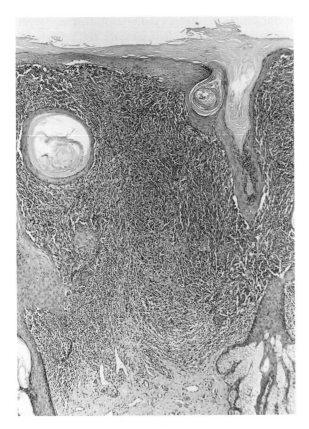

Figure 3.12 *This malignant melanoma of the vulva shows a predominantly spindle cell morphology with dermal invasion and a very prominent lymphoid infiltrate. (Reproduced from* CPD Bulletin – Cellular Pathology, vol. 1, 1998, pp 19–25, with the permission of Rila Publications, London.)

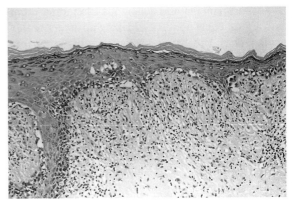

Figure 3.13 *At higher magnification the radial growth phase of the melanoma shows similarities to acral lentiginous melanoma (the so-called mucosal lentiginous variant of vulvar melanoma). (Reproduced from* CPD Bulletin – Cellular Pathology, vol. 1, 1998, pp 19–25, with the permission of Rila Publications, London.)

It has been suggested that the FIGO staging system used for squamous carcinoma does not correlate well with survival in malignant melanoma of the vulva,[75] but others disagree.[67,76,79] Mitotic rate has been said, by some, to be of prognostic importance,[67,76] as have the presence or absence of ulceration and the cell type.[67,80] Morphometry has not been shown to be clearly useful.[80] Recently, it has been suggested that ploidy studies may be important,[81] although confirmation of this is at present lacking.

EPITHELIAL TUMOURS OF GLANDS AND ADNEXAL STRUCTURES

Carcinoma of Bartholin's glands

More than 200 cases of this tumour have been reported[82–84] and the histological type varies widely. Mean age at diagnosis is the mid-50s but the age range is very wide. Presentation is usually with a mass, pain or discharge. Three criteria have been demanded in order to accept that a tumour originates in a   Bartholin's gland:

1 The tumour must arise in the usual area of Bartholin's gland.
2 A transition from non-neoplastic to neoplastic tissue must be seen.
3 No primary tumour of similar type must be present at another site.

the invasive zone). There is disagreement in the literature about the prognostic usefulness of melanoma typing in malignant melanomas of the vulva.[67,75,76]

As with other skin sites, prognosis appears to be closely determined by tumour depth, which is best assessed by direct measurement, as described by Breslow, rather than by Clark's levels. By inference from other sites, the likely relevant depths will be up to 0.76 mm (prognosis excellent), 1.5 mm (intermediate group) and over 1.5 mm (prognosis poor). This hypothesis gains support from studies using depth measurement[76] and older studies using Clark's levels.[77,78] A considerable practical problem, however, with the utilization of such depths for prognosis and treatment in vulvar tumours is that they tend to present late and prognostic bands of greater overall thickness may also have some value at this site.[67]

Adenocarcinoma and squamous carcinoma occur with almost equal frequency, making up 80 per cent of malignancies. Variants of adenocarcinoma, e.g. papillary and mucinous carnicomas, are well described. Adenoid cystic carcinoma possibly makes up a further 8–15 per cent of carcinomas (there are more than 45 cases in the literature showing the characteristic histological pattern of cords and nests of cells, with a prominent myoepithelial cell layer, arranged around a dense hyaline core). The remaining tumours are transitional (with eight cases in the literature up until 1994),[85] adenosquamous and undifferentiated carcinomas, and malignant melanomas.

The aetiology of tumours arising in the gland has not been studied in depth but recent work suggests a role for HPV infection in squamous carcinoma and further proposes that squamous and adenocarcinomas at this site may arise in the transition zone between epithelial types in Bartholin's duct, whereas adenoid cystic tumours may arise from myoepithelial cells.[86] Tumours of Bartholin's gland typically spread locally and to regional nodes.

Adenoid cystic tumours are slow growing with only 15 per cent being metastatic at the time of diagnosis, compared with 20–50 per cent for adeno- and squamous carcinomas, but local recurrence is common. For squamous, adenosquamous and adenocarcinomas the 5-year survival rate is approximately 50 per cent with no nodal involvement, but less than 20 per cent with two or more nodes involved.[82,83]

Sweat gland and other tumours

The great majority of these tumours are benign and the most common at this site is the simple papillary hidradenoma. Clear cell hidradenomas are also described,[87] as are trichoepitheliomas, trichilemmomas and syringomas. Syringomas may be multiple and associated with pruritus. Proliferating trichilemmal tumours at this site may be mistaken histologically and clinically for squamous carcinomas.[88] Rare malignant examples of sweat gland tumours unassociated with Paget's disease have been described, including eccrine and apocrine variants,[89] although the histological appearance of the cases illustrated is not always convincing. Sebaceous carcinoma is also described[90] as is carcinoma arising from Skene's glands.[91] Benign and malignant mixed tumours occur and probably arise from sweat glands or Bartholin's glands.[92]

Ectopic mammary-type tissue may be seen in the vulvar connective tissues. A range of mammary-type tumours, benign and malignant, are also described,[93] and a proportion of cases of vulvar Paget's disease may arise in such structures. Adenocarcinomas in the breast-type tissue are very rare but appear usually to be small; they are really impossible to separate histologically from sweat gland carcinomas.

SARCOMAS AND RELATED CONDITIONS

Leiomyosarcoma

This appears to be the most common of the vulvar sarcomas, which are rare tumours accounting for only approximately 1–2 per cent of all vulvar malignancies.[94,95] Most appear to represent *de novo* tumours rather than malignant change in a leiomyoma, and have usually presented as rapidly growing masses larger than 5 cm in diameter in women in their 20s and 30s. Those cases not cured by wide local excision appear to have a protracted course with local recurrences, but widespread metastases may occur.

Diagnosis of malignancy at this site has in the past been based on tumour size, the presence of mitotic counts over 10 per 10 high power fields (h.p.f.), pleomorphism, infiltrative margins and abnormal mitoses. Tavassoli and Norris[94] reviewed 32 smooth muscle tumours of the vulva, and found large size and high mitotic rate to be the best predictors of recurrence, although none of their series metastasized; this is in contrast to the outcome seen by others.[96,97] Nielsen and colleagues[98] suggest that tumours showing three of the following features should be considered malignant:

- ≥5 cm in diameter
- infiltrative margins
- ≥5 mitoses per 10 h.p.f.
- moderate-to-severe cellular atypia.

It has been traditional to consider vulvar smooth muscle tumours (benign and malignant) as cutaneous leiomyomas/sarcomas, but Newman and Fletcher[99] question this viewpoint because they appear to be clinicopathologically distinct in that they are much larger tumours and commonly show myxoid and hyaline change. Epithelioid differentiation is also seen more frequently in the vulvar tumours.

Fibrosarcoma

Tumours previously classified as fibrosarcomas have occurred over a wide age range[96,97] and appear to have a poor prognosis. Most of these tumours would now be reclassified as other types of sarcoma, e.g. schwannoma, monophasic synovial sarcoma, etc., and immunocytochemistry is imperative in excluding alternative diagnoses before acceptance of a tumour as a fibrosarcoma. Even allowing for their historical over-diagnosis, they have been rarely reported.

Malignant fibrous histiocytoma

Said to be the second most common vulvar sarcoma,[97] this tumour occurs in various subtypes of highly variable histological pattern, but generally contains a fibroblast-like component together with histiocytic cells and often large bizarre cells. As for fibrosarcomas, histological criteria for diagnosis and opinions on these tumours have changed and they appear, in reality, to represent a morphological pattern shared by a number of anaplastic sarcomas, including liposarcoma, leiomyosarcoma and rhabdomyosarcoma. Historically, they have classically presented as a large mass in a middle-aged woman. Widespread metastases have been reported in a proportion of cases.[97,100]

Ten cases of dermatofibrosarcoma protuberans, a low-grade malignant tumour often in the past put in the fibrous histiocytoma tumour group, recurring locally and rarely metastasizing, have been described in the vulva.[101] It is composed of spindle cells in an interweaving 'storiform' (rush mat-like) pattern with infiltrative margins.

Aggressive angiomyxoma and angiomyofibroblastoma

Aggressive angiomyxoma was first described by Steeper and Rosai[102] and in women shows a predilection for the vulva and paravaginal tissues of young adults. Up to 1992 26 cases had been reported in the vulva, vagina, pelvic floor and perineum of women.[103] It is characterized by slow growth and extensive local recurrences, and is locally infiltrative with very poorly defined margins. Most recurrences occur within 3–4 years of primary surgery. Metastases are not described and this condition does not appear to be a true sarcoma.

Macroscopically, the tumours are usually large (up to 60 cm), gelatinous and sticky (Fig. 3.14). Histologi-

cally, they show an abundant myxoid stroma with scattered collagen bundles and numerous vessels present, some of which are thick walled (Figs 3.15 and 3.16). Glandular elements have been described. Some workers have favoured a myofibroblast origin and immunocytochemistry tends to support this, with immunohistochemical positivity for vimentin, actin and S100 protein,[103] but other studies by electron microscopy favour a purely fibroblast origin.[104]

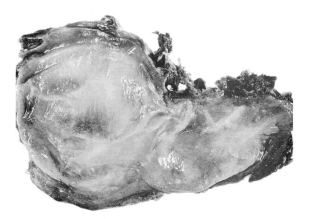

Fig 3.14 *Photograph of a recurrent aggressive angiomyxoma involving the paravaginal tissues. The tumour measured more than 20 cm in its maximum diameter. The cut surface shows the typical gelatinous appearance and the tumour margins are irregular and poorly defined.*
(Reproduced from CPD Bulletin – Cellular Pathology, *vol. 1, 1998, pp 1–36, with the permission of Rila Publications, London.)*

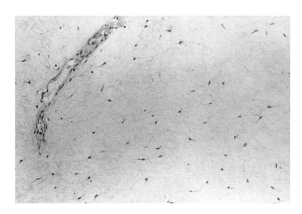

Figure 3.15 *Aggressive angiomyxoma. The tumour shows stellate and spindled cells in an abundant 'myxoid' matrix. (Reproduced from* CPD Bulletin – Cellular Pathology, *vol. 1, 1998, pp 19–25, with the permission of Rila Publications, London.)*

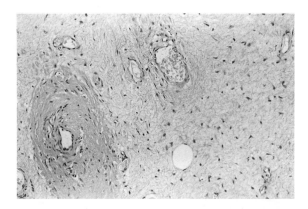

Figure 3.16 *Aggressive angiomyxoma. Vessels are numerous and some are thick walled. (Reproduced from* CPD Bulletin – Cellular Pathology, *vol. 1, 1998, pp 1–36, with the permission of Rila Publications, London.)*

Angiomyofibroblastoma is described almost exclusively in the vulva of premenopausal women.[105,106] Although benign and not producing local recurrences after complete removal, it is described here because of the difficulty in differentiating it from aggressive angiomyxoma. It presents as a circumscribed mass, usually less than 5 cm in diameter, and may be mistaken clinically for a Bartholin's cyst. Histologically, the tumour shows ovoid, round or spindled cells in an oedematous background with evidence of numerous capillaries. Occasionally, cellular aggregates and solid areas are seen and an adipocytic component or epithelioid pattern of differentiation may be evident. A single example of malignant transformation of angiomyofibroblastoma to sarcoma has been described.[107]

Rhabdomyosarcoma

The embryonal variant typically seen in the vagina has been described on only a few occasions in the vulva;[108–110] in two cases the disease was fatal. It should be remembered that benign vulvar and vaginal fibroepithelial (pseudosarcomatous) polyps may superficially histologically resemble embryonal rhabdomyosarcoma[111] and care should be taken not to confuse the two. Several cases of the alveolar variant of rhabdomyosarcoma have been described at this site.[112–115] Other reports of rhabdomyosarcoma exist where their type was not stated. Prognosis generally appears to be poor.

Other sarcomas

Malignant granular cell tumours,[116] alveolar soft part sarcoma,[117] malignant schwannoma,[115,118] Kaposi's sarcoma,[119,120] synovial sarcoma,[121] malignant rhabdoid tumour[122] and epithelioid sarcoma (including a 'proximal' variant)[123,124] have all been described on the vulva. Most essentially appear similar to those at the more common sites of occurrence, although epithelioid sarcomas here may be more aggressive.[125] Occasional cases are reported of vascular tumours, including haemangiopericytomas[118] and haemangiosarcomas.[126]

Liposarcomas of the vulva are rare; most have had the appearances of well-differentiated liposarcoma/atypical lipomatous tumour and have arisen in middle-aged women. Clinical outcome appears to be favourable, although the tumours may show unusual histological appearances, which are possibly unique to this site.[127]

It should be borne in mind that postoperative spindle cell nodules may also occur on the vulva and may be misdiagnosed as sarcomas.[128,129] Diagnostic difficulties may also be experienced with nodular fasciitis at this site (11 cases in the literature to date).[130]

MISCELLANEOUS PRIMARY TUMOURS

Yolk sac (endodermal sinus) tumours occur rarely as primary vulvar tumours[131] as do mesotheliomas.[118] Davos and Abell[118] also reported an 'embryonal stromal sarcoma'. A suggested case of adenosarcoma arising in endometriosis has been described.[132]

Primary lymphomas are very rare but this site has been stated to be the second most common site in the female genital tract site after the cervix.[133,134] Most appear to be of a diffuse, large-cell type. They tend to occur in women of reproductive age and present as an erythematous mass.

Merkel's cell tumours have occasionally been described and may be associated with VIN or invasive squamous carcinoma. They usually present as solitary or multiple intradermal nodules in elderly women and have a high risk of early metastasis to regional nodes.[135,136] Histologically they typically show the small-cell pattern of neuroectodermal tumours, but may show trabecular, intermediate or small-cell differentiation. They are reactive with neuroendocrine markers such as anti-chromogranin, but may be misdiagnosed as basal cell carcinomas, lymphomas or metastatic small-cell bronchial or cervical carcinomas.

A phyllodes tumour with postsurgical recurrence has been reported arising in 'aberrant breast tissue'.[137]

METASTATIC TUMOURS

The vulva is an uncommon site for metastases (Fig. 3.17). Most come from the female genital tract. In a series of more than 260 cases of vulvar malignancy, Dehner found that 8 per cent of tumours were metastatic.[138] Out of 22 cases 10 were metastatic cervical squamous carcinomas. Metastatic endometrial carcinoma was next in frequency. Other metastases described are transitional cell carcinomas of urethra and bladder,[138,139] carcinoma of breast,[138,140] vagina, stomach, lung, ovary, kidney and lymphoma. Metastatic choriocarcinomas, sarcomas and malignant melanomas have also been seen. Most metastases are seen within the labia majora. Bartholin's glands may be involved. The metastasis usually presents within 18 months of diagnosis of the primary tumour and few patients survive for more than 12 months.

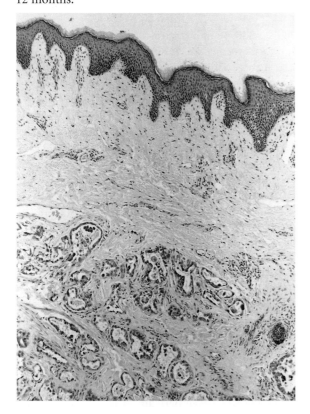

Figure 3.17 *In the deep dermis and subcutis, there is a metastatic clear-cell carcinoma of tubulopapillary type (possibly a metastasis from the ovary).*

REFERENCES

1 Wilkinson EJ. Superficially invasive carcinoma of the vulva. In: Wilkinson EJ (ed). *Pathology of the vulva and vagina*. New York: Churchill Livingstone, 1987: 103–17.

2 Wharton J, Gallagher S, Rutledge FN. Microinvasive carcinoma of the vulva. *Am J Obstet Gynecol* 1974; **118**: 159–62.

3 Buscema J, Stern JL, Woodruff JD. Early invasive carcinoma of the vulva. *Am J Obstet Gynecol* 1981; **140**: 563–9.

4 Donaldson ES, Powell DE, Hanson MB, van Nagell JR. Prognostic parameters in invasive vulvar cancer. *Cancer* 1981; **11**: 184–90.

5 Hacker NF, Berek JS, Lagasse LD et al. Individualisation of treatment for stage I squamous cell vulvar carcinoma. *Obstet Gynecol* 1984; **63**: 155–62.

6 Yoonessi M, Goodell T, Satchidanand S et al. Microinvasive squamous carcinoma of the vulva. *J Surg Oncol* 1983; **24**: 315–21.

7 Pickel H, Haas J. Microcarcinoma of the vulva. *J Reprod Med* 1986; **31**: 831–5.

8 Dvoretsky PM, Bonfiglio TA, Helmkamp BF et al. The pathology of superficially invasive thin vulvar squamous carcinoma. *Int J Gynecol Pathol* 1984; **3**: 331–42.

9 Van der Velden J, Kooyman CD, Van Lindert ACM, Heintz APM. A stage Ia vulvar carcinoma with an inguinal node recurrence after local excision. A case report and literature review. *Int J Gynecol Cancer* 1992; **2**: 157–9.

10 Kurman RJ, Norris HJ, Wilkinson E. Tumors of the vulva. In: *Tumors of the cervix, vagina and vulva*. Washington, DC: Armed Forces Institute of Pathology, 1992: 179–255.

11 Barnes AE, Crissman JD, Schellhas HF, Azoury RS. Microinvasive carcinoma of the vulva: a clinicopathological evaluation. *Obstet Gynecol* 1980; **56**: 234–8.

12 Wilkinson EJ, Rico MJ, Pierson KK. Microinvasive carcinoma of the vulva. *Int J Gynecol Pathol* 1982; **1**: 29–39.

13 Zaino RJ. Carcinoma of the vulva, urethra and Bartholin's glands. In: Wilkinson EJ (ed). *Pathology of the vulva and vagina*. New York: Churchill Livingstone, 1987: 119–53.

14 Sedlis A, Homesley H, Bundy BN et al. Positive groin lymph nodes in superficial squamous cell vulvar cancer. A gynecologic oncology group study. *Am J Obstet Gynecol* 1987; **156**: 1159–64.

15 Andreasson B, Bock JE, Weberg E. Invasive cancer in the vulvar region. *Acta Obstet Gynecol Scand* 1982; **6**: 113–19.

16 Green TH, Ulfelder H, Meigs J V. Epidermoid carcinoma of the vulva: an analysis of 238 cases. I. Etiology and diagnosis. *Am J Obstet Gynecol* 1958; **75**: 834–47.

17 Jones RW, Baranyai J, Stables S. Trends in squamous cell carcinoma of the vulva: the influence of vulvar intraepithelial hyperplasia. *Obstet Gynecol* 1997; **90**: 448–52.

18 Carter J, Carlson J, Fowler J et al. Invasive vulvar tumors in young women – A disease of the immunosuppressed? *Gynecol Oncol* 1993; **51**: 307–10.

19 Crum CP. Carcinoma of the vulva: epidemiology and pathogenesis. *Obstet Gynecol* 1992; **79**: 448–54.

20 Toki T, Kurman RJ, Park JS, Kessis T, Daniel RW, Shah KV. Probable nonpapillomavirus etiology of squamous cell carcinoma of the vulva in older women: a clinicopathologic study using in situ hybridization and polymerase chain reaction. *Int J Gynecol Pathol* 1991; **10**: 107–25.

21 Trimble CL, Hildesheim A, Brinton LA, Shah KV, Kurman RJ. Heterogeneous etiology of squamous carcinoma of the vulva. *Obstet Gynecol* 1996; **87**: 59–64.

22 Monk BJ, Burger RA, Lin F, Parham G, Vasilev SA, Wilczynski SP. Prognostic significance of human papillomavirus DNA in vulvar carcinoma. *Obstet Gynecol* 1995; **85**: 709–15.

23 Japaze H, Garcia Bunuel R, Woodruff JD. Primary vulvar neoplasia. A review of in-situ and invasive carcinoma 1935–1972. *Obstet Gynecol* 1977; **49**: 404–11.

24 Herod JJO, Shafi MI, Rollason TP et al. Vulvar intra-epithelial neoplasia: long term follow up of treated and untreated women. *Br J Obstet Gynaecol* 1996; **103**: 446–52.

25 Green TH. Carcinoma of the vulva – a reassessment. *Obstet Gynecol* 1978; **52**: 462-9.

26 Hay DM, Cole FM. Primary invasive carcinoma of the vulva in Jamaica. *J Obstet Gynecol Br Commonwealth* 1969; **76**: 821–30.

27 Brinton LA, Nasca PC, Mallin K, Baptiste MS, Wilbanks GD, Richart RM. Case–control study of cancer of the vulva. *Obstet Gynecol* 1990; **75**: 859–66.

28 Boyce J, Fruchter RG, Kasambilides E et al. Prognostic factors in carcinoma of the vulva. *Gynecol Oncol* 1985; **20**: 364–77.

29 Rowley KC, Gallion HH, Donaldson ES et al. Prognostic factors in early vulvar cancer. *Gynecol Oncol* 1988; **31**: 43–9.

30 Hopkins MP, Reid GC, Vettrano I, Morley GW. Squamous cell carcinoma of the vulva: prognostic factors influencing survival. *Gynecol Oncol* 1991; **43**: 113–17.

31 Bjerregaard B, Andreasson B, Visfeldt J, Bock JE. The significance of histology and morphometry in predicting lymp node metastases in patients with squamous cell carcinoma of the vulva. *Gynecol Oncol* 1993; **50**: 323–9.

32 Iversen T, Abeler V, Aalders J. Individualized treatment of Stage 1 carcinoma of the vulva. *Obstet Gynecol* 1981; **57**: 85–9.

33 Dolan JR, McCall AR, Gooneratne S, Walter S, Lansky DM. DNA ploidy, proliferation index, grade and stage as prognostic factors for vulvar squamous carcinomas. *Gynecol Oncol* 1993; **48**: 232–5.

34 Ballouk F, Ambros RA, Malfetano JH, Ross JS. Evaluation of prognostic indicators in squamous carcinoma of the vulva including nuclear DNA content. *Mod Pathol* 1993; 6: 371–5.

35 Drew PA, AL-Abbadi MA, Orlando CA, Hendricks JB, Kubilis PS, Wilkinson EJ. Prognostic factors in carcinoma of the vulva: a clinicopathologic and DNA flow cytometric study. *Int J Gynecol Pathol* 1996; **15**: 235–41.

36 Isaacs JH. Verrucous carcinoma of the female genital tract. *Gynecol Oncol* 1976; **4**: 259–69.

37 Japaze H, Van Dinh T, Woodruff JD. Verrucous carcinoma of the vulva: study of 24 cases. *Obstet Gynecol* 1982; **60**: 462–6.

38 Brisigotti M, Moreno A, Murcia C, Matias-Guia X, Prat J. Verrucous carcinoma of the vulva. A clinicopathologic and immunohistochemical study of five cases. *Int J Gynecol Pathol* 1989; **8**: 1–7.

39 Partridge EE, Murad T, Shingleton HM et al. Verrucous lesions of the female genitalia. 2. Verrucous carcinoma. *Am J Obstet Gynecol* 1980; **137**: 412–18.

40 Baird PJ, Elliot P, Stening M, Korda A. Giant condyloma acuminatum of the vulva and anal canal. *Aust NZ J Obstet Gynaecol* 1979; **19**: 119–22.

41 Downey GO, Okagaki T, Ostrow RS et al. Condylomatous carcinoma of the vulva with special reference to human papillomavirus DNA. *Obstet Gynecol* 1988; **72**: 68–73.

42 Wolber RA, Talerman A, Wilkinson EJ, Clement PB. Vulvar granular cell tumours with pseudocarcinomatous hyperplasia: a comparative analysis with well differentiated squamous carcinoma. *Int J Gynecol Pathol* 1991; **10**: 59–66.

43 Hording U, Daugaard S, Junge J, Lundvall F. Human papillomaviruses and multifocal genital neoplasia. *Int J Gynecol Pathol* 1996; **15**: 230–4.

44 Kurman RJ, Toki T, Schiffman MH. Basaloid and warty carcinomas of the vulva. Distinctive types of squamous cell carcinoma frequently associated with human papillomaviruses. *Am J Surg Pathol* 1993; **17**: 133–45.

45 Copas P, Dyer M, Comas FV, Hall DJ. Spindle cell carcinoma of the vulva. *Diag Gynecol Obstet* 1982; **4**: 235–41.

46 Underwood J-W, Adcock LL, Okagaki T. Adenosquamous carcinoma of skin appendages (adenoid squamous cell carcinoma, pseudoglandular squamous carcinoma, adenoacanthoma of sweat gland of Lever) of the vulva. A clinical and ultrastructural study. *Cancer* 1978; **42**: 1851–8.

47 Lasser A, Cornorg JL, Morris JM. Adenoid squamous cell carcinoma of the vulva. *Cancer* 1974; **33**: 224–7.

48 Cruz-Jimenez PR, Abell MR. Cutaneous basal cell carcinoma of the vulva. *Obstet Gynecol* 1975; **36**: 1860–8.

49 Benedet JL, Miller DM, Ehlen TG, Bertrand MA. Basal cell carcinoma of the vulva: clinical features and treatment results in 28 patients. *Obstet Gynecol* 1997; **90**: 765–8.

50 Feakins RM, Lowe DG. Basal cell carcinoma of the vulva: a clinicopathologic study of 45 cases. *Int J Gynecol Pathol* 1997; **16**: 319–24.

51 Breen JL, Neubecker RD, Greenwald E, Gregori CA. Basal cell carcinoma of the vulva. *Obstet Gynecol* 1975; **46**: 122–9.

52 Palladino VS, Duffy JL, Bures GJ. Basal cell carcinoma of the vulva. *Cancer* 1969; **24**: 460–76.

53 Perrone T, Twiggs LB, Adcock LL, Dehner LP. Vulvar basal cell carcinoma: an infrequently metastasising neoplasm. *Int J Gynecol Pathol* 1987; **6**: 152–65.

54 Gleeson NC, Ruffolo EH, Hoffman MS, Cavanagh D. Basal cell carcinoma of the vulva with groin node metastases. *Gynecol Oncol* 1994; **53**: 366–8.

55 Merino MJ, Livolsi VA, Shwartz PE, Rudnicki J. Adenoid basal cell carcinoma of the vulva. *Int J Gynecol Pathol* 1982; **1**: 299–306.

56 Taylor PR, Stenwig JT, Klausen H. Paget's disease of the vulva. *Gynecol Oncol* 1975; **3**: 46–60.

57 Baehrendtz H, Einhom N, Pettersson F, Silfverswiird C. Paget's disease of the vulva, the Radiumhemmet series 1975–1990. *Int J Gynecol Cancer* 1994; **4**: 1–6.

58 Olson DJ, Fujimura M, Swanson P, Okagaki T. Immunohistochemical features of Paget's disease of the vulva with and without adenocarcinoma. *Int J Gynecol Pathol* 1991; **10**: 285–95.

59 Jones RE, Austin C, Ackerman AB. Extramammary Paget's disease: a critical re-examination. *Am J Dermatopathol* 1979; **1**: 101–32.

60 Fishman DA, Chambers SK, Shwartz PE, Kohorn EI, Chambers JT. Extramammary Paget's disease of the vulva. *Gynecol Oncol* 1995; **56**: 266–70.

61 Kodama S, Kaneko T, Saito M, Yoshiya N, Honma S, Tanaka K. A clinicopathologic study of 30 patients with Paget's disease of the vulva. *Gynecol Oncol* 1995; **56**: 63–70.

62 Molinie V, Paniel BJ, Lessana-Leibowitch M, Moyal-Barracco M, Pelisse M, Escande JP. Paget's disease of the vulva. 36 cases. *Ann Dermatol Venereol* 1993; **120**: 522–7.

63 Ariel IM. Malignant melanoma of the female genital system: A report of 48 patients and review of the literature *J Surg Oncol* 1981; **16**: 371–83.

64 Chung AF, Woodruff JM, Lewis JL. Malignant melanoma of the vulva: a report of 44 cases. *Obstet Gynecol* 1975; **45**: 638–46.

65 Ragnarssonolding B, Johanson H, Rutgvist LE, Ringborg U. Malignant melanoma of the vulva and vagina: trends in incidence, age distribution and long term survival among 245 consecutive cases in Sweden 1960–1984. *Cancer* 1993; **71**: 1893–7.

66 Edington PT, Monaghan JM. Malignant melanoma of the vulva and vagina. *Br J Obstet Gynaecol* 1980; **87**: 422–4.

67 Bradgate M, Rollason TP, McConkey CC, Powell J. Malignant melanoma of the vulva: A clinico-pathological study of 50 cases. *Br J Obstet Gynaecol* 1990; **97**: 124–33.

68 Morrow CP, Rutledge FN. Melanoma of the vulva. *Obstet Gynecol* 1972; **39**: 745–52.

69 Friedman RJ, Ackerman AB. Difficulties in the histologic diagnosis of melanocytic nevi on the vulvae of premenopausal women. In: Ackerman AB (ed). *Pathology of malignant melanoma*. New York: Masson, 1981: 119–27.

70 Rogers RS III, Gibson LE. Mucosal, genital and unusual clinical variants of melanoma. *Mayo Clin Proc* 1997; **72**: 362–6.

71 Clark WH Jr, Hood AF, Tucker MA, Jampel RM. Atypical melanocytic nevi of the genital type with a discussion of reciprocal parenchymal–stromal interactions in the biology of neoplasia. *Hum Pathol* 1998; **29**(Suppl 1): S1–24.

72 Mulvany NJ, Sykes P. Desmoplastic melanoma of the vulva. *Pathology* 1997; **29**: 241–5.

73 Benda JA. Neurotropic desmoplastic melanoma of the vulva. *Gynecol Oncol* 1997; **64**: 180.

74 Kendall Pierson K. Malignant melanomas and pigmented lesions of the vulva. In: Wilkinson EJ (ed). *Pathology of the vulva and vagina*. New York: Churchill Livingstone, 1987: 155–79.

75 Podratz KC, Gaffey TA, Symmonds RE, Johansen KL, O'Brien PC. Melanoma of the vulva: an update. *Gynecol Oncol* 1983; **16**: 153–68.

76 Johnson TL, Kumar NB, White CD, Morley GW. Prognostic features of vulvar melanoma: a clinicopathological analysis. *Int J Gynecol Pathol* 1986; **5**: 110–18.

77 Morrow CP, DiSaia PJ. Malignant melanoma of the female genitalia: A clinical analysis. *Obstet Gynecol Surv* 1976; **31**: 233–71.

78 Jaramillo BA, Ganjei P, Averette HE et al. Malignant melanoma of the vulva. *Obstet Gynecol* 1985; **66**: 398–401.

79 Raber G, Mempel V, Jackish C et al. Malignant melanoma of the vulva. Report of 89 patients. *Cancer* 1996; **78**: 2353–8.

80 Tasseron EWK, Van der Esch EP, Hart AAM, Brutel de la Riviere G, Aartson EJ. A clinicopathological study of 30 melanomas of the vulva. *Gynecol Oncol* 1992; **46**: 170–5.

81 Scheistroen M, Trope C, Kaern J, Abeler VM, Pettersen EO, Kristensen GB. Malignant melanoma of the vulva FIGO stage 1: Evaluation of prognostic factors in 43 patients with emphasis on DNA ploidy and surgical treatment. *Gynecol Oncol* 1996; **61**: 253–8.

82 Leuchter RS, Hacker NF, Voet RL et al. Primary carcinoma of the Bartholin gland: a report of 14 cases and review of the literature. *Obstet Gynecol* 1982; **60**: 361–7.

83 Wheelock JB, Goplerud DR, Dunn LJ, Oates JF. Primary carcinoma of the Bartholin gland: a report of 10 cases. *Obstet Gynecol* 1984; **63**: 820–4.

84 DePasquale SE, McGuiness TB, Mangan CE, Husson M, Woodland MB. Adenoid cystic carcinoma of Bartholin's gland: a review of the literature and report of a patient. *Gynecol Oncol* 1996; **61**: 122–5.

85 Forster H, Till A, Martin H. Transitional cell carcinoma of Bartholin's glands. *Zentralbl Gynakol* 1994; **116**: 289–94.

86 Felix JC, Cote RJ, Kramer EE, Saigo P, Goldman GH. Carcinomas of Bartholin's gland. Histogenesis and the etiological role of human papillomavirus. *Am J Pathol* 1993; **142**: 925–33.

87 Nielsen NC. Hidradenoma of the vulva. *Acta Obstet Gynecol* 1973; **52**: 387–9.

88 Avinoach I, Zirkin HJ, Glezerman M. Proliferating trichilemmal tumor of the vulva. Case report and review of the literature. *Int J Gynecol Pathol* 1989; **8**: 163–8.

89 Wick MR, Goellner JR, Wolfe JT, Su WPD. Vulvar sweat gland carcinomas. *Arch Pathol Lab Med* 1985; **109**: 43–7.

90 Jacobs DM, Sandles LG, Leboit PE. Sebaceous carcinoma arising from Bowen's disease of the vulva. *Arch Dermatol* 1986; **122**: 1191–3.

91 Taylor RN, Lacey CG, Shuman MA. Adenocarcinoma of Skene's duct associated with a systemic coagulopathy. *Gynecol Oncol* 1985; **22**: 250–6.

92 Rorat E, Wallach RC. Mixed tumours of the vulva: clinical outcome and pathology. *Int J Gynecol Pathol* 1984; **3**: 323–8.

93 van der Putte SCJ. Mammary-like glands of the vulva and their disorders. *Int J Gynecol Pathol* 1994; **13**: 150–60.

94 Tavassoli FA, Norris FJ. Smooth muscle tumours of the vulva. *Obstet Gynecol* 1979; **53**: 213–24.

95 Audet-Lapointe P, Paquin F, Guerard MJ et al. Leiomyosarcoma of the vulva. *Gynecol Oncol* 1980; **10**: 350–5.

96 DiSaia PJ, Rutledge F, Smith JP. Sarcoma of the vulva: report of 12 patients. *Obstet Gynecol* 1971; **38**: 180–4.

97 Davos I, Abell M. Soft tissue sarcomas of the vulva. *Gynecol Oncol* 1976; **4**: 70–86.

98 Nielsen GP, Rosenberg AE, Koerner FC, Young RH, Scully RE. Smooth-muscle tumors of the vulva. A clinicopathological study of 25 cases and review of the literature. *Am J Surg Pathol* 1996; **20**: 779–93.

99 Newman PL, Fletcher CD. Smooth muscle tumours of the external genitalia: clinicopathological analysis of a series. *Histopathology* 1991; **18**: 523–9.

100 Hensley GT, Friedrich EG. Malignant fibroxanthoma: a sarcoma of the vulva. *Am J Obstet Gynecol* 1973; **116**: 289–91.

101 Karlen JR, Johnson K, Kashkari S. Dermatofibrosarcoma protuberans of the vulva. A case report. *J Reprod Med* 1996; **41**: 267–9.

102 Steeper T, Rosai J. Aggressive angiomyxoma of the female pelvis and perineum. *Am J Surg Pathol* 1983; **7**: 463–76.

103 Elchalal U, Lifschitz-Mercer B, Dgani R, Zalel Y. Case report. Aggressive angiomyxoma of the vulva. *Gynecol Oncol* 1992; **47**: 260–2.

104 Begin LR, Clement PB, Kirk ME et al. Aggressive angiomyxoma of pelvic soft parts: a clinicopathologic study of nine cases. *Hum Pathol* 1985; **16**: 621–8.

105 Fletcher CDM, Tsang WY-W, Fisher C et al. Angiomyofibroblastoma of the vulva. A benign neoplasm distinct from aggressive angiomyxoma. *Am J Surg Pathol* 1992; **16**: 373–82.

106 Hiruki T, Thomas MJ, Clement PB. Vulvar angiomyofi-broblastoma. *Am J Surg Pathol* 1993; **17**: 423–4 (letter).

107 Nielsen GP, Young RH, Dickersin GR, Rosenberg AE. Angiomyofibroblastoma of the vulva with sarcomatous transformation ('angiomyofibrosarcoma'). *Am J Surg Pathol* 1997; **21**: 1104–8.

108 Talerman A. Sarcoma botryoides presenting as a polyp on the labium majus. *Cancer* 1973; **32**: 994–9.

109 Hildebrand HF, Krivosic I, Grandier-Vazeille X et al. Perineal rhabdomyosarcoma in a newborn child: pathological and biochemical studies with emphasis on contractile proteins. *J Clin Pathol* 1980; **33**: 823–9.

110 Copeland LJ, Gershenson DM, Saul PB et al. Sarcoma botryoides of the female genital tract. *Obstet Gynecol* 1985; **66**: 262–6.

111 Mucitelli DR, Charles EZ, Kraus FT. Vulvovaginal polyps. Histologic appearances, ultrastructure, immunohistochemical characteristics and clinicopathologic correlations. *Int J Gynecol Pathol* 1990; **9**: 20–40.

112 Copeland LJ, Sneige N, Stringer A et al. Alveolar rhabdomyosarcoma of the female genitalia. *Cancer* 1985; **56**: 849–55.

113 Imachi M, Tsukamoto N, Kamura T et al. Alveolar rhabdomyosarcoma of the vulva. Report of two cases. *Acta Cytol* 1991; **35**: 345–9.

114 Bond SJ, Seibel N, Kapur S, Newman KD. Rhabdomyosarcoma of the clitoris. *Cancer* 1994; **73**: 1984–9.

115 Maldonado A, Fradera J, Velez-Garaia E. Carcinocythemia in a patient with rhabdomyosarcoma. *Bol Assoc Med PR* 1991; **83**: 13–16.

116 Robertson AJ, McIntosh W, Lamont P, Guthrie W. Malignant granular cell tumour (myoblastoma) of the vulva: report of a case and review of the literature. *Histopathology* 1981; **5**: 69–79.

117 Shen JT, D'Ablang G, Morrow CP. Alveolar soft part sarcoma of the vulva: report of first case and review of the literature. *Gynecol Oncol* 1982; **13**: 120–8.

118 Davos I, Abell M. Soft tissue sarcomas of the vulva. *Gynecol Oncol* 1976; **4**: 70–86.

119 Hall DJ. Kaposi's sarcoma of the vulva: a case report and brief review. *Obstet Gynecol* 1979; **54**: 478–83.

120 LiVolsi VA, Brookes JJ. Soft tissue tumours of the vulva. In: Wilkinson EJ (ed). *Pathology of the vulva and vagina*. New York: Churchill Livingstone, 1987: 209–38.

121 Nielsen GP, Shaw PA, Rosenberg E et al. Synovial sarcoma of the vulva: report of two cases. *Mod Pathol* 1996; **9**: 970–4.

122 Perrone T, Swanson PE, Twiggs L, Ulbright TM, Dehner LP. Malignant rhabdoid tumor of the vulva: is distinction from epithelioid sarcoma possible? A pathologic and immunohistochemical study. *Am J Surg Pathol* 1989; **13**: 848–58.

123 Hall DJ, Grimes MM, Goplerud DR. Epithelioid sarcoma of the vulva. *Gynecol Oncol* 1980; **9**: 237–46.

124 Guillou L, Wadden C, Coindre JM et al. 'Proximal-type' epithelioid sarcoma, a distinctive aggressive neoplasm showing rhabdoid features. Clinicopathologic, immunohistochemical, and ultrastructural study of a series. *Am J Surg Pathol* 1997; **21**: 130–46.

125 Ulbright TM, Brokaw SA, Stehman FB, Roth LM. Epithelioid sarcoma of the vulva: evidence suggesting a more aggressive behaviour than extra-genital epithelioid sarcoma. *Cancer* 1983; **52**: 1462–9.

126 Nirenberg A, Ostor AG, Slavin J et al. Primary vulvar sarcomas. *Int J Gynecol Pathol* 1995; **14**: 55–62.

127 Nucci MR, Fletcher CD. Liposarcoma (atypical lipomatous tumors) of the vulva: a clinicopathologic study of six cases. *Int J Gynecol Pathol* 1998; **17**: 17–23.

128 Proppe KH, Scully RE, Rosai J. Postoperative spindle cell nodules of the genitourinary tract resembling sarcomas: a report of eight cases. *Am J Surg Pathol* 1984; **8**: 101–8.

129 Manson CM, Hirsch PJ, Coyne JD. Post-operative spindle cell nodule of the vulva. *Histopathology* 1995; **26**: 571–4.

130 O'Connell JX, Young RH, Nielsen GP et al. Nodular fasciitis of the vulva: a study of six cases and literature review. *Int J Gynecol Pathol* 1997; **16**: 117–23.

131 Dudley AG, Young RH, Lawrence WD, Scully RE. Endodermal sinus tumour of the vulva in an infant. *Obstet Gynecol* 1983; **61**: 76S–9s.

132 Brooks JJ, Wheeler JE. Malignancy arising in extragonadal endometriosis. A case report and summary of the world literature. *Cancer* 1977; **40**: 3065–73.

133 Young RH, Harris NL, Scully RE. Lymphoma-like lesions of the lower female genital tract: a report of 16 cases. *Int J Gynecol Pathol* 1985; **4**: 289–99.

134 Plouffe L, Tulandi T, Rosenberg A, Ferenzy A. Non-Hodgkins lymphoma in Bartholin's gland: A report and review of the literature. *Am J Obstet Gynecol*. 1984; **148**: 608.

135 Copeland LJ, Cleary K, Sneige N, Edwards CL. Neuroendocrine (Merkel cell) carcinoma of the vulva: a case report and review of the literature. *Gynecol Oncol* 1985; **22**: 367–78.

136 Husseinzadeh N, Whesseler T, Newman N, Shbaro I, Ho P. Neuroendocrine (Merkel cell) carcinoma of the vulva. *Gynecol Oncol* 1988; **29**: 105–12.

137 Tbakhi A, Cowan DF, Kumar D, Kyle D. Recurring phyllodes tumor in aberrant breast tissue of the vulva. *Am J Surg Pathol* 1993; **17**: 946–50.

138 Dehner LP. Metastatic and secondary tumours of the vulva. *Obstet Gynecol* 1973; **42**: 47–57

139 Powell CS, Jones PA. Carcinoma of the bladder with metastasis in the clitoris. *Br J Obstet Gynaecol* 1983; **90**: 380–1.

140 Mader MH, Friedrich EG Jr. Vulvar metastasis of breast carcinoma – A case report. *J Reprod Med* 1982; **27**: 169–71.

4

Molecular and viral pathogenesis of vulvar cancer

AP PINTO, MC LIN, CP CRUM

Cancer of the vulva is a relatively uncommon disease with an incidence of approximately 1.8 per 100 000, but increasing significantly to 20 per 1 000 000 after the age of 75.[1–3] Risk factors for vulvar cancer include other genital carcinomas, chronic vulvar inflammatory disorders, smoking, prior history of genital warts and vulvar carcinoma in situ (vulvar intraepithelial neoplasm or VIN.)[4–9]

Clinical, pathological, molecular and epidemiological data accrued over the past 20 years support the concept that vulvar squamous carcinoma, unlike its counterpart in the cervix, arises via at least two pathogenic routes (Fig. 4.1 and Table 4.1): the first consists of human papillomavirus (HPV) infection leading to a vulvar pre-cancer (VIN) which, in a proportion of women, progresses to invasive carcinoma. Other risk factors associated with this process include immunological factors, age and cigarette smoking. The other pathway is less well understood, but presumably entails the development of host gene alterations, which accumulate in the vulvar squamous epithelium. Participants in this scenario include vulvar inflammatory disorders, such as lichen sclerosus or epithelial hyperplasia, increasing age and the development of cytological atypia. Considering both morphological

and clinical data, approximately 30 per cent of vulvar carcinomas are associated with HPV and classic forms of VIN, while an equal proportion is associated with epithelial abnormalities that demonstrate atypia in the setting of lichen sclerosus and hyperplasia (differentiated VIN). Another third arise in the absence of a conspicuous precursor lesion.[10] The purpose of this chapter is to update the reader on the potential mechanisms influencing the development of vulvar cancer along these two pathways.

PAPILLOMAVIRUSES

HPV-mediated neoplastic transformation

In recent years, HPV has been proposed as an aetiological agent for a large spectrum of genital tract diseases, among them vulvar squamous neoplasia.[11–13] As in cervical carcinoma, HPV is closely associated with a subset of vulvar carcinomas and presumably operates via the initial development of a precursor (VIN) lesion.

The following summarizes the molecular mechanisms of HPV cell transformation and the application

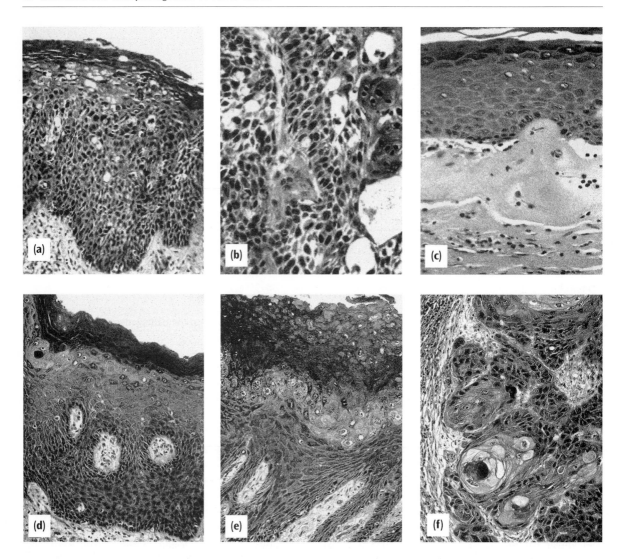

Figure 4.1 *Morphological phenotypes of vulvar cancer. Group I consists of tumours associated with HPV nucleic acids, including those associated with classic VIN (a) and demonstrating morphology resembling intraepithelial lesions, including warty and basaloid (b) forms. Lesions in group II are associated with lichen sclerosus (c) or hyperplasia (d), including atypical keratinizing hyperplasias (e) (differentiated VIN) and exhibit keratinizing histology (f).*

of this information to clinical disease. The viral life-cycle of HPVs is intimately associated with the pro-gramme of differentiation of the host epithelial cell.[14] Papillomaviruses infect the epithelium via defects in the squamous mucosa, presumably entering the basal cells. Proposed receptors for entry of the virus include α_6- and β_4-integrins, which are attached to the extra-cellular matrix and upregulated during wound healing and may facilitate entry of the virus into the cells via endocytosis. Once in the cells, expression of the virus is tightly controlled and replication is initiated as a function of epithelial maturation. This process is asso-

ciated with expression of late (structural) genes and the production of viral capsids, late (Ll, L2) proteins or both in the surface epithelium. As the surface cells are committed to differentiation, neoplastic transforma-tion cannot occur in this cell population. Moreover, the regulatory influences of certain HPV open reading frames (El, E2), in the context of the normal viral life cycle, may preclude expression of sequences critical to neoplastic transformation within replicating cells (Fig. 4.2).

Cancer-associated papillomaviruses, specifically HPV type 16, typically do not progress through the

Table 4.1 *Categories of patients with vulvar carcinoma*

Characteristic	Group I	Group II
Age (years)	Relatively younger (35–65)	Relatively older (55–85)
Previous condyloma	Common	Uncommon
Previous sexually transmitted disease	Common	Uncommon
Smoking history	Common	Uncommon
Coexisting lesions	Classic VIN (Bowen's disease, bowenoid papulosis)	Lichen sclerosus, vulvar hyperplasia, atypical hyperplasia (differentiated VIN)
Cofactors in development	Age, immune status, high-risk HPV type, viral integration, chromosomal amplification at 3q	Age, progressive mutations in host genes within the squamous epithelium
Cervical neoplasia	High association	Low association
Histopathology	Intraepithelial like (wart or basaloid)	Keratinizing or well differentiated

orderly process of viral maturation and assembly in infected epithelium. In this scenario, it is assumed that unregulated expression of viral oncogenes, specifically of *E6* and *E7*, occurs in the replicating cell population (parabasal cells) and irreversibly alters their growth characteristics (Fig. 4.2).[15] Recent studies have shown that the *E7* of HPV 18 stimulates cell proliferation and decreases growth factor requirements. Moreover, *E6* and *E7* oncogenes of HPV 16 have the capacity to delay terminal differentiation in keratinocytes. Similar to the oncoproteins of other DNA viruses, such as adenovirus and simian virus 40 (SV40), the HPV E6 and E7 proteins interact with cell regulatory proteins such as p53 and the retinoblastoma protein (pRb).[16,17] It

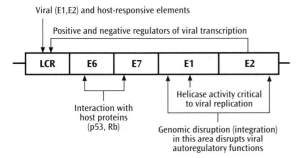

Figure 4.2 *Schematic of viral factors influencing papillomavirus oncogenesis, including expression of oncogenes E6 and E7, and viral integration, which dissociates these open reading frames from control by downstream regulatory elements in E1 and E2.*

was shown also that, under the control of a strong promoter, the *E7* gene alone could immortalize cells,[18] and that the efficiency of this viral oncoprotein on binding pRb was reflected in the capacity of different 'high- and low-risk' HPVs to immortalize or transform.[18,19]

At some point in the pathogenesis of carcinoma, usually at the changeover point between intraepithelial and invasive disease, the virus is frequently covalently bound to the chromosomal DNA. Integration of the viral genome into the DNA of the host's carcinoma cells appears to be non-random and often occurs within El and E2, resulting in loss or alteration of E2 (Fig. 4.2), although other regions of the viral genome remain intact.[20–22] E2 is a DNA-binding protein that has an indirect role in transformation by regulating transcription from the E6/E7 promoter of HPV 16 and HPV 18.[23–25] Thus, integration and loss of E2 function result in overproduction of E6 and E7 protein.[26] El has helicase activity which positively influences DNA replication, hence the functional loss of both genes may contribute, directly or indirectly, to the loss of normal viral function and development of immortalization.[27] Although the site of integration of the HPV genome is consistently located between *E1* and *E2* open reading frames (ORFs) as described before, integration into the host chromosome is apparently random. Although this statement appears to be true in many anogenital carcinomas, however, integration of viral sequences was consistently found in cell lines and may coincide with proto-oncogene loci[28] or with chromosomal fragile sites.[28–30]

The cell cycle and papillomaviruses

The genes involved in the cell cycle have not been fully elucidated, but there is evidence that the HPV E6 and E7 proteins influence several points in the transition from the Gl to the S phase. This occurs via both the direct and indirect effects of the E6 and E7 gene products on tumour suppressor genes (*Rb* and *p53*), cyclins and cyclin-dependent kinases (Fig. 4.3).

A critical juncture in the cell cycle is the G1–S phase checkpoint, which governs the initiation of DNA synthesis. This checkpoint is important in the regulation of both normal cell division and, particularly, cell division in the face of unrepaired DNA damage, the control of which is critical. In brief, expression of *p53* upregulates p21, a cell cycle inhibitory protein; p21 then binds to cyclin-dependent kinases and inhibits DNA synthesis. The E6 protein of HPV 16 binds to *p53* and enhances *p53* degradation, with the net effect being a loss of cell cycle inhibition. As *p53* mediates cell cycle arrest in response to DNA damage, continued cell division with unrepaired DNA may explain the subsequent marked karyotypic abnormalities characteristic of neoplasia.[27,31]

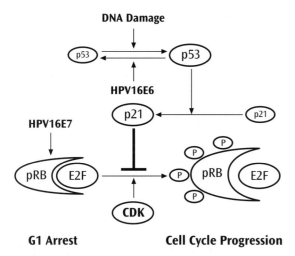

Figure 4.3 *Schematic of host genes, including cell cycle proteins, influenced by the E6 and E7 gene products. E6 effectively reduces p53 protein levels via degradation, whereas E7 effectively releases the E2F transcription factor by binding Rb, promoting cell cycle progression.*

The Rb gene product normally binds to the E2F–DPl complex, which if unbound activates the transcription of the genes responsible for the S phase. The E7 protein of HPV 16 binds Rb, effectively permitting the transition to the S phase. Other positive influences on S-phase transition include upregulation of cyclins A and E by E7, with activation of cyclin-dependent kinases. The net effect of E7 expression is therefore the bypassing of the Gl–S transition checkpoint.[27,31]

HPV detection in vulvar cancer and precursors

The prevalence of HPV DNA in squamous carcinomas of the vulva has varied widely in published reports.[32,33] This range in HPV positives reflects several variables, including assay sensitivity, sample sizes and demographic issues (see Chapter 1). In relation to the type of HPV involved in both precursor lesions and invasive tumours, the studies agree that HPV 16 is the one most frequently found, followed distantly by HPV 33 and HPV 18 (Fig. 4.4).[34–37] HPV 16 is the prototypical high-risk HPV type in vulvar neoplasia, occurring in approximately 80 per cent of HPV-positive tumours. Intraepithelial neoplasms of the classic type (Bowen's disease, bowenoid papulosis, etc.) and invasive carcinomas with growth patterns resembling intraepithelial disease (intraepithelial like, warty or basaloid) frequently test positive for HPV, reaching up to 80 per cent by polymerase chain reaction (PCR) amplification.[12,37,38] In contrast, tumours composed of well-differentiated keratinizing epithelium, or that are associated with vulvar hyperplasia, lichen sclerosus or atypias associated with these entities (differentiated VIN), score positive in 13.3–16.4 per cent of cases.

A detailed morphological analysis of VINs found the following: a high frequency of HPV DNA among the lesions presenting histopathological parameters that characterize classic VINs, including veruccopapillary morphology (69.2 per cent), koilocytotic atypia (70.8 per cent), multinucleation (72.3 per cent), absence of maturation (79.2 per cent), and presence of nuclear atypia extending up through at least two-thirds of the epithelial thickness (79.3 per cent).[35] There is a lower rate of HPV nucleic acids among lesions that present characteristics related to differentiated variants of VIN, specifically those with preservation of normal maturation in which the atypia was confined to the lower epithelial layers (14.2 per cent).

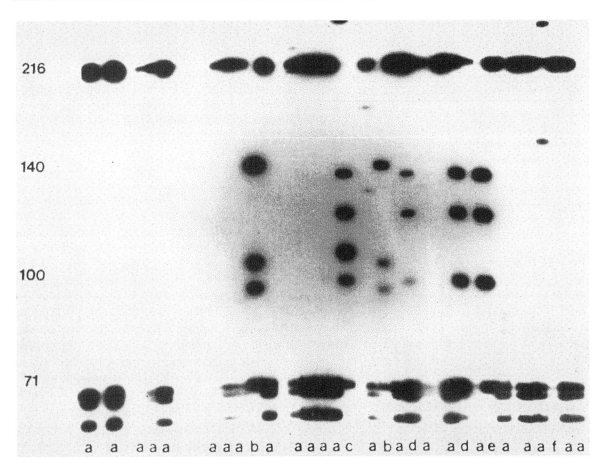

Figure 4.4 *Restriction fragment length polymorphism analysis of PCR-amplified HPV DNA from VIN lesions. Numbers at the left depict the approximate molecular weight; letters at the bottom denote the following HPV types: (a) HPV 16; (b) HPV 33; (c) HPV 31 and unknown type; (d) HPV 31 and 16; (e) HPV 31; (f) HPV 16 and unknown type. (Reproduced with permission from Haefner and colleagues.[35])*

Karyotypical abnormalities associated with HPV-related neoplasia

Chromosome 1 appears to be the one most frequently involved in structural and numerical alterations in carcinomas of the cervix and in HPV-immortalized cell lines.[39–44] These alterations most commonly result in the duplication of the long arm material, and may be associated with the progression of all forms of cancer, occurring at a late stage in the carcinogenesis process.[45] However, in the case of cervical neoplasms, the lq duplication appears to be associated with immortality or transition to the malignant phenotype. Other chromosomes identified as potentially involved with HPV-induced carcinogenesis are chromosomes 11 and 3, among others.[29,30] An extensive study on cervical squamous carcinomas and their

precursor lesions, using comparative genomic hybridization, DNA cytometry, immunohistochemical proliferative marker (Ki-67) and HPV genotyping, revealed a gain of chromosome 3q that occurs in HPV-16-infected aneuploid cells, representing a potentially critical genetic aberration in the transition from severe dysplasia/carcinoma in situ to invasive cervical carcinoma.[46] Previously, a singular cytogenetic study using short-term cultures from vulvar cancers established six cell lines. Multiple karyotypic abnormalities were found, among which were seven that were consistently present in five of the six tumours: losses of 3p14-cen, 8pter-p11, 22q 13.1-q 13.2 and the short arm of the inactive X; gains involving 3q25-qter and 11 q21; and rearrangement breakpoints at 5cen-q12.[47] The gains at 3q were subsequently shown to be connected with HPV-16-

associated tumours, confirming this cervical relationship.

HOST FACTORS

In this section, specific genetic changes associated with vulvar cancers, specifically HPV-negative tumours (p53), are addressed, genetic alterations between HPV-negative and -positive tumours are compared, and comments about the HPV-negative 'precursor' lesion made, including data from studies of clonality and allelic loss.

The *p53* tumour suppressor gene

Mutations in the tumour suppressor gene *p53* are common in malignant human neoplasms, including squamous cell carcinomas of diverse sites. Initial studies of cervical carcinoma cell lines and tumour specimens suggested that there was a distinct subset of HPV-negative cervical carcinomas that were associated with mutations in *p53*.[48] Because, as detailed above, *p53* function may be directly altered by E6 proteins of HPV 16, investigators postulated that *p53* mutations provided an alternative mechanism for tumorigenesis in HPV-negative tumours.[48] However, subsequent reports have confirmed neither an HPV-negative subgroup of cervical tumours nor the consistent presence of *p53* mutations in these tumours.[49,50] Rather, the balance of studies indicates that *p53* mutations are relatively uncommon in cervical cancer and may be present in tumours testing positive or negative for HPV nucleic acids. It is now assumed that most 'HPV-negative' cervical carcinomas are as likely to signify insensitive HPV assays as a unique pathogenesis.

As vulvar cancers include a group that are clearly HPV negative, these tumours are ideal for studying the potential role of *p53* mutations. Based on morphological data, this HPV-negative group would comprise those neoplasms associated with lichen sclerosus or vulvar hyperplasia, and exhibiting keratinizing morphology. These tumours would be the most likely to harbour mutations in *p53* and, in fact, molecular genetic studies have associated *p53* mutations with the HPV-negative vulvar carcinomas. These studies have addressed two issues: (1) the relationship between *p53* mutations and HPV status; and (2) expression of *p53* antigens as a function of HPV status. Three papers carefully correlated *p53* mutation and HPV status. A

strong correlation between *p53* mutations and HPV-negative vulvar cancers was found in these studies.[51–53] HPV-positive tumours, like their counterparts in the cervix, uncommonly displayed mutations. Expression studies using immunohistochemistry have not discriminated HPV-negative tumours by *p53* immunostaining, consistent with the fact that *p53* overexpression may reflect phenomena other than genetic mutation.[54,55]

Although immunohistochemical studies of *p53* expression in cervical and vulvar neoplasms have not corroborated data on *p53* mutations, a recent report is likely to prompt additional study of the interactions between HPV and *p53* in these neoplasms.[56] In this study, a common polymorphism of *p53*, containing an arginine at amino acid 72 of exon 4, was strongly associated with invasive carcinoma in contrast to normal controls. This finding not only suggests, for the first time, a pre-existing genetic condition predisposing HPV-infected women to cervical cancer, but also strengthens the role of *p53* in both HPV-negative and -positive vulvar cancers. However, this study has yet to be verified and it should be emphasized that variability in the frequency of the arginine polymorphism is considerable, depending on the population.

Studies of allelic loss (loss of heterozygosity)

As mentioned above, one study has confirmed a high frequency of karyotypic abnormalities in vulvar squamous cell carcinomas.[47] Previous publications have found consistent correlations between chromosomal losses, detected by cytogenetic methods, and the results of molecular approaches, using microsatellite or restriction fragment length polymorphism markers, in squamous cell carcinomas of the head and neck and squamous and adenocarcinomas of the lung.[57–62]

A study comparing allelic losses in HPV-positive and -negative tumours was recently concluded in our laboratory (Table 4.2 and Fig. 4.5).[63] In contrast to the study by Worsham and colleagues,[47] this study identified a wider range of allelic losses, including loss of heterozygosity (LOH) at more than 30 per cent of informative cases on chromosomes 1p, 5q, 10p, 10q, 11q, 15q, 21q (on two different loci) and 22q. The highest prevalence of LOH was seen on chromosome 17p (58.3 per cent). Consistent genetic losses on this chromosomal arm had also been described in many solid tumours and in squamous cell carcinomas of the

Table 4.2 *Comparison of studies showing karyotypic losses in vulvar cancer[47] versus the current study of loss of heterozygosity (LOH)[63]*

Karyotypic losses[47]	N/T (%)	LOH[63]	Percentage
		2q	50.0
3p	5/6 (83.3)	3p	50.0
5q	4/6 (66.6)	5q	42.9
8p	5/6 (83.3)	8p	50.0
		8q	57.1
		10p	44.4
10q	4/6 (66.6)	10q	44.4
15q	3/6 (50.0)	15q	35.7
		17p	58.3
18q	4/6 (66.6)		
19p	4/6 (66.6)	nt	
		21q	46.2
		21q	42.9
		21q	50.0
22q	5/6 (83.3)	22q	40.0
Xp	5/6 (83.3)		

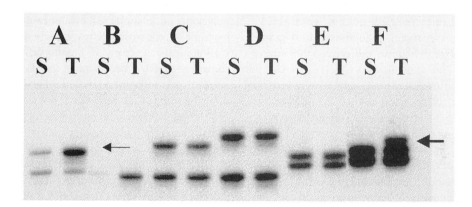

Figure 4.5 *Polyacrylamide gel depicting PCR-amplified polymorphic loci of stromal (S) or tumour (T) DNA, from samples A to F. Products are interpreted as either heterozygous, with balanced product intensity, homozygous, with a single product (uninformative), heterozygous with a dominant product (small arrow, loss of heterozygosity), and novel, with additional or displaced bands (large arrow, microsatellite instability).*

head, neck, lung and oesophagus.[59,62,64–66] Conversely, a low incidence of LOH at this site has been reported in cervical squamous tumours.[67,68] This chromosome arm is the site of a known gene with demonstrated tumour suppressor function (*p53*), and mapping studies of chromosome 17 in carcinomas of the head and neck have shown consistent involvement of this gene locus, the TP53 at 17p13.1, as well as the CHRNB 1 locus at 17p12–p11.1.[69,70] One of these studies also indicated 17p12–p11 as a potential site for a novel tumour suppressor gene.[69] In this study, a higher pro-

portion of HPV-negative versus HPV-positive tumours (four of five versus three of seven) contained allelic losses on chromosome 17p, but this finding was not statistically significant and indicates that LOH on 17p will not discriminate between the two tumour types. However, it does not exclude the possibility that specific alterations in 17p, such as *p53* mutations, are more common in HPV-negative vulvar squamous cell carcinomas.

High prevalences ($\geq$ 50 per cent) of LOH in our study were found on chromosomes 2q, 3p, 8p, 8q, 17p and 21q (on a third locus) (Table 4.2). Allelic losses in 8p were also described in squamous cell carcinomas of the head and neck, and the lung, and are consistent with previous cytogenetic findings in short-term culture of vulvar carcinoma cells.[47,57,71–73] Surprisingly, LOH on 8q, the second most frequent site of losses in our study (53.3 per cent), has not been verified in squamous cell carcinomas of any other site except for the cervix. Allelic losses on 3p are in accordance with previous investigations. According to previous LOH studies, this chromosome appears to play an important role in the carcinogenesis and progression of squamous epithelium-derived tumours of any previously studied site, including the head and neck, oesophagus, lung, skin, anus and cervix, as well as in other solid tumours.[57–59,62,64–66,74–78] Losses on 3p were also detected at a high frequency (five of six) on squamous vulvar carcinoma cell cultures using cytogenetic approaches.[47] Although this region is of interest for identifying additional genes critical to the development of lower genital tract tumours, there is, however, no evidence from this study that allelic loss in this region will distinguish HPV-positive from HPV-negative tumours. A recent unpublished study examining 3p in vulvar squamous cell cancers has found similar results.

Losses in both arms of chromosome 10 were verified in 44.4 per cent of the cases studied. Some previous studies detected 10p allelic losses in 40–60 per cent of head and neck and 33 per cent of oesophageal squamous cancers.[57,64] Losses on 10q were reported on cytogenetic studies of cell lines derived from squamous cell carcinoma of the head and neck and the vulva.[47,79]

The determination of consistent LOH on the short arm of chromosome 21 by three different markers – CHLCGATA129D11 (46.2 per cent), CHLCGATA188F04 (42.9 per cent) and D21S1446 (50 per cent) – strongly suggests that important genes related to vulvar carcinogenesis and progression are located on this region. An interesting fact is the absence of similar verifications in tumours of other sites, including squamous carcinomas. This region seems to be potentially specific to vulvar squamous carcinoma and merits further study. Additional allelic losses of interest, found at a lower frequency in this study and which have not been strongly associated with non-genital squamous cell carcinomas, include 2q (50 per cent), 10q (44.4 per cent), 15q (35.7 per cent) and 22q (40 per cent). Losses on 10q and 22q have also been reported.[47]

In summary, both HPV-positive and HPV-negative vulvar squamous cell carcinomas (VSCCs) exhibit a broad range of allelic losses, some of which (3p, 5q, 8p, 10p, 11q, 17p) are shared with squamous carcinomas at other sites, whereas others (2q, 8q, 10q, 15q and 22q) appear more closely associated with VSSCs. Such loci identified by this and prior reports may be useful targets in the study of pre-cancerous squamous lesions associated with HPV-positive and HPV-negative tumours.[80]

Clonal studies of HPV-positive and HPV-negative precursor lesions

The occurrence of mutations in the vulvar epithelium with the ageing process, similar to what occurs in sun-exposed skin, is the most probable explanation for the significant increase in vulvar cancer incidence after the age of 75.[1–3] One method that has been developed recently to characterize this epithelium is the clonal assay, based on inactivation (methylation) of the androgen receptor gene.[81] As inactivation is random, polyclonal populations will exhibit roughly equal proportions of cells with inactivation of either allele. Populations arising from a single cell will exhibit consistent inactivation of one of the alleles. As methylated DNA is resistant to enzyme digestion, predigestion of androgen receptor DNA, followed by selective PCR amplification, will discriminate between polyclonal tissues, in which both alleles will be amplified following digestion, and monoclonal tissues, in which one of the two alleles will not be amplified because of prior enzymatic disruption. As the length of the amplified region varies between the two X chromosomes in most cases, PCR-based assays are frequently successful in determining whether cell populations are monoclonal in origin.[82] Monoclonality has been held to be synonymous with squamous neoplasia, and has been demonstrated in cervical intraepithelial neoplasia (CIN) in recent studies. Studies of endometrium using cytogenetic and clonal assays have determined that endometrial polyps and endometrial 'hyperplasias' are clonal in origin.[81,83,84] In the case of the vulvar epithelium, the questions that have been addressed have concerned not only whether VIN lesions were monoclonal, but whether other abnormalities associated with carcinoma, including lichen sclerosus and hyperplasia, were also monoclonal.

In a recent study carried out at our laboratory, VINs of the classic type were virtually always monoclonal using this assay.[85] This is consistent with a monoclonal origin for these lesions and corroborates parallel studies of squamous intraepithelial lesions of the cervix, most of which have been scored as monoclonal.[86] However, this does not exclude the possibility that some VINs are polyclonal, as was found in one case in our study. In particular, the multicentric nature of VIN supports the existence of multiple cells of origin, and it is conceivable that cells in close proximity may give rise to lesions that are polyclonal. This may be partly explained by studies of allelic loss in these lesions (see later). The possibility that some VINs behave as an 'infection', with involvement of multiple stem cells as observed in condylomata, cannot be excluded.

HPV-negative tumours are preceded by a spectrum of epithelial alterations, including lichen sclerosus, hyperplasia and either entity with associated atypia (differentiated VIN).[10] As these alterations place individuals at a greater risk for cancer, and because they may exhibit cellular atypia, their clonal status is central to our understanding of the pathogenesis of these carcinomas. In one study of vulvar hyperplasias and one case of lichen sclerosus associated with invasive carcinomas, approximately half of the hyperplasias and the lichen sclerosus were monoclonal.[85] In contrast, vulvar hyperplasias from four HPV-negative vulvar carcinomas were found to be polyclonal and exhibited no evidence of *p53* mutations in the study by Kim and colleagues.[87] Based on these studies, it is clear that vulvar hyperplasias are a heterogeneous entity, which may or may not be related to the carcinomas with which they are juxtaposed. The presence of clonality in lichen sclerosus is intriguing, but few studies have been performed on these lesions to determine whether monoclonality is a constant or rare phenomenon, or whether it is a marker for neoplastic progression.

Is there a genetic link between HPV-negative non-invasive and invasive mucosa?

Assays for allelic loss have emerged as an alternative method for determining the genetic relationship between invasive carcinomas and adjacent epithelial changes. A recent report examining LOH, in a spectrum of squamous lesions of the head and neck ranging from hyperplasia to cancer, identified it in 31 per cent of histologically benign squamous hyperplasias and almost all squamous dysplasias and carcinomas in situ.[88] The authors proposed a model for head and neck tumorigenesis in which progressive genetic alterations (allelic loss) accompany the evolution of squamous neoplasia. In this scenario, allelic loss in some benign-appearing hyperplasias identifies these alterations as potential precursor lesions.[88]

In a recent study using this methodology, Lin and colleagues[80] analysed four cases of vulvar carcinoma and their adjacent epithelium at 10 chromosomal loci.[80] LOH was detected in both HPV-positive and HPV-negative tumours, and in adjacent non-invasive epithelium, including classic and differentiated VIN and hyperplastic epithelium. The most revealing observation was the chromosomal heterogeneity of allelic loss, with both VINs and hyperplasias exhibiting LOH that was not shared by the invasive carcinoma (Fig. 4.6).[80] These findings suggest that the vulvar mucosa plays host to many genetic alterations which are not directly related to invasive carcinoma. It remains to be determined whether these alterations necessarily precede the neoplastic phenotype, occur at random and are inconsequential, or they reflect a greater susceptibility of the host epithelium for neoplasia.

UNRESOLVED ISSUES IN THE PAPILLOMAVIRUS/HOST MUTATION DICHOTOMY

The previous descriptions detail two distinct scenarios in the pathogenesis of vulvar cancer, which may include different aetiological agents, precursor lesions and invasive carcinomas. However, both HPV-positive and HPV-negative tumours share several features in common, as detailed below.

Association of HPV and lichen sclerosus

Although lichen sclerosus does not exhibit cytological atypia, there is an association between this disorder and vulvar cancer. Approximately one-third of cancers are associated with lichen sclerosus in the adjacent epithelium.[89] Moreover, lichen sclerosus increases the risk of vulvar cancer by 10–100-fold, with approximately 1–4 per cent of women with this disease developing cancer.[89] The relationship between vulvar maturation disorders and cancer is discussed in detail in Chapter 6.

Studies have shown that, in cancers associated with lichen sclerosus, there was either no epithelial abnor-

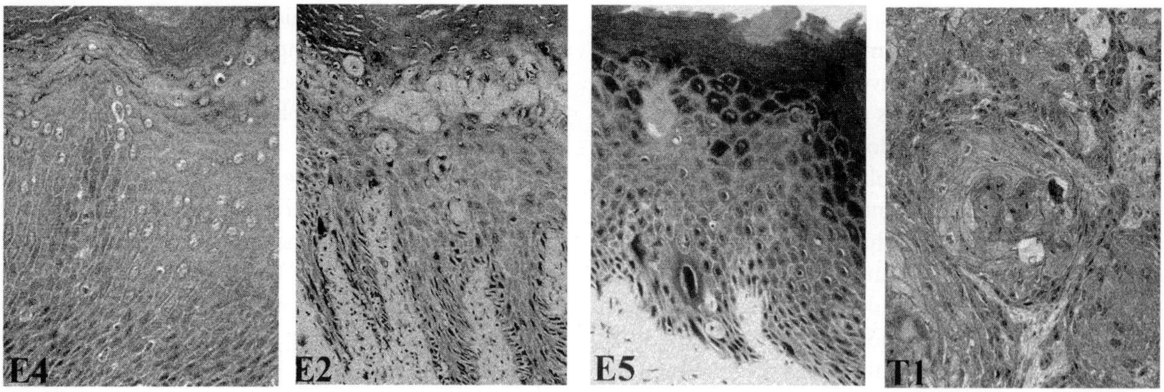

Sample	Tissue	1.2	2.3	2.4	5.2	5.3	8.2	21.1
N1–N3	Stroma							
E3	Normal Epith							
E1	Hyper	L						
E4	Hyper						L	
E6	DVIN							
F2	DVIN			L				
F5	DVIN			L		L		
T1–T3	MDCa		L	L	L			L

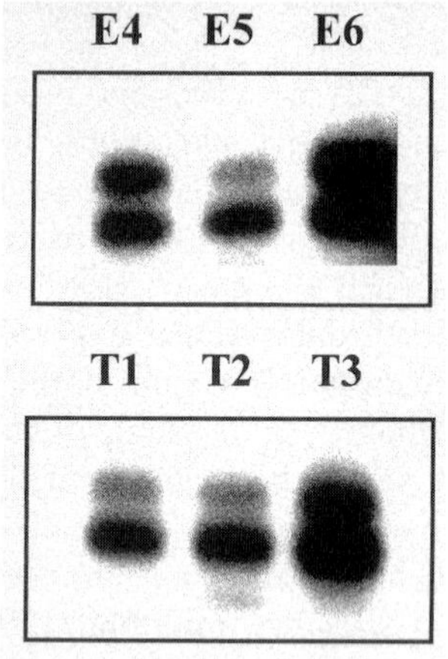

Figure 4.6 *Heterogeneity of allelic loss in an HPV-negative vulvar cancer and adjacent squamous mucosa. Note that several hyperplastic, atypical (differentiated VIN) and invasive foci contain loss of heterozygosity (L) in different chromosomal loci, with variable overlap. This is consistent with a heterogeneous population of mucosal epithelia with allelic loss, some of which are not directly related to the adjacent invasive carcinoma. (Reproduced with permission from Lin and colleagues.*[80]*)*

mality or the abnormality consisted of the differentiated variant of VIN.[10] This is consistent with the development of a non-HPV-related precursor lesion in the setting of lichen sclerosus, possibly as a result of a cellular gene mutation(s). One study of six differentiated VIN lesions occurring in association with lichen sclerosus and vulvar carcinoma detected no HPV.[90] A study of vulvar cancers associated with lichen sclerosus likewise did not identify HPV in the tumours.[10] These studies suggested that intraepithelial and invasive squamous lesions, arising in association with lichen sclerosus, develop via mechanisms other than HPV infection. It would be consistent with a scenario in which *p53* mutations or other host mutations operated, similar to that of sun-exposed skin.[91]

Although the pathogenic mechanisms of vulvar cancer associated with HPV and lichen sclerosus appear to be distinct, recent studies have challenged this dichotomy with reports of HPV in lesions associated with lichen sclerosus. For example, one study has identified HPV nucleic acids in four of 18 cases of lichen sclerosus by PCR.[92] Three of the four HPV-DNA-positive patients were premenopausal, and in none of the cases could HPV nucleic acids be demonstrated directly in the lichen sclerosus by in situ hybridization.[92] A more recent study using PCR identified HPV nucleic acids in seven of 19 vulvar carcinomas associated with lichen sclerosus.[93] In a recent study from our laboratory, PCR analysis identified HPV 16 in three of six VIN lesions associated with lichen sclerosus, and the tissue distribution of all three was verified by in situ hybridization (Fig. 4.7).[35] All three positives occurred in older women (aged 67, 80 and 81 years) and one was associated with an invasive carcinoma. Interestingly, all three cases contained a classic VIN.[35] Thus, there are data to support two different forms of epithelial neoplasia associated with lichen sclerosus, including one associated with and

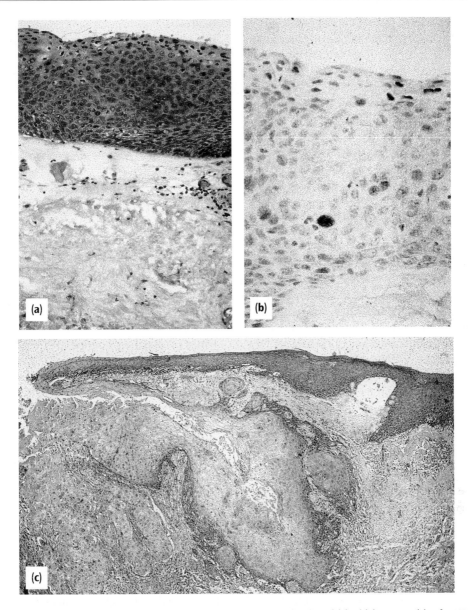

Figure 4.7 *An unusual case of lichen sclerosus in which a classic VIN has developed (a) which was positive for HPV 16 by PCR and in situ hybridization (b). This is adjacent to an invasive carcinoma (c). (Reproduced with permission from Haefner and colleagues.[35])*

one without HPV nucleic acids. These recent studies are provocative, implying that HPV and vulvar lichen sclerosus may cooperate in the genesis of vulvar neoplasms in some older women.

Age as a factor in both groups

The fact that papillomavirus-related vulvar neoplasms frequently occur in older women, including women in their 60s and 70s, is at odds with the scenario commonly observed with cervical neoplasia. The risk of vulvar neoplasia increases as a function of age and the coexistence of a number of age-related epithelial alterations (such as vulvar hyperplasia, lichen sclerosus or differentiated VIN) suggests that age plays an important role in the pathogenesis of this disease.

Despite the findings by some that older women with vulvar neoplasia are less likely to harbour HPV nucleic acids, the data from others indicate a strong association between HPV and cancers in older women as well.[35,94] Thus, it appears that both HPV status and ageing itself operate independently in the genesis of vulvar neoplasia. Conceivably, the ageing process makes women more susceptible to this disease. Whether hormonal, immunological, environmental or behavioural factors conspire to place certain women at risk is unclear, although the strong association between smoking and classic VIN is of interest.[95]

Molecular markers and natural history

Differences in biological behaviour between HPV-positive and HPV-negative tumours have been suggested, and the role of HPV as a prognostic marker in vulvar cancer has been addressed for different groups in the literature. Ansink and colleagues[93] and Monk and colleagues,[96] analysing archival tissues for HPV via PCR, reported a significantly longer survival for HPV-positive neoplasms.[93,96] The second group found HPV to be the only independent prognostic factor after multivariate analysis. Contrary to this finding, in one other study,[97] a higher rate of metastatic disease was associated with HPV positivity. In a large series of cases ($n = 78$) tested by a similar methodology, no difference in prognosis between HPV-positive and HPV-negative vulvar carcinomas was found.[98] Two other groups also failed to show a significant relationship between HPV status and prognosis.[99,100] We recently tested a Brazilian population of 158 cases of invasive vulvar carcinoma treated by radical surgery.[37] After modelling risk of death from cancer as a function of several variables, including age, stage and histopathological features, we found no significant association between HPV status and prognosis.[37] However, this negative evidence of association between the presence of HPV DNA and the prognosis of vulvar carcinoma does not exclude an influence of HPV status on natural history, inasmuch as the associated precursor lesions, timing of invasion and opportunity for early clinical detection may differ between HPV-positive and HPV-negative tumours.

The prognostic significance of p53 immunopositivity is also unclear. Kagie and colleagues[55] and Gordinier and colleagues[101] found no association between p53 immunostaining and adverse prognosis, whereas Kohlberger and colleagues[102] associated it with poorer overall survival. Most studies do associate p53 mutations with either nodal metastases or invasive, rather than with non-invasive epithelium,[87] consistent with the assumption that p53 mutations do not precede invasion.[103]

One study showed a significantly worse survival in tumours with p53 mutations, consistent with other studies of HPV-negative vulvar cancers, which showed a worse prognosis for this group.[95,96,104] However, as for p53 expression, the association is not consistent, because other studies have failed to link poor outcome with HPV negativity.[55,98–100] In fact, one study has shown a worse prognosis for subsets of neoplasia often associated with HPV.[55]

OTHER FACTORS RELATED TO THE PATHOGENESIS OF VULVAR CARCINOMAS

Cigarette smoking

Exposure, age of start, period and frequency of cigarette smoking all appear to influence the incidence of CIN and cervical cancer.[105] The two principal mechanisms by which smoking contributes to cervical neoplasia include the direct exposure to nicotine and cotinine, and adducts of the type expected from the reaction of polycyclic aromatic hydrocarbons and aromatic amines – other compounds of tobacco smoke – with the DNA in the cervical epithelial cells of smokers.[106,107] The associations among different genotypes of carcinogen-metabolizing enzymes, smoking and cervical neoplasia were investigated in two studies by Warwick and colleagues.[108,109] They first found that smokers with phase 1 cytochrome P450 detoxifying enzyme (CYP2D6) with the wild-type, extensive, metabolizer genotype (EM), are at increased risk of high-grade CIN but at reduced risk of squamous cell carcinoma (SCC).[110] This finding accords with the fact that certain tobacco-specific N-nitrosamines are substrates for CYP2D6 and may therefore be involved in the pathogenesis of CIN.[110] However, the carcinogen(s) required for progression to SCC, which are presumably effectively detoxified by CYP2D6 EM subjects, is not known. The second study by Warwick and colleagues[109] found no significant association between other genotypes, the theta class glutathione S-transferase (GSTT1) and cervical neoplasia. These findings are similar to those previously found with the phase 2 glutathione S-transferase (GSTMI) genotype.[108,109]

A second mechanism for tobacco-related carcinogenesis is immunosuppression. Smoking-related changes in the peripheral immune system of humans have included elevated blood cell counts, increased cytotoxic/suppresser and decreased inducer/helper T-cell numbers, slightly suppressed T-lymphocyte activity, significantly decreased natural killer (NK) cell activity and reduced circulating immunoglobulin titres, except for the immunoglobulin IgE which is elevated.[111] Decreased counts for the cells of Langerhans in the cervix of female smokers have also been verified by several studies.[112–114] These experimental data are supported by clinical studies that reveal the association between smoking and history of immunosuppressive conditions in young patients with vulvar invasive disease.[115] In this publication, the authors propose that smoking leads to immunosuppression and that this condition could be responsible for activation of any viruses remaining latent in the tissues. With an immunosuppressed condition, there would be development of clinical HPV-related lesions (VIN) and subsequent invasive cancer in a young population.

There are no experimental studies that address the role of smoke components in anogenital tumours, other than cervical carcinoma, in the literature. However, population-based case–control studies have addressed the role of smoking, among other factors, in the aetiology of vulvar cancers (see Chapter 1). Daling and colleagues[116] showed that cigarette smoking has a late stage or promotional effect in the aetiology of squamous cancer of all anogenital sites, including vulva, anus and penis, but not the vagina. Andersen and colleagues[12] noted a significant association between smoking and HPV-negative vulvar cancers in an uncontrolled study. Brinton and colleagues[95] found a significant interaction between smoking and genital warts, with subjects who reported both having 35 times the risk of non-smokers without a history of condylomata.[95] This last finding most probably reflects characteristics that are shared by cervical cancer and the group of vulvar cancers mediated by the same viral factor. These epidemiological studies support the possible synergism between HPV and smoking in the genesis of other squamous anogenital cancers, including the cervix.[117] Finally, a recent study addressed the role of smoking in the outcome of patients with squamous cell carcinoma of the vulva.[118] These preliminary data indicate a decreased survival in patients who were current or former smokers at the time of diagnosis of vulvar cancer.

Immunological factors

Several studies in the literature support a close association between HPV-related tumorigenesis/progression and the immune system. However, the exact mechanisms that trigger the induction of an efficient immune response against HPV-related lesions are still unknown. They are equally important in the activation of the immune system and to the genetic composition of the host. As there is no direct exposure of HPV proteins to immunocompetent cells (macrophages or Langerhans' cells), it is conceivable that the development of antibodies to virus proteins may well depend upon secondary infection through small wounds, resulting in the exposure of viral proteins to these cells. In HPV-related cancer, this mechanism depends on cell necrosis among invasively growing tissues.[119]

The presence of mononuclear cells, mostly CD4 cells and macrophages, has been demonstrated in regressing papillomas.[120] The role of local immune response in cervical carcinogenesis was quantitatively studied with immunoperoxidase staining.[121] There was a significant association of the increase in number of immunocompetent cells, such as NK cells, macrophages, cells of Langerhans, memory T cells and especially CD4-positive cells, with the increase of the grade of cervical dysplasia. However, these cell populations decrease significantly in number in high-grade lesions or carcinoma in situ. These findings indicate that the local immune response may play an important role in surveillance against the development and progression of cervical cancer. On the other hand, a decrease in counts of Langerhans' cell in low-grade CIN and in smokers and pregnant women was verified in another study.[114] Similar findings have also been demonstrated previously by others, and may show the interaction between immune elements and agents such as HPV, steroid hormones and smoking in the aetiology of cervical neoplasia.[113]

The role of the humoral immune response in controlling HPV infection and related lesions is also far from being completely understood; nevertheless, it seems to be able to prevent papillomavirus infection. The association of serum antibodies to HPV proteins with HPV-related diseases was established by several studies.[122] Most of them were based on the use of recombinant or synthetic antigens, which resemble, in function and immunogenicity, the authentic early (non-structural) and late (structural) HPV proteins, and were detected in several assays, including enzyme-linked immunosorbent assay (ELISA), Western blotting and, more recently, immunoprecipitation. From the antigens used in these studies, recombinant HPV late proteins, which assemble into virus capsids – called virus-like particles (VLPs) – were the most impressively documented. Despite their relatively low sensitivity, these studies have found antibodies to viral capsids (measured using VLP) and some early viral proteins in a significant proportion of patients with benign and malignant HPV-related diseases. A small number of patients are, however, devoid of detectable antibodies, even when tested by combinations of assays that would increase the predicted value of the serological test. This fact could be related to differences in antigen presentation during the course of infection or even to other unknown factors of biological significance.

Immunological factors were also found to be significant in determining the outcome of squamous cell carcinoma of the vulva, independent of HPV status and other clinical and pathological factors, in a series of experiments by Price.[123] Marked plasmalymphocytic infiltration, particularly of B lymphocytes producing IgA, indicated good prognosis in a retrospective investigation. Prospective studies in smaller but similar populations, investigated by the same author, revealed that a marked degree of infiltration with T lymphocytes, as the predominant cell type, was also associated with other favourable prognostic indicators. However, the immunological interplay between host and squamous carcinoma of the vulva still needs clarification.

Immunosuppressed women are at increased risk of developing intraepithelial and invasive squamous neoplasia of the lower genital tract. This includes patients who have undergone organ transplantation and are taking immunosuppressive medications, have Hodgkin's disease or are HIV positive.[119] The link between HPV-related diseases and HIV positivity is even stronger because both conditions, HPV and HIV infection, are sexually transmitted and their risk population share several demographic characteristics. Nevertheless, large case–control studies have shown that, despite these associations, HPV infection and HIV seropositivity are independent risk factors for the development of CIN. HIV seropositivity is also an independent risk factor for HPV infections, both latent and clinically expressed. The same studies had showed that a low CD4-positive T-lymphocyte count (under 200 T cells/μl) is also specifically associated with HPV infections and the development of CIN, and

that the ratio of the latent HPV infections to clinically expressed infections increases with the increase of CD4-positive T-lymphocyte counts from less than 200 T cells/μl to normal levels in HIV-negative patients. However, whether HPV and HIV are directly associated or indirectly linked to HIV immunosuppression remains unclear. As the two viruses do not co-infect or co-localize in cervical tissues, if molecular interactions occur between HIV and HPV they are probably mediated by extracellular factors. Enhanced HPV gene expression in HIV-infected women can potentially be explained by interactions involving the transactivator protein of HIV-1 (tat 1) and the HPV 16 promoter (P97), leading to reversal of E2 repression. On the other hand, the same HIV protein has also been shown to inhibit T-cell proliferation in vitro. Renal transplant recipients have a higher risk of developing cancer of the vulva than of the cervix – a 100-fold increase compared with the general population.[119] Case reports about the development of invasive vulvar squamous cell carcinomas in HIV-infected women have also been reported.[123]

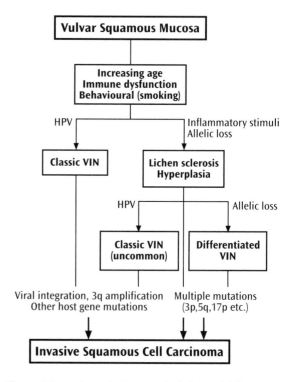

Figure 4.8 *A schematic diagram depicting multiple pathways to invasive vulvar cancer (refer to text).*

CONCLUSIONS

The pathogenesis of vulvar cancer involves the interplay of viral and environmental exposures, host genetic and immune factors, and the wide range of variables probably explains the diverse morphological phenotypes observed in these tumours. Fig. 4.8 attempts to place some of these factors in perspective, and outlines scenarios that take into account risk factors and molecular pathways. Nevertheless, a more complete understanding of the pathogenesis of vulvar cancer will require attention to the ageing process and the interaction of host, viral and other factors in the context of time.

REFERENCES

1 Silverberg E. *Statistical and epidemiological information on gynecologic cancer*. Atlanta, GA: American Cancer Society, 1980: 9.
2 Cramer DW, Cutler SJ. Incidence and histopathology of malignancies of the female genital organs in the United States. *Am J Obstet Gynecol* 1974; **118**: 443–60.
3 Krain LS. Carcinoma of the vulva in California 1942–1969. The California Tumor Registry experience. *Oncology* 1973; **28**: 110–16.
4 Zaino RJ. Carcinoma of the vulva, urethra, and bartholin's glands. In: Wilkinson EJ (ed) *Pathology of the vulva and vagina*. New York: Churchill Livingstone, 1987: 119–53.
5 Henson D, Tarone R. An epidemiologic study of cancer of the cervix, vagina, and vulva based upon the Third National Cancer Survey in the United States. *Am J Obstet Gynecol* 1977; **129**: 525–32.
6 Gosling JRG, Abell MR, Drolette BM, Loughrin TD. Infiltrative squamous cell (epidermoid) cancer of vulva. *Cancer* 1961; **14**: 330–43.
7 Cramer DW. Epidemiology of the gynecologic cancers. *Compr Ther* 1978; **4**: 9–17.
8 Peters RK, Mack TM, Bemstein L. Parallels in the epidemiology of selected anogenital carcinomas. *J Natl Cancer Inst* 1984; **72**: 609–15.
9 Sengupta BS. Carcinoma of the vulva in Jamaican women. *Acta Obstet Gynecol Scand* 1981; **60**: 537–44.
10 Leibowitch M, Neill S, Pelisse M, Moyal-Baracco M. The epithelial changes associated with squamous cell carcinoma of the vulva; a review of the clinical, histological and viral findings in 78 women. *Br J Obstet Gynaecol* 1990; **97**: 1135–9.
11 zur Hausen H. Papillomaviruses in human cancer. *Cancer* 1987; **59**: 1692–6.
12 Andersen WA, Franquemont DW, Williams J, Taylor PT, Crum CP. Vulvar squamous cell carcinoma and papillomaviruses: two separate entities? *Am J Obstet Gynecol* 1991; **165**: 329–36.
13 Crum CP. Carcinoma of the vulva: epidemiology and pathogenesis. *Obstet Gynecol* 1992; **79**: 448–54.
14 Taichman LB, LaPorta RF. The expression of papillomaviruses in epithelial cells. In: Salzman NP, Hoeley PM (eds). *The Papovaviridae*. New York: Plenum Press, 1987.
15 Munger K, Phelps WC, Bubb V, Howley M, Schlegel R. The E6 and E7 genes of the human papillomavirus type 16 together are necessary and sufficient for transformation of primary human keratinocytes. *J Virol* 1989; **63**: 4417.
16 Dyson NP, Howley K, Munger K, Harlow E. The human papillomavirus-16 E7 oncoprotein is able to bind to the retinoblastoma gene product. *Science* 1989; **243**: 934.
17 Werness BA, Levine AJ, Howley PM. Association of human papillomavirus types 16 and 18 E6 proteins with p53. *Science* 1990; **248**: 76–9.
18 Halbert CL, Demers GW, Galloway DA. The E7 gene of human papillomavirus type 16 is sufficient for immortalization of human epithelial cells. *J Virol* 1991; **65**: 473–8.
19 Heck DV, Yee CL, Howley PM, Munger K. Efficiency of binding the retinoblastoma protein correlates with the transforming capacity of the E7 oncoproteins of the human papillomaviruses. *Proc Natl Acad Sci USA* 1992; **89**: 4442–6.
20 Schwarz E, Freese UK, Gissmann L et al. Structure and transcription of human papillomavirus sequences in cervical carcinoma cells. *Nature* 1985; **314**: 111–14.
21 Baker CC, Phelps WC, Lindgren V, Braun MJ, Gonda MA, Howley PM. Structural and translational analysis of human papillomavirus type 16 sequences in cervical carcinoma cell lines. *J Virol* 1987; **61**: 962–71.
22 Shirasawa H, Tomita Y, Kubota K et al. Transcriptional differences of the human papillomavirus type 16 genome between precancerous lesions and invasive carcinomas. *J Virol* 1988; **62**: 1022.
23 Thierry F, Yanif M. The BPV-1 E *trans*-acting protein can be either an activator or repressor of the HPV 18 regulatory region. *EMBO J* 1987; **6**: 3391–7.
24 Bernard BA, Bailly C, Lenoir M-C, Darmon M, Thierry F, Yaniv M. The human papillomavirus type 18 (HPV 18) E2 gene product is a repressor of the HPV 18 regulatory region in human keratinocytes. *J Virol* 1989; **63**: 4317–24.

25 Romanczuk H, Thierry F, Howley PM. Mutational analysis of *cis* elements involved in E2 modulation of human papillomavirus type 16 p97 and type m18 p105 promoters. *J Virol* 1990; **64**: 2849–59.

26 Vousden KH, Wrede D, Crook T. HPV oncoprotein function: releasing the brakes on cell growth control. *Papillomavirus Report* 1991; **2**: 1–3.

27 Alani PM, Munger K. Human papillomaviruses and associated malignancies. *J Clin Oncol* 1998; **16**: 330–7.

28 Couturier J, Sastre-Garau X, Schneider-Maunoury S, Labib A, Orth G. Integration of papillomavirus DNA near myc genes in genital carcinomas and its consequences for proto-oncogene expression. *J Virol* 1991; **65**: 4534–8.

29 Popescu NC, DiPaolo JA. Preferential sites for viral integration on mammalian genome. *Cancer Genet Cytogenet* 1989; **42**: 157–71.

30 Smith PP, Friedman CL, Bryant EM, McDougall JK. Human papillomavirus viral integration and fragile sites in HPV immortalized human keratinocyte cell lines. *Genes Chrom Cancer* 1992; **5**: 150–72.

31 Vousden KH. Regulation of the cell cycle by viral oncoproteins. *Cancer Biol* 1995; **6**: 109–16.

32 Brandenberger AW, Rudinger R, Hanggi W, Bersinger NA, Dreher E. Detection of human papillomavirus in vulvar carcinoma: A study by in situ hybridization. *Arch Gynecol Obstet* 1992; **252**: 31–5.

33 Park JS, Jones RW, McLean NM et al. Possible etiologic heterogeneity of vulvar intraepithelial neoplasia. A correlation of pathologic characteristics with human papillomavirus detection by in situ hybridization and polymerase chain reaction. *Cancer* 1991; **67**: 1599–607.

34 Buscema J, Naghashfar Z, Sawada E, Daniel R, Woodruff JD, Shah K. The predominance of human papillomavirus type 16 in vulva neoplasia. *Obstet Gynecol* 1988; **71**: 601–6.

35 Haefner H, Tate J, McLachlin CM, Crum CP. Vulvar intraepithelial neoplasia: Age, morphological phenotype, papillomavirus DNA and coexisting invasive carcinoma. *Hum Pathol* 1995; **26**: 147–54.

36 Hording U, Kringsholmn B, Andreasson B, Visfeld J, Daugaard S, Bock JE. Human papillomavirus in vulvar squamous-cell carcinoma and in normal vulvar tissues: a search for a possible impact of HPV on vulvar cancer prognosis. *Int J Cancer* 1993; **55**: 394–6.

37 Pinto AP, Signorello LB, Crum CP, Harlow BL, Abrao F, Villa LL. Squamous cell carcinoma of the vulva in Brazil: Prognostic importance of host and viral variables. *Gynecol Oncol* 1999 **74**(1): 61–7.

38 Toki T, Kurman RJ, Park JS et al. Probable nonpapillomavirus etiology of squamous cell carcinoma of the vulva in older women: a clinicopathologic study using in situ hybridization and polymerase chain reaction. *Int J Gynecol* 1991; **10**: 107–25.

39 Atkin BN. Chromosome changes in preneoplastic and neoplastic genital lesions. *Branbury Rep* 1986a; **21**: 303.

40 Sreekantaiah C, Braekeleer NM, Hass O. Cytogenetic findings in cervical carcinoma. A statistical approach. *Cancer Genet Cytogenet* 1991; **53**: 75.

41 DiPaolo JA, Woodworth NC, Popescu NC, Notario V, Doniger J. Induction of human cervical squamous cell carcinoma by sequential transfection with human papillomavirus 16 DNA and viral *ras*. *Oncogene* 1989; **4**: 395.

42 Smith PP, Bryant EM, Kaur P, McDougall JK. Cytogenetic analysis of eight human papillomavirus immortalized human keratinocyte cell lines. *Int J Cancer* 1989; **44**: 1124–31.

43 Popescu NC, DiPaolo JA. Integration of human papillomavirus 16 DNA and genomic rearrangements in immortalized human keratinocyte lines. *Cancer Res* 1990; **50**: 1316.

44 Debiec-Rychter M, Zukowski K, Wang CY, Wen WN. Chromosomal characterizations of human nasal and nasopharyngeal cells immortalized by human papillomavirus type 16 DNA. *Cancer Genet Cytogenet* 1991; **52**: 51.

45 Atkin BN. Chromosome 1 aberrations in cancer. *Cancer Genet Cytogenet* 1986; **21**: 279.

46 Hesehneyer K, Schrock E, Manoir S, Blegen H et al. Gain of chromosome 3q defines the transition from severe dysplasia to invasive carcinoma of the uterine cervix. *Proc Natl Acad Sci USA* 1996; **93**: 479–84.

47 Worsham MJ, Van Dyke DL, Grenman SE et al. Consistent chromosome abnormalities in squamous cell carcinoma of the vulva. *Genes, Chromosomes Cancer* 1991; **3**: 420–32.

48 Scheffner M, Munger K, Byrne JC, Howley PM. The state of the p53 and retinoblastoma genes in human cervical carcinoma cell lines. *Proc Natl Acad Sci USA* 1991; **88**: 5523–7.

49 Fujita M, Inoue M, Tanizawa O, Iwamoto S, Enomoto T. Alterations of the p53 gene in human primary cervical carcinoma with and without human papillomavirus infection. *Cancer Res* 1992; **52**: 5323.

50 Ikenberg H, Matthay K, Schmitt B et al. p53 mutation and NMM2 amplification are rare even in human

papillomavirus negative cervical carcinomas. *Cancer* 1995; **76**: 57–66.

51 Kim YT, Thomas NF, Kessis TD, Wilkinson EJ, Hedrick L, Cho KR. p53 mutations and clonality in vulvar carcinomas and squamous hyperplasias suggesting that squamous hyperplasias do not serve as direct precursors of human papillomavirus-negative vulvar carcinomas. *Hum Pathol* 1996; **27**: 389–95.

52 Lee YY, Wilczynski SP, Chumakov A, Chih D, Koeffler HP. Carcinoma of the vulva: HPV and p53 mutations. *Oncogene* 1994; **9**: 1655–9.

53 Milde-Langosch K, Albrecht K, Joram S, Schlechte H, Giessing M, Loning T. Presence and persistence of HPV infection and p53 mutation in cancer of the cervix uteri and the vulva. *Int J Cancer* 1995; **63**: 639–45.

54 Walts AE, Koeffler HP, Said JW. Localization of the p53 protein and human papillomavirus in anogenital squamous lesions: immunohistochemical and in situ hybridization studies in benign, dysplastic, and malignant epithelia. *Hum Pathol* 1993; **24**: 1238–42.

55 Kagie MJ, Kenter GG, Tollenaar RA, Hermans J, Trimbos JP, Fleuren GJ. p53 protein overexpression, a frequent observation in squamous cell carcinoma of the vulva and in various synchronous vulvar epithelia, has no value as a prognostic marker. *Int J Gynecol Pathol* 1997; **16**: 124–30.

56 Storey A, Thomas M, Kalita A et al. Role of a p53 polymorphism in the development of human papillomavirus-associated cancer. *Nature* 1998; **393**: 229–34.

57 Carey TE, Van Dyke DL, Worsham MJ. Nonrandom chromosome aberrations and clonal populations in head and neck cancer. *Anticancer Res* 1993; **13**: 2561–7.

58 Bockmuhl U, Petersen I, Schwendel A, Dietel M. Genetic screening of head and neck carcinomas using comparative genomic hybridization (CGH). *Laryngorhinootologie* 1996; **75**: 408–14.

59 Ah-See KW, Cooke TG, Pickford IR, Soutar D, Balmain A. An allelotype of squamous carcinoma of the head and neck using microsatellite markers. *Cancer Res* 1994; **54**: 1617–21.

60 Sakurai M, Tamada J, Maseki N et al. Chromosomal deletions in non-small cell lung carcinomas. *Proc Annu Meet Am Assoc Cancer Res* 1991; **32**: A1176.

61 Petersen I, Bujard M, Cremer T, Dietel M, Ried T. Comparative genomic hybridization reveals multiple DNA gains and losses in non-small cell lung carcinomas. *Proc Annu Meet Am Assoc Cancer Res* 1995; **36**: A3289.

62 Sato S, Nakamura Y, Tsuchiya E. Difference of allelotype between squamous cell carcinoma and adenocarcinoma of the lung. *Cancer Res* 1994; **54**: 5652–5.

63 Pinto AP, Lin MC, Mutter GL, Sun D, Crum CP. Allelic loss in HPV positive and negative vulvar carcinomas. *American Journal of Pathol* 1999; **154(4)** : 1009–1015.

64 Aoki T, Mori T du X, Nisihira T, Matsubara T, Nakamura Y. Allelotype study of esophageal carcinoma. *Genes Chromosom Cancer* 1994; **10**: 177–82.

65 Quinn AG, Sikkink S, Rees JL. Basal cell carcinomas and squamous cell carcinomas of human skin show distinct patterns of chromosome loss. *Cancer Res* 1994; **54**: 4756–9.

66 Lasko D, Cavenee W, Nordenskjdld M. Loss of constitutional heterozygosity in human cancer. *Annu Rev Genet* 1991; **25**: 281–314.

67 Busby-Earle RMC, Steel CM, Bird CC. Cervical carcinoma: low frequency of allele loss at loci implicated in other common malignancies. *Br J Cancer* 1993; **67**: 71–5.

68 Mitra AB, Murty VV, Li-RG, Pratap M, Luthra UK, Chaganti RS. Allelotype analysis of cervical carcinoma. *Cancer Res* 1994; **54**: 4481–7.

69 Adamson R, Jones AS, Field JK. Loss of heterozygosity studies on chromosome 17 in head and neck cancer using microsatellite markers. *Oncogene* 1994; **9**: 2077–82.

70 Wu CL, Sloan P, Read A, Harris R, Thakker N. Deletion mapping on the short arm of chromosome 3 in squamous cell carcinoma of the oral cavity. *Cancer Res* 1994; **54**: 6484–8.

71 Van Dyke DL, Worsham MJ, Benninger MJ, Carey TE. The recurrent chromosome changes in 29 squamous cell carcinomas of the head and neck region. Fifth International Workshop on Chromosomes in Solid Tumors. 10–12 January 1993, Tucson, AZ, A28, 1993 (Meeting Abstract).

72 el Naggar AK, Hurr K, Luna MA, Geopfert H, Batsakis JG. Sequential loss of heterozygosity at microsatellite motifs in preinvasive and invasive (HNSC). *Proc Annu Meet Am Assoc Cancer Res* 1995; **36**: A3253 (Meeting Abstract).

73 Ohata H, Emi M, Fugiwara Y et al. Deletion mapping of the short arm of chromosome 8 in non-small cell lung carcinoma. *Genes Chromosom Cancer* 1993; **7**: 85–8.

74 Ogasawara S, Maesawa C, Tamura G et al. Frequent microsatellite alterations on chromosome 3p in esophageal squamous cell carcinoma. *Proc Annu Meet Am Assoc Cancer Res* 1995; **36**: A3262.

75 Cheng JQ, Crepin M, Hamelin R. Loss of heterozygosity on chromosomes lp, 3p, 11p and 11q in human non-

small cell lung cancer. *Serono Symp Publ Raven* 1990; **78**: 357–64.

76 Muleris M, Sahnon RJ, Girodet J, Zafrani B, Dutrillaux B. Recurrent deletions of chromosomes 11q and 3p in anal canal carcinoma. *Int J Cancer* 1987; **39**: 595–8.

77 Srivatsan ES, Misra BC, Venugopalan M, Wilczynski SP. Loss of heterozygosity of alleles on chromosome 11 in cervical carcinoma. *Am J Hum Genet* 1991; **49**: 868–77.

78 Wistuba IL, Montellano FD, Milchgrub S et al. Deletions of chromosome 3p are frequent and early events in the pathogenesis of uterine cervical carcinoma. *Cancer Res* 1997; **57**: 3154–87.

79 Sreektantaiah C, Rao PH, Xu L, Sacks PG, Schantz SP, Chaganti RS. Consistent chromosomal losses in head and neck squamous cell carcinoma cell lines. *Genes Chromosom Cancer* 1994; **11**: 29–39.

80 Lin Ming-Chieh, Mutter GL, Trivijisilp P, Boynton KA, Sun D, Crum CP. Patterns of allelic loss (LOH) in vulvar squamous carcinomas and adjacent noninvasive epithelia. *Am J Pathol* 1998; **152**: 1313–8.

81 Allen RC, Zoghbi HY, Moseley AB, Rosenblatt HM, Belmont JW. Methylation of HpaII and HhaI sites near the polymorphic CAG repeat in the human androgen-receptor gene correlates with X chromosome inactivation. *Am J Hum Genet* 1992; **51**: 1229–39.

82 Vogelstein B, Fearon ER, Hamilton SR, Feinberg AP. Use of restriction fragment length polymorphisms to determine the clonal origin of human tumors. *Science* 1985; **227**: 642–5.

83 Mutter GL, Chaponot ML, Fletcher JL. A RCP assay for nonrandom X chromosome inactivation identifies monoclonal endometrial cancers and precancers. *Am J Pathol* 1995; **146**: 501–8.

84 Fletcher J, Pinkus J, Lage J, Morton C, Pinkus G. Clonal 6p21 rearrangement is restricted to the mesenchymal component of an endometrial polyp. *Genes Chromosom Cancer* 1992; **5**: 260–3.

85 Tate JE, Mutter GL, Boynton K, Crum CP. Monoclonal origin of vulvar intraepithelial neoplasia and some vulvar hyperplasias. *Am J Pathol* **150**(1): 315–22.

86 Park TW, Richart RM, Sun XW, Wright TC Jr. Association between human papillomavirus type and clonal status of cervical squamous intraepithelial lesions. *J Natl Cancer Inst* 1996; **88**: 355–8.

87 Kim YT, Thomas NF, Kessis TD, Wilkinson EJ, Hedrick L, Cho KR. p53 mutations and clonality in vulvar carcinomas and squamous hyperplasias suggesting that squamous hyperplasias do not serve as direct precursors of human papillomavirus-negative

vulvar carcinomas. *Hum Pathol* 1996; **27**: 389–95.

88 Califano J, van der Riet P, Westra W et al. Genetic progression model for head and neck cancer: implications for field cancerization. *Cancer Res* 1996; **56**: 2488–92.

89 Rodke J, Friedrich EG Jr, Wilkinson EJ. Malignant potential of mixed vulvar dystrophy (lichen scleroses with squamous cell hyperplasia). *J Reprod Med* 1988; **33**: 545–50.

90 Neill SM, Lessanaleibowitch M, Pelisse M, Moyal-Barracco M. Lichen sclerosus, invasive squamous cell carcinoma and human papillomavirus. *Am J Obstet Gynecol* 1990; **162**: 1633–4.

91 Ziegler A, Jonason AS, Leffell DJ et al. Sunburn and p53 in the onset of skin cancer. *Nature* 1994; **372**: 773–6.

92 Kiene P, Milde-Langosch K, Loning T. Human papillomavirus infection in vulvar lesions of lichen scleroses et atrophicus. *Arch Dermatol Res* 1991; **283**: 445–8.

93 Ansink AC, Krul MRL, De Weger RA et al. Human papillomavirus, lichen sclerosus, and squamous cell carcinoma of the vulva: detection and diagnostic significance. *Gynecol Oncol* 1994; **52**: 180–4.

94 Park JS, Jones RW, McLean NM et al. Possible etiologic heterogeneity of vulvar intraepithelial neoplasia. A correlation of pathologic characteristics with human papillomavirus detection by in situ hybridization and polymerase chain reaction. *Cancer* 1991; **67**: 1599–607.

95 Brinton LA, Nasca PC, Mallin K, Baptiste MS, Wilbanks GD, Richart RM. Case–control study of cancer of the vulva. *Obstet Gynecol* 1990; **75**: 859–66.

96 Monk BJ, Burger RA, Lin F, Parham G, Vasilev SA, Wilcynski SP. Prognostic significance of human papillomavirus DNA in vulvar carcinoma. *Obstet Gynecol* 1995; **85**: 709–15.

97 Nuovo GJ, Delvenne P, MacConnell PBA et al. Correlation of histology and detection of human papillomavirus DNA in vulvar cancers. *Gynecol Oncol* 1991; **43**: 275–80.

98 Hording U, Kringsholm B, Andreasson B, Visfeld J, Daugaard S, Bock JE. Human papillomavirus in vulvar squamous-cell carcinoma and in normal vulvar tissues: a search for a possible impact of HPV on vulvar cancer prognosis. *Int J Cancer* 1993; **55**: 394–6.

99 Bloss JD, Liao SY, Wilczynski SP et al. Clinical and histologic features of vulvar carcinomas analyzed for human papillomavirus status: Evidence that squamous cell carcinoma of the vulva has more than one etiology. *Hum Pathol* 1991; **22**: 711–18.

100 Brandenberger AW, Rudinger R, Hanggi W, Bersinger NA, Dreher E. Detection of human papillomavirus in vulvar carcinoma: A study by in situ hybridization. *Arch Gynecol Obstet* 1992; **252**: 31–5.

101 Gordinier AW, Steinhoff M, Hogan JW et al. S-phase fraction, p53, and Her-2/Neu status as predictors of nodal metastasis in early vulvar carcinoma. *Gynecol Oncol* 1997; **67**: 200–2.

102 Kohlberger P, Kainz C, Breiteneeker G et al. Prognostic value of immunohistochemically detected p53 expression in vulvar carcinoma. *Cancer* 1995; **76**: 1786–9.

103 Pilotti S, D'amato L, Della Torre G et al. Papillomavirus, p53 and primary carcinoma of the vulva. *Diagn Mol Pathol* 1995; **4**: 239–48.

104 Sliutz G, Schmidt W, Tempfer C et al. Detection of p53 point mutations in primary human vulvar cancer by PCR and temperature gradient electrophoresis. *Gynecol Oncol* 1997; **64**: 93–8.

105 Gram IT, Austin H, Stalsberg H. Cigarette smoking and the incidence of cervical intraepithelial neoplasia, grade III, and cancer of the cervix uteri. *Am J Epidemiol* 1992; **135**: 341–6.

106 Hellberg D, Nilsson S, Haley NJ, Hoffman D, Wynder E. Smoking and cervical intraepithelial neoplasia: nicotine and cotinine in serum and cervical mucus in smokers and nonsmokers. *Am J Obstet Gynecol* 1988; **158**: 910–13.

107 Simons AM, Phillips DH, Coleman DV. Damage to DNA in cervical epithelium related to smoking tobacco. *BMJ* 1993; **306**: 1444–8.

108 Warwick AP, Redman CW, Jones PW et al. Progression of cervical intraepithelial neoplasia to cervical cancer: interactions of cytochrome P450 CYP2D6 EM and glutathione S-transferase GSTM1 null genotypes and cigarette smoking. *Br J Cancer* 1994; **70**: 704–8.

109 Warwick A, Sarhanis P, Redman C et al. Theta class glutathione S-transferase GSTT1 genotypes and susceptibility to cervical neoplasia: interactions with GSTM1, CYP2D6 and smoking. *Carcinogenesis* 1994; **15**: 2841–5.

110 Crespi CL, Penman BW, Gelboin HV, Gonzales FJ. A tobacco smoke-derived nitrosamine, 4-(methylnitrosamino)-1-(3-pyridyl)-1-butanone, is activated by multiple human cytochrome P450s including the polymorphic human cytochrome P4502D6. *Carcinogenesis* 1991; **12**: 1197–201.

111 Johnson JD, Houchens DP, Kluwe WM, Craig DK, Fisher GL. Effects of mainstream and environmental tobacco smoke on the immune system in animals and humans: a review. *Crit Rev Toxicol* 1990; **20**: 369–90.

112 Tay SK, Jenkins D, Maddox P, Campion M, Singer A. Subpopulations of Langerhans' cells in cervical neoplasia. *Br J Obstet Gynaecol* 1987; **94**: 10–15.

113 Barton SE, Hollingworth A, Maddox PH et al. Possible cofactors in the etiology of cervical intraepithelial neoplasia. An immunopathologic study. *J Reprod Med* 1989; **34**: 613–16.

114 Poppe WA, Drijkoningen M, Ide PS, Laweryns JM, Van Assche FA. Langerhans' cells and L1 antigen expression in normal and abnormal squamous epithelium of the cervical transformation zone. *Gynecol Obstet Invest* 1996; **41**: 207–13.

115 Carter J, Carlson J, Fowler J et al. Invasive vulvar tumors in young women – A disease of the immunosuppressed? *Gynecol Oncol* 1993; **51**: 307–10.

116 Daling JR, Sherman KJ, Hislop TG et al. Cigarette smoking and the risk of anogenital cancer. *Am J Epidemiol* 1992; **135**: 180–9.

117 zur Hausen H. Human genital cancer: synergism between two virus infections or synergism between a virus infection and initiating events? *Lancet* 1982; **ii**: 1370.

118 Kirschner CV, Yordan EL, Geest KD, Wilbanks GD. Smoking, obesity, and survival in squamous cell carcinoma of the vulva. *Gynecol Oncol* 1994; **56**: 79–84.

119 Gissmann L. Immunologic responses to human papillomavirus infection. In: Lorincz AT, Reid R (guest eds), Masse S (ed). *Obstetrics and gynecology clinics of North America human papillomavirus* I, Vol 23. Philadelphia: WB Saunders Co, 1996: 625–39.

120 Stanley MA, Coleman N, Chambers M. The host response to lesions induced by human papillomavirus. In: Mindel A (ed). *Genital warts and human papillomavirus infection*. London: Edward Arnold, 1994: 21–44.

121 Takehara K. Local immune responses in uterine cervical carcinogenesis. *Nippon Sanka Fujinka Gakkai Zasshi* 1996; **48**: 1063–70.

122 Wright TC, Sun XW. Anogenital papillomavirus

infection and neoplasia in inununodeficient women. In: Lorincz AT, Reid R (guest eds), Baniewicz C (ed). *Obstetrics and gynecology clinics of North America – human papillomavirus II*, Vol. 23 Philadelphia: WB Saunders Co, 1996: 861–93.

123 Price JH. Local immune response in the prognosis of vulval cancer: an immunohistological study. *Dis Abstr Int* 1991; **52**: 419.

5

Is vulvar intraepithelial neoplasia a precursor of cancer?

RW JONES

> ... the final answer to the question of whether vulvar atypias or carcinoma in situ are likely to undergo progression to invasion will not be known until a sufficient number of untreated patients have been observed over many years[1]

In the classic original review of vulvar intraepithelial neoplasia (VIN), Knight observed that 'considerable discussion has arisen as to the nature of Bowen's disease (of the vulva) over a period of 20 years'.[2] The natural history of VIN remains a contentious issue more than five decades later.

Two important factors need to be taken into account when addressing the biological nature of VIN. First, the heterogeneous and evolving nature of VIN has often not been appreciated. For example, does the less common, unifocal, slightly raised, red lesion seen in older women (and reported in the past as Bowen's disease) have the same neoplastic potential as the multifocal pigmented lesion seen commonly in younger women today? Second, when addressing the natural history of 'intraepithelial neoplasia' one needs to define the outcome between those cases where the object has been to eliminate the lesion by treatment and those where residual disease is present after inadequate treatment or representative biopsy.

Knight concluded in the original literature review in 1943, that the lesion should be regarded as a slowly growing epithelioma.[2] A decade later Gardiner noted that intraepithelial carcinoma of the vulva could initially exist alone and later become invasive (reporting two such cases), early invasion could be found in a field of VIN, or VIN could be present at the border of an invasive squamous cell carcinoma.[3]

By the 1960s, the concept of VIN as a premalignant condition of the vulva appeared to be firmly established as 'a form of intraepithelial carcinoma that may progress to infiltrative squamous cell carcinomas'.[4]

The literature written by the leaders in the field (which accompanied the dramatic increase in the reported frequency of VIN) in the 1970s and 1980s began to question whether the lesion should always be regarded as a true precursor of cancer.[5,6] Friedrich, the doyen of vulvar disease at this time, stated that 'progression of the disease to invasive carcinoma has not been documented with frequency sufficient to justify the term carcinoma in situ'.[7] What caused the dramatic reversal of opinion? First, a number of large studies appearing at this time reported 'low progression rates to invasion' of 0–4 per cent (Table 5.1). It was not fully appreciated by many (and still not fully recognized by some today) that the biological behaviour of VIN was

Table 5.1 *Progression of VIN 3 to invasive vulvar carcinoma longitudinal studies since 1970 (minimum 25 cases)*

Ref.	Year	No. of patients	No. progressing[a]	Percentage	Comment
Collins[8]	1970	41	1	2.4	3-year transit time to invasion
Forney[9]	1977	27	0	0	
Japaze[10]	1977	71	2	2.8	Both cancers at anal margin; one patient immunosuppressed
Buscema[11]	1980	102	4	4	Progression in two young immunosuppressed patients, both at the anal margin
Friedrich[6]	1980	50	1	2	21 year old, immunosuppressed, progressed without treatment to invasion in 1 year; regression in five cases
Iversen[12]	1981	29	1	3.5	Invasion at incomplete resection margin; 9-year transit time to invasion
Benedet[13]	1982	81	3	3.7	2-, 3- and 6-year transit times to invasion
Caglar[14]	1982	50	0 (5[a])	–	[b]Invasion missed in original biopsy in three cases; invasion noted within 4 months of treatment in two cases
di Paola[15]	1982	28	0	0	
Bernstein[16]	1983	65	0	0	Spontaneous regression in 5 of 13 cases within 6 months
Crum[17]	1984	41	2 (5[c])	4.9	[c]Invasion within 12 months in three cases; 3- and 10-year transit times One anal cancer
Leuchter[18]	1984	142	0	0	One spontaneous regression
Andreasson[19]	1985	49	1	2.0	
Powell[20]	1986	50	0[d]	–	[d]Superficial invasion in excised specimen in four (8%)
Ragnarsson[21]	1987	74	3	4.0	Two cases previously irradiated
Wilkinson[22]	1988	93	2	2.1	
Husseinzadeh[23]	1989	33[e]	0[f]	–	[e]47% lost to follow-up [f]Invasion missed in original biopsy in three cases
Barbero[24]	1990	27	0	0	
Jones[25]	1994	105 treated	4	3.8	Four cases under 50 years
		8 untreated	7	87.5	Four cases at external urethra or anal margins Four cases previously irradiated; transit time to invasion 2–8 years in 10 of 11 cases One anal carcinoma in an immunosuppressed patient One spontaneous regression
Hording[26]	1995	73	5 (12[g])	6.8	[g]Microinvasion in 7 of 12 initial excision specimens
Herod[27]	1996	92	9	10.0	Five cases under 50 years; transit time to invasion 1–8 years in 8 of 9 cases. One perianal cancer
Van Beurden[28]	1998	47	0	0	Expectant management of asymptomatic multifocal lesions

[a] Figures in brackets refer to the number of cases of progression quoted by the author(s). Those not in brackets represent the revised number of cases of progression.

largely destroyed by treatment. Second, a number of studies reported regression of lesions with the histological appearance of VIN. Third, there appeared to be an unacceptably long transit time between the in situ phase and invasion. Finally, it was suggested that VIN may not represent a cancer precursor but simply an epithelial proliferative event as a response to viral infection.[5] The challenge by Friedrich and others to the historical viewpoint has been the basis of the confusion of the 1990s.

MORPHOLOGICAL EVIDENCE

The early observations that vulvar carcinoma in situ could be seen at the margin of an invasive squamous cell carcinoma or the presence of 'microinvasion' in a field of VIN provided persuasive evidence pointing to the invasive nature of the lesion. Several recent studies have noted that VIN 3 can be demonstrated adjacent to about 30 per cent of squamous cell carcinomas of the vulva.[29] In addition, studies confirm that most stage Ia carcinomas of the vulva arise in a field of VIN 3.[30]

The introduction of the VIN 1–3 histology grading system carried the implicit inference of a biological continuum that may end with the development of invasive carcinoma. Only rarely has there been documented evidence of progression of VIN 1 to VIN 3.[24] Thus, in contrast to a similar grading system in the cervix, there are no data on progression rates of the various grades of VIN. The VIN grading system should therefore be seen as a convenient histological description of a spectrum of intraepithelial changes, and it should not be inferred that it is a biological continuum. This chapter therefore principally addresses the question of VIN 3 as a precursor of vulvar carcinoma.

Difficulty may be encountered in cases of lichen sclerosus with or without squamous hyperplasia, in which basal epithelial atypia is noted adjacent to an invasive carcinoma. Although some may regard these changes as representing a low-grade VIN, the features do not always fulfil the criteria for a differentiated VIN.

The uncommon differentiated variant of VIN has been noted occasionally to have a very short progression interval to invasive carcinoma.[31]

VIN lesions display a morphological heterogeneity that can be subclassified into warty, basaloid, mixed warty/basaloid and uncommonly differentiated types (for further discussion see Chapter 2). One study

reported progression occurring in warty, basaloid and mixed warty/basaloid VIN types to the corresponding carcinomas.[32]

Over the past two decades there has been increasing evidence to implicate human papillomavirus (HPV) infection as an aetiological factor in VIN, with studies demonstrating that up to 90 per cent of VIN lesions are HPV positive, usually HPV 16.[33] Although HPV positivity is often considered to be more relevant in younger women with VIN, two studies have reported HPV positivity in older women with VIN 3, who have subsequently progressed to invasive vulvar carcinoma.[32,34] The role of oncogenic HPVs in vulvar oncogenesis is further discussed in Chapter 4.

An important step in tumour development is the switch to an angiogenic phenotype. Compared with VIN 1 and VIN 2, VIN 3 lesions demonstrate a dense network of microvessels under the dysplastic epithelium and an intense expression of angiogenic peptide (vascular endothelial growth factor).[35]

Karyotype analysis of VIN 3 lesions shows aneuploid DNA content in most, suggesting a malignant potential.[36] Nevertheless, spontaneous regression of some cases of VIN demonstrating aneuploidy has been reported.[6]

CLINICAL CONSIDERATIONS

Clinicians faced with the management of women presenting with high-grade VIN may be falsely reassured by the low progression rates quoted in the literature (see Table 5.1). Careful examination of the evidence reveals that the reported low progression rates reflect the outcome following treatment, and not the true natural history of the untreated lesion.

The only direct evidence to assist the clinician is the very small number of reported cases of untreated VIN 3.[6,16,25,37] Here the evidence is conflicting. Earlier studies emphasized the possibility of regression.[6,16] More recently, a series of untreated cases of VIN 3 reported progression to invasion in seven of eight cases, including three women in their 30s. The remaining case had the clinical features of bowenoid papulosis and regressed spontaneously.[25] This study points to the significant invasive potential of VIN. Ostor reported a case of progression in a woman who received treatment with bleomycin alone.[37]

A summary of most reported series (minimum of 25 cases) of VIN 3 since 1970 is shown in Table 5.1.[6,8–28]

In collating this material, every attempt has been made to exclude cases presented in serial publications. Potential deficiencies in the histology of some earlier studies needs to be taken into account. In some studies there has been inappropriate inclusion of cases with early invasion, for example, unsuspected invasion was noted in the excised specimen, or invasion has been recorded within 1 year of the diagnosis of VIN, raising the possibility of missed invasion at the outset. The surprisingly high incidence of invasion (18.8 per cent) noted in the subsequently excised specimens of 69 women in whom a pre-treatment biopsy had reported VIN 3 alone, suggests that all cases of invasion occurring within a defined period (e.g. 1 or 2 years) should be excluded whenever the question of progression of VIN to invasive cancer is being investigated.[38] Insufficient clinical data and inadequate follow-up limit the usefulness of many of the studies.

Taking these factors into account, a number of general observations can be made. Most studies report that between 2 per cent and 5 per cent (range 0–10 per cent) of treated cases develop invasive vulvar carcinoma during follow-up. Those who regard such a progression rate (actually an 'outcome') as low[7] should note that this is more than ten times the rate of invasive cervical cancer after treatment of cervical intraepithelial neoplasia (CIN) 3.

The transit time of VIN 3 to invasion is recorded in only six studies. (Cases of invasion occurring within 1 year of the diagnosis of VIN 3 have been excluded in order to avoid the criticism of possible 'missed invasion'.) These studies report invasion occurring within 10 years of the diagnosis and/or treatment of VIN 3 in 25 of 27 cases (93 per cent).[8,12,13,17,25,27] The transit time to invasion appears to be identical in both treated and untreated VIN 3.[25] This suggests that cases of invasive vulvar cancer that follow treatment for VIN may represent inadequate primary treatment of the VIN.[12] It has already been noted that the differentiated variant of VIN may demonstrate an aggressive course to invasion.[31] The transit time to invasion noted above provides a strong case against those who have argued that there is unlikely to be a direct causal relationship between VIN and invasive vulvar cancer, as a result of the 30-year difference in the mean ages of women presenting with VIN and invasive vulvar cancer.[5] A recent study suggests that the increasing incidence of VIN seen over the past 20–30 years may now be responsible for a changing pattern in squamous cell carcinoma of the vulva.[39] It also supports the evidence presented above for the transit time of VIN to invasion. In this study,[39] two cohorts of women with squamous cell carcinoma of the vulva, separated by at least two decades, were reviewed. In the earlier cohort, only one of 56 (1.8 per cent) patients was aged under 50, whereas in the recent cohort 12 of 57 (21 per cent) patients were aged under 50. Ten of the 13 (77 per cent) women aged under 50, compared with 13 of 100 (13 per cent) women aged over 50 had a warty or basaloid VIN associated with the invasive carcinoma. This evidence, although indirect, is a strong argument in favour of the concept of VIN as a precursor of vulvar cancer, especially in younger women.

A number of studies report an apparent excess of cases occurring at the anal margin or at the external urethral meatus.[10,11,25] It is notable that five of the cases in these studies report the development of anal carcinoma in young immunosuppressed women. The most likely explanation for carcinoma developing at these orifices is incomplete excision of VIN at these more difficult surgical sites.[6]

Early studies pointed to increasing age, immunosuppression and previous pelvic radiotherapy as factors influencing the likelihood of invasive vulvar cancer after treatment of VIN.[3,11,17,40] More recent reports have demonstrated that invasion can occur in healthy women of any age. Jones and Rowan[25] and Herod et al[27] report that almost half (9 of 20) of their reported cases of VIN that progressed to invasive carcinoma were in women aged under 50. This fits with the trend, already noted, of an increasing proportion of vulvar carcinomas occurring in younger women.[39] A history of previous pelvic radiotherapy does not appear to be a contributing factor influencing cases of progression reported today.[25,27]

Immunosuppressed patients have an increased risk of developing lower genital tract neoplasia.[41] Although recent studies of VIN report only a very small number of immunosuppressed cases, there is no doubt that this group is particularly at risk of developing vulvar or perianal cancer.[42]

The increased incidence of human immunodeficiency virus (HIV) noted in some series of VIN has to date not been associated with invasive vulvar cancer, but follow-up is limited.[40] As survival of HIV-infected women improves, one might anticipate an increasing frequency of invasive vulvar cancer in this group of women.

The behaviour of VIN 1 and VIN 2 lesions is poorly documented. VIN 2 is a relatively uncommon histological diagnosis and, like its counterpart in the cervix, should at present probably be regarded for management purposes as a biological high-grade abnormality.

VIN 1 is only a histological diagnosis and most reported cases probably represent viral or reactive changes. Herod and colleagues[27] noted that the percentage diagnosis of VIN 1 was markedly different between the two participating centres in his study (15 per cent versus 30 per cent), which suggests that this histological diagnosis is highly subjective. It has already been noted that there may be diagnostic difficulty in some women who have lichen sclerosus with squamous hyperplasia, in which basal epithelial atypia may be misinterpreted as a low-grade VIN, but in which the features do not fulfil the criteria for a differentiated VIN.

Two recent studies have, in a limited way, examined the outcome in VIN 1 and VIN 2. Barbero and colleagues[24] recorded progression of VIN 1 to invasion in a 69-year-old woman over a 2-year period, and noted a second case of VIN 1 progressing to VIN 3. They also noted 'regression' in 18 cases of VIN 1 and 2 managed medically. In a further study, there were no cases of progression of VIN 1 and 2.[27]

VIN lesions should be considered as part of a contiguous field of risk. First, about a half of all women with VIN have, at some time, preinvasive or invasive disease in the cervix or vagina. Second, the entire vulva and perianal skin remain at risk of further intraepithelial or invasive disease in any woman who has had VIN lesions. Although recurrences of VIN or the development of invasive cancer are more likely to occur at the margins of incompletely resected disease,[12] such events can occur anywhere in a field of previously normal vulvar skin.[43] It has been suggested that invasive disease is more likely to arise in unifocal than in multifocal lesions, but this has yet to be firmly established.[28] The significance of the colour of VIN lesions in relation to their invasive potential is not known.

REGRESSION

Both the International Society for the Study of Vulvar Disease and the International Society of Gynaecological Pathologists have stressed the importance of eliminating eponymous terminology and using only the term 'vulvar intraepithelial neoplasia'. Nevertheless, a clinical variant of VIN 2–3, referred to as bowenoid papulosis, remains firmly in the dermatological and some gynaecological literature. Its clinical importance is that, although the histology is characteristic of the usual high-grade VIN, it may spontaneously regress. The early description was of 'reversible vulvar atypia'.[44,45] The disease is usually seen in young (often teenage), sexually active women, many of whom are non-Caucasian, and it is frequently seen in relation to pregnancy. The lesion is characteristically multifocal, pigmented and papular. Most lesions are positive for HPV 16. An expectant approach to the management of women fitting the criteria noted above is initially appropriate. Although the literature predominantly portrays bowenoid papulosis as a benign condition, caution is necessary because there are reports of such cases progressing to invasion, including in very young women.[46,47]

Spontaneous regression of VIN 3 has been recorded in a number of early studies, and it is not clear whether these cases represented typical examples of bowenoid papulosis or were other clinical variants.[6,11,16] Examples of spontaneous regression are relatively uncommon in the recent literature, presumably because most cases have been treated.

PREVENTION

If the concept of VIN as a precursor of vulvar cancer is accepted, clinicians have a responsibility to become more actively involved in prevention strategies. One study demonstrated significant delays in more than half of all women presenting with VIN 3.[25] This was usually because the patient or her doctor mistakenly assumed that the woman's symptoms were caused by candidiasis or genital condyloma. Delays in presentation may be crucial if the mean transit time from VIN 3 to invasion is about 4 years.[25,27] Another study reported that about a quarter of women presenting with vulvar cancer had had symptoms in excess of 5 years.[48] Deficiencies in both the primary and secondary health care of women with vulvar symptoms expose them unnecessarily to the risk of vulvar cancer. Early recognition and effective treatment of VIN 3 are the responsibility of all clinicians.

What conclusions can be reached on the nature of VIN at the close of the twentieth century? First, it is an increasing and remarkably heterogeneous condition now seen principally in younger women, which has undergone considerable evolution over the past 30 years. Evidence points to the modern lesion being associated with both changing sexual mores (HPV) and social (cigarette smoking) practices. The understandable confusion of clinicians with regard to the biological nature of the lesion is a result of conflicting evidence in relation to regression and progression of the epithelial changes, and the modifying influences of treatment. Attitudes to the invasive potential of the lesion have moved almost through a complete circle during the second half of this century, from those who believed the lesion to be premalignant in nature, to those who seriously questioned its neoplastic potential, and now to an increasing number who accept that, in most cases, VIN is a genuine precursor of cancer. The histological association of VIN 3 with invasive carcinoma, the presence of aneuploidy in most cases of VIN 3, and the presence of oncogenic HPV types in VIN 3 and the corresponding cancer points strongly to VIN 3 as a precursor of invasive disease. Although earlier studies indicated the possibility of spontaneous regression of high-grade VIN, more recent studies have demonstrated that, irrespective of age, untreated lesions have a significant invasive potential. This may explain the observation of an increasing frequency of vulvar carcinoma in younger women. Approximately 2–5 per cent of treated cases will eventually develop invasive cancer. It has become clear that the transit time to invasion is less than 10 years in both treated and untreated lesions.

The elimination of the lesion by treatment removes the opportunity to study the natural history of the disorder and one must now rely on less direct techniques to study it. More detailed enquiry is required into those cases that spontaneously regress, those that progress to invasive cancer and the epidemiology of preinvasive and invasive vulvar cancer. A quarter of a century ago Woodruffe pointed to VIN as a 'Contemporary Challenge'.[5] This challenge is likely to continue well into the next millennium.

REFERENCES

1 Woodruff JD. Vulvar atypia and carcinoma in situ (Editorial Comment). *J Reprod Med* 1976; **17**: 155–63.
2 Knight R. Bowen's disease of the vulva. *Am J Obstet Gynecol* 1943; **46**: 514–24.
3 Gardiner SH, Stout FE, Arbogast JL, Huber CP. Intraepithelial carcinoma of the vulva. *Am J Obstet Gynecol* 1953; **65**: 539–49.
4 Abell MR, Gosling JRG. Intraepithelial and infiltrative

carcinoma of vulva: Bowen's type. *Cancer* 1961; **14**: 318–29.
5 Woodruff JD, Julian C, Puray T, Mermut S, Katayama P. The contemporary challenge of carcinoma in situ of the vulva. *Am J Obstet Gynecol* 1973; **115**: 677–86.
6 Friedrich EG, Wilkinson EJ, Fu YS. Carcinoma in situ of the vulva: a continuing challenge. *Am J Obstet Gynecol* 1980; **136**: 830–43.
7 Friedrich EG. Intraepithelial neoplasia of the vulva. In: Coppleson M (ed). *Gynecological oncology*. Edinburgh: Churchill Livingstone, 1981: 303–19.
8 Collins CG, Roman-Lopez JJ, Lee FYL. Intraepithelial carcinoma of the vulva. *Am J Obstet Gynecol* 1970; **108**: 1187–91.
9 Forney JP, Morrow CP, Townsend DE, DiSaia PJ. Management of carcinoma in situ of the vulva. *Am J Obstet Gynecol* 1977; **127**: 801–6.
10 Japaze H, Garcia-Bunuel R, Woodruff JD. Primary vulvar neoplasia: a review of in situ and invasive carcinoma, 1935–1972. *Obstet Gynecol* 1977; **49**: 404–11.
11 Buscema J, Woodruff JD, Parmley TH, Genadry R. Carcinoma in situ of the vulva. *Obstet Gynecol* 1980; **55**: 225–30.
12 Iversen T, Abeler V, Kolstad P. Squamous cell carcinoma in situ of the vulva. A clinical and histopathological study. *Gynecol Oncol* 1981; **11**: 224–9.
13 Benedet JL, Murphy KJ. Squamous carcinoma in situ of the vulva. *Gynecol Oncol* 1982; **14**: 213–19.
14 Caglar H, Tamer S, Hreshchyshyn MM. Vulvar intraepithelial neoplasia. *Obstet Gynecol* 1982; **60**: 346–9.
15 Di Paola GR, Rueda-Leverone NG, Belardi MG, Vighi S. Vulvar carcinoma in situ: A report of 28 cases. *Gynecol Oncol* 1982; **14**: 236–42.
16 Bernstein SG, Kovacs BR, Townsend DE, Morrow CP. Vulvar carcinoma in situ. *Obstet Gynecol* 1983; **61**: 304–7.
17 Crum CP, Liskow A, Petras P, Keng WC, Frick HC. Vulvar intraepithelial neoplasia (severe atypia and carcinoma in situ). *Cancer* 1984; **54**: 1429–34.
18 Leuchter RS, Townsend DE, Hacker NF, Pretorius RG, Lagasse LD, Wade ME. Treatment of vulvar carcinoma in situ with CO_2 laser. *Gynecol Oncol* 1984; **19**: 314–22.
19 Andreasson B, Bock JE. Intraepithelial neoplasia in the vulvar region. *Gynecol Oncol* 1985; **21**: 300–5.
20 Powell LC, Dinh TV, Rajaraman S et al. Carcinoma in situ of vulva: A clinicopathologic study of 50 cases. *J Reprod Med* 1986; **31**: 808–14.
21 Ragnarsson B, Raabe N, Willems J, Pettersson F.

Carcinoma in situ of the vulva: Long term prognosis. *Acta Oncol* 1987; **26**: 277–80.

22 Wilkinson EJ, Cook JC, Friedrich EG, Massey JK. Vulvar intraepithelial neoplasia: Association with cigarette smoking. *Colposcopy Gynecol Laser Surg* 1988; **4**: 153–9.

23 Husseinzadeh N, Newman NJ, Wesseler TA. Vulvar intraepithelial neoplasia: A clinicopathological study of carcinoma in situ of the vulva. *Gynecol Oncol* 1989; **33**: 157–63.

24 Barbero M, Micheletti L, Preti M et al. Vulvar intraepithelial neoplasia: a clinicopathologic study of 60 cases. *J Reprod Med* 1990; **35**: 1023–8.

25 Jones RW, Rowan DM. Vulvar intraepithelial neoplasia III: A clinical study of the outcome in 113 cases with relation to the later development of invasive vulvar carcinoma. *Obstet Gynecol* 1994; **84**: 741–5.

26 Hording U, Junge J, Poulsen H, Lundvall F. Vulvar intraepithelial neoplasia III: a viral disease of undetermined progressive potential. *Gynecol Oncol* 1995; **56**: 276–9.

27 Herod JJO, Shafl MI, Rollason TP, Jordan JA, Luesley DM. Vulvar intraepithelial neoplasia: long term follow up of treated and untreated women. *Br J Obstet Gynaecol* 1996; **103**: 446–52.

28 Van Beurden M, Van Der Vange N, Ten Kate FJW, de Craen AJ, Schilthuis MS, Lammes FB. Restricted surgical management of vulvar intraepithelial neoplasia 3: Focus on exclusion of invasion and on relief of symptoms. *Int J Gynecol Cancer* 1998; **8**: 73–7.

29 Leibowitch M, Neill S, Pelisse M, Moyal-Baracco M. The epithelial changes associated with squamous cell carcinoma of the vulva: a review of the clinical, histological and viral findings in 78 women. *Br J Obstet Gynaecol* 1990; **97**: 1135–9.

30 Herod JJO, Shafl MI, Rollason TP, Jordan JA, Luesley DM. Vulvar intraepithelial neoplasia with superficially invasive carcinoma of the vulva. *Br J Obstet Gynaecol* 1996; **103**: 453–6.

31 Kaufman RH. Intraepithelial neoplasia of the vulva. *Gynecol Oncol* 1995; **56**: 8–21.

32 Park JS, Jones RW, McLean MR, et al. Possible etiologic heterogeneity of vulvar intraepithelial neoplasia: a correlation of pathologic characteristics with human papillomavirus detection by in situ hybridization and polymerase chain reaction. *Cancer* 1991; **67**: 1599–1607.

33 Junge J, Poulsen H, Horn T, Hording U, Lundvall F. Human papillomavirus (HPV) in vulvar dysplasia and carcinoma in situ. *APMIS* 1995; **103**: 501–10.

34 Van Sickle M, Kaufman RH, Adam E, Adler-Storthz K. Detection of human papillomavirus DNA before and after development of invasive vulvar cancer. *Obstet Gynecol* 1990; **76**: 540–2.

35 Bancher-Todesca D, Obermair A, Bilgi S et al. Angiogenesis in vulvar intraepithelial neoplasia. *Gynecol Oncol* 1997; **64**: 496–500.

36 Fu Y, Reagan JW, Townsend DE, Kaufman RH, Richart RM, Wentz WB. Nuclear DNA study of vulvar intraepithelial and invasive squamous neoplasms. *Obstet Gynecol* 1981; **57**: 643–52.

37 Ostor AG, Sfameni SF, Kneale BL, Fortune DW. Progression of squamous carcinoma in situ of the vulva to invasive carcinoma after systemic bleomycin therapy. *Aust NZ J Obstet Gynaecol* 1984; **24**: 55–8.

38 Chafe W, Richards A, Morgan L, Wilkinson E. Unrecognized invasive carcinoma in vulvar intraepithelial neoplasia VIN. *Gynecol Oncol* 1988; **31**: 154–62.

39 Jones RW, Baranyai J, Stables S. Trends in squamous cell carcinoma of the vulva: The influence of vulvar intrae-pithelial neoplasia. *Obstet Gynecol* 1997; **90**: 448–52.

40 Jones RW, McLean MR. Carcinoma in situ of the vulva: A review of 31 treated and five untreated cases. *Obstet Gynecol* 1986; **68**: 499–503.

41 Penn I. Cancers of the anogenital region in renal transplant recipients. Analysis of 65 cases. *Cancer* 1986; **58**: 611–16.

42 Korn AP, Abercrombie PD, Foster A. Vulvar intraepithelial neoplasia in women infected with human immuno-deficiency virus-1. *Gynecol Oncol* 1996; **61**: 384–6.

43 Friedman M, White RG, Moar JJ, Browde S. Progression of vulval carcinoma in situ. A case report. *S Afr Med J* 1983; **64**: 748–9.

44 Friedrich EG. Reversible vulvar atypia. A case report. *Obstet Gynecol* 1972; **39**: 173–81.

45 Skinner MS, Sternberg YM, Ichinose H, Collins J. Spontaneous regression of Bowenoid atypia of the vulva. *Obstet Gynecol* 1973; **42**: 40–6.

46 Planner RS, Andersen HE, Hobbs JB, Williams RA, Fogarty LF, Hudson PJ. Multifocal invasive carcinoma of the vulva in a 25–year-old woman with Bowenoid papulosis. *Aust NZ J Obstet Gynaecol* 1987; **27**: 291–5.

47 Bergeron C, Naghashfar Z, Canaan C, Shah K, Fu Y, Ferenczy A. Human papillomavirus type 16 in intraepithelial neoplasia (Bowenoid papulosis) and coexistent invasive carcinoma of the vulva. *Int J Gynecol Pathol* 1987; **6**: 1–11.

48 Jones RW, Joura EA. Analysis of the clinical events at presentation in 102 women with carcinoma of the vulva. Evidence of diagnostic delay. *J Reprod Med* 1999 (in press).

6

Are 'non-neoplastic' disorders of the vulva premalignant?

AB MACLEAN

Early descriptions of the association between leukoplakia and malignancy come from members of the staff of the Middlesex Hospital, London. In 1869, John Hulke described a lesion of the tongue – leukoplakia – that was associated with development of cancer, and soon afterwards Sir Henry Morris drew attention to similar appearances that preceded vulvar cancer. Sir Comyns Berkeley and Victor Bonney, both on the consulting staff of the Middlesex Hospital, developed the concept that leukoplakic vulvitis bore a relation to carcinoma 'closer than that of any other pathological lesion with the exception of the entirely modern X-ray dermatitis'. This statement was based on their experience of 58 cases of vulval cancer seen over the previous 10 years; leukoplakic vulvitis had been present in every case.[1]

Their description[1] of leukoplakic vulvitis divided the lesion into the four following stages:

1 reddened, swollen excoriation with a dry vulvar surface;

2 decrease in labial size to become mere ridges, the red becoming pale and the skin semi-opaque;

3 fissuring, cracking, ulceration and bleeding, with progression to cancer;

4 if cancer did not occur, the disease became quiescent, with the surface smooth and shiny white, and the labia minora and clitoris disappearing as a result of contraction of the subepithelial tissues.

The description of pathology of these stages included, for the second stage, that a hyaline zone appeared beneath the epidermis, with disappearance of elastic fibres, and an underlying collection of lymphocytes and plasma cells. Later there was epidermal thinning, altered keratinization and disappearance of the interpapillary downgrowths.

These clinical and histological appearances are consistent with lichen sclerosus. The problems arose in trying to define 'leukoplakic vulvitis'.

TERMINOLOGY

The terminology of vulvar lesions has been confused by a variety of descriptions, in different languages, that often had greater meaning for dermatologists than for gynaecologists or pathologists. 'Ichthyosis' was described by Weir in 1875, 'leukoplakia' by Schwimmer in 1877, 'kraurosis' by Breisky in 1885, and 'lichen plan sclereux' by Hallopeau in 1889.[2,3] These terms were subsequently used by different authors to make associations or define differences, e.g. Berkeley and Bonney[1] described the perceived differences between leukoplakic vulvitis and kraurosis. Much of the confusion was created by most white lesions being called 'leukoplakic'. Bowen's disease of the vulva (first described by Bowen in 1912 but now designated 'vulvar intraepithelial neoplasia') was often associated with or could be mistaken for leukoplakia.[4,5]

Professor Jeffcoate attempted to rescue the situation, certainly for British gynaecologists and trainees by introducing the term 'chronic epithelial dystrophy'[6] and promoting its use within his widely studied textbook.[7]

> There is as yet no evidence to justify the view that leucoplakia, leucoplakic vulvitis, kraurosis (primary atrophy), and lichen sclerosus et atrophicus are separate disease entities. Judged by either macroscopical or microscopical criteria, these represent no more than a variety of skin reactions to adverse factors which, although obscure, are more likely to be 'general' than 'local'. The type of reaction is dependent on the environment of the vulva and not on the underlying cause. It is therefore suggested that all these names be abandoned, since they hinder rather than help the elucidation of their causes. In their place, and pending further knowledge, the non-committal inclusive term of chronic epithelial dystrophy is proposed as one convenient for clinical practice.[6]

Not all British gynaecologists greeted this term with enthusiasm. Professor Charles Douglas of the Royal Free Hospital, London, co-author of the book *Diseases of the vulva*,[3] described lichen sclerosus under 'progressive sclerotic and atrophic processes of the vulva', and did not use 'dystrophy' in their book.

At the Second International Congress of the International Society for the Study of Vulvar Disease, the Committee on Terminology recommended that the terms lichen sclerosus et atrophicus, leukoplakia, neurodermatitis, leukeratosis, Bowen's disease, erythroplasia of Queyrat, carcinoma simplex, leukoplakic vulvitis, hyperplastic vulvitis and kraurosis vulvae should be deleted from the vocabulary of vulval diseases, and should be replaced by:

- vulvar dystrophies
- vulvar atypia
- Paget's disease of the vulva
- squamous cell carcinoma in situ.

The dystrophies were classified according to the following microscopic features:

- Hyperplastic dystrophy:
  – without atypia
  – with atypia
- Lichen sclerosus
- Mixed dystrophy (lichen sclerosus with foci of epithelial hyperplasia):
  – without atypia
  – with atypia.

Atypia was further categorized as mild, moderate or severe, depending on the extent of the change, and it might exist as (A) without dystrophy or (B) with dystrophy.[8]

Although this description of a new nomenclature suggested that the term 'dystrophy' would characterize the many disorders of epithelial growth and nutrition, it does little to enhance our understanding. Dystrophy means a disorder of structure or function of an organ or tissue as a result of perverted nutrition and there are good reasons for abandoning it.[9,10] Therefore the International Society for the Study of Vulvar Disease (ISSVD) and the International Society of Gynaecological Pathologists introduced the terms 'non-neoplastic epithelial disorders of skin and mucosa' to include lichen sclerosus, squamous cell hyperplasia (formerly hyperplastic dystrophy) and other dermatoses, and 'vulvar intraepithelial neoplasia' (VIN) to include atypias and carcinomas in situ. If mixed epithelial disorders were identified, it was recommended that both conditions should be reported, e.g. lichen sclerosus with squamous cell hyperplasia (formerly mixed dystrophy), lichen sclerosus with VIN (formerly mixed dystrophy with atypia) and hyperplastic dystrophy with atypia became VIN.[11]

The term 'non-neoplastic epithelial disorder' is not without its problems, partly because it may coexist with neoplastic lesions, e.g. VIN or squamous cell carcinoma.

Furthermore, the Terminology Committee of the ISSVD has modified it, as of November 1997, into

Table 6.1 *Revised ISSVD classification of vulvar disease*[a]

1. **Infections**
   Parasitic, e.g. pediculosis, scabies
   Protozoal, e.g. amoebiasis
   Viral, e.g. herpes virus infection, condyloma
       acuminatum
   Bacterial
   Fungal, e.g. candidiasis, dermatophytosis
   Others

2. **Inflammatory skin disease**
   Spongiotic disorders
       Contact dermatitis
           Irritant
           Allergic
       Atopic dermatitis (acute and chronic)
       (Seborrhoeic dermatitis)
       Others
   Psoriasiform disorders
       Psoriasis
       Lichenification (lichen simplex)[b]
       Atopic dermatitis (chronic)
       Seborrhoeic dermatitis
       Others
   Lichenoid disorders
       Lichen sclerosus
       Lichen planus
       Fixed drug eruption
       Plasma cell vulvitis
       Lichenoid reaction, not otherwise specified (focal or
           diffuse)[c]
       Lupus erythematosus
       Others
   Vesicobullous disorders
       Pemphigoid
       Pemphigus
       Erythema multiforme
       Stevens–Johnson syndrome
       Others
   Granulomatous disorders
       Non-infectious:
           Sarcoidosis
           Crohn's disease
           (Hidradenitis suppurativa)
           Others
       Infectious:
           Tuberculosis
           Granuloma inguinale
           Others
   Vasculitis or related inflammatory disorders
       Leukocytoclastic
       Urticaria
       Aphthous ulcer

   Lymphoedema
   Behçet's disease
   Pyoderma gangrenosa
   (Fixed drug eruption)
   (Erythema multiforme)
   (Stevens–Johnson syndrome)
   Others

3. **Skin appendage disorders**
   Hidradenitis suppurativa
   Fox–Fordyce disease
   Disorders of sweating
   Others

4. **Hormonal disorders**
   Oestrogen
       Excess:
           Precocious puberty
           Others
       Deficiency:
           Physiological
           Lactation
           Postmenopausal
           Others
       Iatrogenic
   Androgen
       Excess:
           Physiological
           Iatrogenic

5. **Ulcers and erosions**
   (diseases that ulcerate and/or erode are listed
   according to histological findings)
   Trauma
       Obstetric
       Surgical
       Sexual
       Accidental
       Others (include fissures of the fossa navicularis)

6. **Disorders of pigmentation**
   Hyperpigmentation
       Melanin
           Lentigo
           Melanosis vulvae
           (Postinflammatory hyperpigmentation)
       Haemosiderin
           (Postinflammatory hyperpigmentation)
       Vitiligo
       Others
   Hypopigmentation
       Vitiligo
       Postinflammatory hypopigmentation
       Others

Note to Table 6.1

This revised classification replaces the ISSVD classification of non-neoplastic epithelial disorders. It is not intended to be a comprehensive listing of all known dermatological or pathological disorders that may involve the vulva or vagina, but to include the more common disorders that involve the vulva.

[a] Report of the Terminology Committee on Non-Neoplastic and Inflammatory Disorders of the Vulva.

[b] The term 'lichenification' encompasses the former ISSVD terms of 'squamous cell hyperplasia' and 'hyperplastic dystrophy'. Lichenification encompasses the term 'lichen simplex' (lichen simplex chronicus).

[c] What has been interpreted as vulvar vestibular inflammation may represent, in some cases, findings considered as within normal.

Initially submitted by the ISSVD Terminology Committee 17 September 1997. Revisions as of 14 November 1997 are as directed at the ISSVD World Congress Meeting, September 1997.

ISSVD Spring 1998 Newsletter

'non-neoplastic and inflammatory disorders of the vulva' and under 'inflammatory skin condition' is grouped 'lichenoid disorders':

- lichen sclerosus
- lichen planus
- fixed drug eruption
- plasma cell vulvitis
- lichenoid reaction, not otherwise specified
- lupus erythematosus
- others

and under 'psoriasiform disorder':

- Lichenification (lichen simplex) with a footnote: the term lichenification encompasses the former ISSVD terms of 'squamous cell hyperplasia' and 'hyperplastic dystrophy'. Lichenification encompasses the term 'lichen simplex' (lichen simplex chronicus) (Table 6.1).

Although the terminology may be both modern and comprehensive, it does not help our understanding of the link with vulvar cancer.

PATHOLOGY

Using this most up-to-date classification of vulvar lesions, the following are the lesions that are of principal interest in having a pre-neoplastic role.

LICHEN SCLEROSUS

The prevalence of this pathology in women is estimated to be between 1 in 300 and 1 in 1000.[12,13] It accounts for up to a quarter of women seen in our vulvar clinic.[14] It is usually bilateral and symmetrical in its involvement of the anogenital area, but in 20 per cent extragenital lesions will occur. The skin is parchment-like, thin, wrinkled and dry. Histology shows flattened or absent rete ridges, a thin prickle-cell layer and basal layer liquefaction. The upper dermis becomes oedematous and later shows hyalinization with an underlying chronic inflammatory cell infiltrate.

LICHEN PLANUS

This lesion is found in mucosal surfaces, e.g. within the mouth, and in the vestibule and vagina where it may be 'erosive', later showing a white, spongy, slightly elevated surface with a trabecular or web-like appearance. The epidermis may be involved as a red or violet, flat-topped papule or as an area of 'hypertrophic' lichen planus. It is claimed that malignant change in the skin may occur with hypertrophic lichen planus, and in the mouth with erosive lichen planus (see later).[13,15] Histology shows marked hyperkeratosis and increase or hypertrophy of the granular and prickle-cell layers. The rete ridges become pointed in outline to give a saw-tooth appearance. There is a dense lymphocytic infiltrate in the upper dermis up to the epidermis, and this may invade the basal layers causing liquefaction and partial destruction to make the dermis–epidermis junction indistinct. Mucosal lesions are similar but, as there is no granular layer, there is little hypertrophy, and erosion of the epithelium above the basal layer occurs.

Lichenification

The skin is thickened and white with accentuated markings, cracks and fissures, and ill-defined margins. Histology consists of hyperkeratosis (thickening of the stratum corneum, usually with hypertrophy of the granular layer) or parakeratosis (abnormal keratinization, where cells of the stratum corneum retain their nuclei and are swollen or more loosely attached to each other; the granular layer may be absent), acanthosis, and irregular elongation and widening of the rete ridges. There is no epidermal cell atypia. It may be seen with lichen sclerosus and lichen planus, but also with psoriasis and condyloma acuminatum. If the superficial dermis has an infiltrate of mainly lymphocytes, but some plasma cells and macrophages, the term 'lichen simplex chronicus' is used.[16,17]

Further description of the histology is given in Chapter 2. Fox and Buckley[18] make the distinction that premalignant lesions are not neoplastic, but in a proportion there will be progression or change to a neoplastic lesion, whereas preinvasive lesions are neoplastic but intraepithelial, and a proportion will invade later.

WHAT IS THE EVIDENCE THAT VULVAR CANCER MIGHT BE PRECEDED BY PREMALIGNANT LESIONS?

One of the difficulties in disentangling the information in the literature is to determine whether patients presented with cancer and an associated lesion, e.g. lichen sclerosus, concurrently, or whether there were serial observations of lichen sclerosus followed by the development of cancer. In addition, some authors are positive in supporting the association, advocating treatment by vulvectomy for all cases of leukoplakia; others do not support the association and are very critical of the value of prophylactic vulvectomy.

Taussig[19] supported Berkeley and Bonney about the importance of leukoplakic vulvitis but disagreed about kraurosis. The British pair argued that kraurosis affected only the introitus and, was associated with contracture and atrophy, and that cancer never supervened. Taussig believed that kraurosis complicated 10–20 per cent of cases of leukoplakia, and attributed as many vulvar cancers to pre-existing kraurosis as to leukoplakia. He described leukoplakic vulvitis in 72 of 104 cases of vulvar cancer, and pre-existing syphilis in nine of 11 vestibular cancers.[19] Bibby,[20] in a review of 71 cases of vulval cancer seen in Leeds, described preceding leukoplakia in 60 per cent.

Langley et al[21] followed 122 patients who had been treated by simple or partial vulvectomy for leukoplakia: 72 had a recurrence of leukoplakia or pruritus, but only one developed cancer, 12 years after her vulvectomy. McAdams and Kistner[22] suggested that 10 per cent of women with leukoplakia would progress to carcinoma.

Woodruff and Baens[23] reviewed 80 cases of leukoplakia: 44 patients were traced and three had developed carcinoma of the vulva, with fatal outcome in two. Leukoplakia was diagnosed when microscopy showed hyperkeratosis plus one or more out of the following: epithelial atrophy, epithelial hypertrophy, collagen zone in the subepithelial dermis, enlargement and deepening of the rete pegs, and evidence of epithelial hyperactivity. They suggested that white atrophic areas resulting from lichen sclerosus rarely became malignant, but that 25 per cent of hypertrophic lesions would eventually become malignant. They noted, however, that atrophic and hypertrophic changes could coexist on the same vulva; carcinoma could then develop, but adjacent to an area of hypertrophy. They recommended that if the term 'leukoplakia' were to be used by the pathologist, it should be modified so as to inform the clinician of the anaplastic activity and potential.

In a subsequent paper from the Johns Hopkins group,[24] there was a discussion from Dr Arthur Hunt who refers to a series of 232 women with lichen sclerosus seen by Perry and Homme at the Mayo Clinic: three women had concurrent squamous cell carcinoma; 184 responded to subsequent questionnaires and none had developed carcinoma. Jeffcoate and Woodcock[6] include a description of 103 women seen with chronic epithelial dystrophy. Histological examination of biopsies in 65 cases found early invasion in one and intraepidermal cancer in four. The remaining 98 women were followed for up to 25 years. Four developed invasive cancer 2 years, 7 months, 10 years, and 4½ years after originally being seen.

Wallace[12] reported that 12 women developed carcinoma out of 290 (4 per cent) with lichen sclerosus who were followed over a 12½-year period.

Hart and colleagues[25] studied 107 patients with lichen sclerosus to determine malignant potential. Five patients had invasive squamous cell carcinoma diagnosed when the initial diagnosis of lichen sclerosus was made, and a sixth had an intraepithelial carcinoma on the clitoris. Follow-up information was obtained for 92, for intervals from 1 month to 22 years; 50 per cent were followed for a minimum of 10 years. One patient had developed multifocal invasive squamous carcinoma 12 years after excision biopsies of bilateral lichen sclerosus. Areas of squamous hyperplasia and dysplasia were present in the original biopsies. This paper includes a table with patient details from 10 series; 16 patients of 465 (3 per cent) developed carcinoma with lichen sclerosus.

Friedrich[13] collected 17 articles describing 1356 patients with lichen sclerosus in whom the combined incidence of carcinoma was only 4.1 per cent. If only the reports published within the previous 17 years (and with better defined terminology) were included, the incidence of concurrent and subsequent carcinoma dropped to only 2.6 per cent. Rodke reported on 50 women who were seen in Friedrich's unit at the University of Florida between 1980 and 1986.[26] Three patients were seen with squamous cell carcinoma, developing 16 years, 21 years and 11 years after first symptoms or management of lichen sclerosus. The cancers were diagnosed at first visit to the Vulvovaginal Referral Unit, or 12 and 24 months, respectively, after first being seen. The areas of invasion occurred adjacent to mixed dystrophy in two and to hyperplastic dystrophy with atypia in the third. Meffert and colleagues[27] collected 5207 published cases of lichen sclerosus and found an incidence of vulvar cancer of 5.4 per cent.

Meyrick-Thomas and colleagues[28] published details on 350 women with lichen sclerosus; again 5 per cent had squamous cell carcinoma. In a subsequent review, on follow-up of 357 women who originally had anogenital lichen sclerosus, 19 had squamous cell carcinoma. Three patients had no symptoms at presentation (suggesting that scratch damage is not causative), two had received radiotherapy 23 and 31 years previously, and three had earlier undergone vulvectomy to control the symptoms of lichen sclerosus. It is difficult to determine how many of these 19 presented with lichen sclerosus and with concurrent cancer, and how many later developed carcinoma.[29]

There is also a series of reports of single cases in which lichen sclerosus appears to have preceded the development of carcinoma. Eng and Jacobs[30] reported on a 91-year-old woman with a 10-year history of pruritus, hypopigmented and white perianal and vulvar skin, and a carcinoma 2 cm in diameter.

August and Milward[31] reported on 12 patients with lichen sclerosus who were treated by cryotherapy. One patient who had had a radium implant 15 years earlier continued to have pruritus and leukoplakia, and eventually squamous carcinoma developed.

Di Paola and colleagues[32] reported on a 64-year-old woman whose first biopsy showed lichen sclerosus; the second, 6 years after the first, showed mild atypia. Two years later a squamous cell carcinoma of one labium majus was found with adjacent carcinoma in situ, but with lichen sclerosus elsewhere; radical vulvectomy was performed, but 6 months later a new squamous carcinoma was found near the introitus.

Cario and colleagues[33] reported on an 18 year old who presented with a 1-month history of a painful lump. Examination found lichen sclerosus and a raised ulcerated lesion, and excision biopsy confirmed squamous carcinoma arising in an area of lichen sclerosus plus hyperplasia with focal atypia.

Lindeque and colleagues[34] reported on a 26-year-old woman with several years of pruritus vulvae, extensive dystrophy, and random biopsies that showed hyperplastic dystrophy with severe atypia and areas of squamous carcinoma.

Roman and colleagues[35] reported on a 22-year-old woman with a 3-month history of pruritus, and a painful lesion; 2 months later multiple biopsies found squamous carcinoma and lichen sclerosus.

LICHEN SCLEROSUS AND CHANGES IN THE EPITHELIUM ADJACENT TO CANCER

It would seem likely that there is an association between the development of cancer and the pathology found in the epidermis immediately adjacent to the area of invasion. This seems to be true for the cervix, where the various terms that have been used include 'carcinomatous transformation', 'carcinomatous layer', 'incipient carcinoma' and 'carcinoma in situ'.[36]

The British Gynaecological Cancer Society established a small group to investigate the association between cancer and pre-cancers of the vulva – the Vulval Invasion and Premalignancy (VIP) Project. Part of this study involved a retrospective review of 171 cases of vulvar squamous cell carcinoma collected in Glasgow, Manchester, Birmingham and Leeds, where the reporting of vulvar histology was performed or reviewed by pathologists with a specific interest. Information was available on the epithelium/epidermis adjacent to 142 cancers: VIN was adjacent to 54 (38 per cent), VIN plus lichen sclerosus in 22 (16 per cent) and lichen sclerosus, squamous hyperplasia or both in 61 (43 per cent).[37] When invasion occurred with lichen sclerosus it was sometimes immediately adjacent (Fig. 6.1), but in others there was lichen sclerosus – hyperplasia – cancer in sequence (Fig. 6.2), and in others lichen sclerosus – intraepithelial neoplasia – cancer. Some of the difficulties in this study were the strict definition of squamous hyperplasia, and when hyperplasia was typical without atypia, i.e. intraepithelial neoplasia. There are similar studies, but comparisons are frustrated by the various classifications and terminology (Table 6.2). It appears that many cancers arise in a background of lichen sclerosus, but with intervening changes – hence the concepts of mixed dystrophy,

Table 6.2 *Changes in the epidermis adjacent to vulvar cancer*

Reference	Year	CA	VIN (%)	AHD (%)	THD (%)	MD (%)	LS (%)	N (%)
Buscema [38]	1980	98	33	19	32	8	4	2
Choo [39]	1982	2	22				33	
Zaino [40]	1982	60	32	53	23	7	25	–
Podratz [41]	1983	–			Dystrophic changes in 58%			
Hacker [42]	1984	–	67	37		12	6	–
Hewitt [43]	1988	–	<10				Majority <3	
Borgno [44]	1988	111	24 (21.6)[a]	Dystrophy 64 (57.6)[a]; HD 53[a]		7	4	
Leibowitch [45]	1990	78	31				61	8
Gomez-Rueda [46]	1994	64	19 (30)[a]		NNED 38 (59)[a]		6 (9)[a]	7 (11)[a]
MacLean [37]	1995	171 (142)	38		NNED 43; NNED + VIN 15			
Walkden [47]	1997	28	–				8 (28.5)[a]	
Scurry [48]	1997	132	32 (24)[a]		SCH 92 (70)[a]; DVIN 52 (39)[a]		63 (48)[a]	9 (7)[a]

[a] In these studies the number of cases are given, with the percentage in brackets.

CA, no. of cases of cancer; VIN, vulvar intraepithelial neoplasia; AHD, atypical hypertrophic dystrophy; THD, typical hypertrophic dystrophy; MD, mixed dystrophy; LS, lichen sclerosus; N, normal; HD, hypertrophic dystrophy; NNED, non-neoplastic epithelial disorder; SCH, squamous cell hyperplasia; DVIN, differentiated VIN.

dystrophy with atypia, or atypical hyperplastic hyperplasia to neoplasia.[26,38,40] The apparent differences between the studies by Hacker and colleagues[42] and Hewitt,[43] where the former found VIN most frequently and the latter found lichen sclerosus, may reflect trans-Atlantic differences in pathology interpretations, and perhaps referral patterns. However, more recent publications[45,46] have divided VIN 3 into VIN 3-undifferentiated (i.e. full-thickness VIN or carcinoma in situ) and VIN 3-differentiated (cellular atypia confined to the lower part of the epidermis with almost normal maturation) types. In Leibowitch's series, 48 of 78 had adjacent lichen sclerosus; 28 had atypia (lichen sclerosus plus VIN 3-differentiated), 12 had upper dermal hyalinization and hyperplasia (lichen sclerosus plus squamous hyperplasia), and eight had an upper dermal band of hyalinization with epidermal changes (lichen sclerosus).[45]

Walkden and colleagues[47] reviewed 28 cases of vulvar squamous cell carcinoma (SCC) seen in a district general hospital. In eight of the cases there was evidence of lichen sclerosus. In one case, the lichen sclerosus was only in the area of the cancer, in two cases in the area of invasion and the surrounding skin, and in three in the adjacent skin only. In two cases there was no evidence of lichen sclerosus in the cancer or in the surrounding skin, but it was found elsewhere on the vulvectomy specimens. Four women had had biopsies taken some time before the development of cancer and had histological evidence of lichen sclerosus, although this was not evident in their vulvectomy specimens.

ARE THERE OTHER CHANGES ADJACENT TO THE NEOPLASTIC CHANGE?

In the past there have been debates over the use of 'et atrophicus' in association with lichen sclerosus. It was assumed that the epidermal appearances were of reduced cell activity, but Clark and colleagues[49] found ^{32}P uptake 1.9–2.4 times higher than the normal mean, and Woodruff and colleagues[24] found increased radio-labelling of epidermal cells of lichen sclerosus, after the injection of tritiated thymidine.

What is the role of the hyperplastic changes associated with lichen sclerosus and cancer? Scurry and colleagues[48] examined sections of 132 cases of squamous cell carcinoma, and found lichen sclerosus in the adjacent skin in 63 of these (48 per cent). In 61 of these 63 there was significant epidermal thickening, in 21 there were changes consistent with lichen simplex chronicus, and among the other 40 the principal changes were of differentiated VIN (basal atypia). They also analysed sections from 86 cases of lichen sclerosus without carcinoma: 73 had associated epidermal thickening and, in 69, these were consistent with lichen simplex chronicus; only two showed differentiated VIN. Although there seemed to be a difference in the changes seen with or without cancer (e.g. the epidermal thickening was greater – 0.71 mm – in patients with cancer compared with those without – 0.41 mm), the authors were unhappy about using histology to distinguish between lichen simplex chronicus and squamous cell hyperplasia.

The term 'squamous cell hyperplasia' has been recommended for use by the ISSVD in two instances, either alone when it refers to a hyperplastic process of unknown aetiology or when associated with lichen sclerosus (previously termed 'mixed dystrophy').

'Squamous cell hyperplasia' when used alone reflects diagnostic failure. In our view, it is likely that many of the cases termed 'squamous cell hyperplasia' are unrecognized hyperplastic lichen sclerosus in a fibrotic phase, without the diagnostic feature of hyaline material in the dermis.[48]

Karram and colleagues[50] used Southern blot hybridization to probe for the presence of human papillomavirus (HPV) types 6, 11, 16 and 18 in 16 women with 'vulvar dystrophy'. Five of the hyperplastic dystrophies were classified as atypical and HPV was found in three; in none of the dystrophies without atypia was HPV DNA detected. Leibowitch and colleagues[45] were unable to find HPV 16 DNA among specimens from invasive carcinoma associated with lichen sclerosus. It seems unlikely that HPV acts as a co-factor in the association between lichen sclerosus and carcinoma.

Kim and colleagues[51] from the departments of pathology at the Johns Hopkins University and the University of Florida, divided a series of squamous cell cancers of the vulva into HPV positive or negative, based on Southern blotting and the polymerase chain reaction (PCR). They observed that HPV-negative cancers were usually associated with squamous hyperplasia. Among the 11 HPV-negative tumours, there were four in which *p53* gene mutations were identified. Adjacent epidermis was microdissected and DNA separately isolated from normal squamous epithelium, invasive squamous carcinoma and associated squamous hyperplasia. In each specimen, the *p53* mutation was found in the invasive tumour tissue but was absent in the normal and hyperplastic epithelium. By using a PCR-based assay for X-chromosome inactivation, they were able to demonstrate monoclonality of the informative invasive tumours, although the adjacent hyperplastic epidermis was polyclonal.

Our group has studied the expression of p53 in lichen sclerosus, using immunohistochemistry.[52] We found that 55 per cent of vulvar cancers have p53 protein overexpression, suggestive of potential mutation. These findings are consistent with those of others. Kohlberger and colleagues[53] found that keratinizing squamous cell carcinoma in older women overexpressed p53 in approximately 50 per cent. Kagie and colleagues[54] also found that about half of vulvar

cancers (53 per cent) overexpressed p53. They showed overexpression of p53 in 27 per cent of synchronous lichen sclerosus, but it is not clear whether p53 was expressed by the lichen sclerosus immediately adjacent to the cancer. We found that cancers arising within a field of lichen sclerosus and the lichen sclerosus immediately adjacent to the cancer all showed p53 overexpression (Fig. 6.3). We found that only 23 per cent of cases of lichen sclerosus (without cancer) expressed this protein.

Tan and colleagues[55] studied p53 expression in vulvar lichen sclerosus, non-genital lichen sclerosus (which appears to have no malignant potential) and normal vulvar skin. There was a significant increase in p53 immunoreactivity in vulvar lichen sclerosus [32.13 (15.11 for mean [SD] epidermal cells per 100 basal cells] compared with vulvar skin [7.52 (5.04)]. It is difficult to interpret these findings of p53 overexpression for vulval lichen sclerosus, because most do not progress to carcinoma. It suggests that p53 is not the only factor in any neoplastic association.

Soini and colleagues[56] confirmed that p53 was not found in normal skin, but demonstrated its presence in benign pathology, e.g. psoriasis and lichen planus. Thus the presence of p53 must not be assumed to represent mutation, or neoplastic potential; it may be the result of accumulation of wild-type protein.

WHAT IS THE ASSOCIATION WITH LICHEN PLANUS?

Occasionally, long-standing vulvar lesions of lichen sclerosus become increasingly symptomatic, and vaginal or vestibular erosions are found. This has occurred among three of 243 patients with lichen sclerosus whom we have been following,[14] where subsequent biopsy confirmed the presence of lichen planus. Hallopeau's description of lichen sclerosus in 1889 was as a variant of lichen planus, and the histological appearances may be similar or overlap.[2]

Therefore, it is not surprising that lichen planus has been found in association with vulvar cancer. In one of the studies that describe epithelial changes adjacent to vulvar cancer, Zaki and colleagues[57] reported on 61 cases of squamous cell carcinoma: lichen sclerosus was associated with 24, VIN 3 with 20 and lichen planus with three. Dwyer and colleagues[58] describe a 58-year-old woman with a 3-year history of pruritus and typical features of lichen planus; she presented with a plaque on the clitoral hood and the excised specimen showed both cancer and lichen planus. Carcinoma in situ (now called VIN 3) is reported developing in a vulvar erosive lichen planus lesion.[15]

As mentioned earlier, it was believed that carcinoma can develop in hypertrophic (cutaneous) and erosive (e.g. oral) lesions.[59] The risks of skin cancer associated with lichen planus may be exaggerated; Sigurgeirsson[60] followed 2071 patients with lichen planus for an average of 10 years, to document the appearance of six skin lesions (four in hypertrophic areas) and eight oral cancers. Fulling[61] and Harland and colleagues[62] suggest that the development of oral cancer complicating lichen planus is likely to be 1 per cent rather than 10 per cent. Mention is made of penile cancers developing within lichen planus[63] but little has been published on malignant changes in vulvar lichen planus.

The converse has been reported i.e. that lichen planus can develop coincidentally or after a diagnosis of cancer; five cases have been described by Helm and colleagues[64] but did not involve the vulva.

CONCLUSION

This chapter has described historical associations with vulvar cancer, and the confusion surrounding both old and new terminology. Even now the histopathological differences, e.g. those between squamous cell hyperplasia and lichen simplex, or the concept of differentiated VIN associated with lichen sclerosus (the previous mixed dystrophy with atypia), seems to evolve.

There is no doubt that vulvar cancer frequently occurs on a background of lichen sclerosus, and we all have small numbers of patients with well-documented

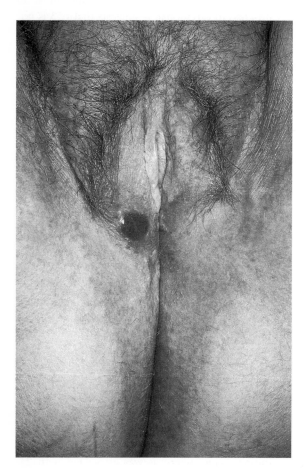

Figure 6.1 *Early cancer in a field of lichen sclerosus. This figure also appears in the colour plate section.*

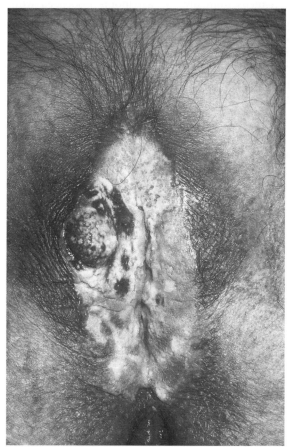

Figure 6.2 *Larger cancer in a field of lichen sclerosus plus squamous hyperplasia. This figure also appears in the colour plate section.*

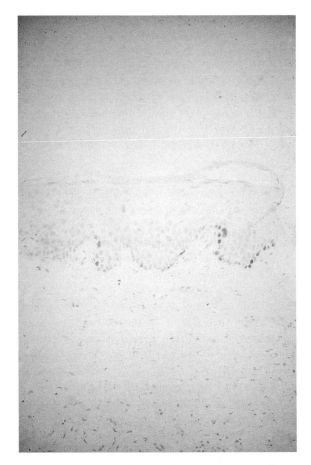

Figure 6.3 *Overexpression of protein P53 in the basal cells of an area of lichen sclerosus; to the right P 53 is seen immediately adjacent to invasive carinoma while, on the left and away from the cancer, P53 expression is absent or reduced. This figure also appears in the colour plate section.*

lichen sclerosus who have subsequently developed carcinoma. Scratch 'damage' can be implicated for many, but some patients present with little or only recent symptoms. The role of long-term use of topical potent corticosteroid therapy and the potential that altered cell-mediated immunity might contribute to an increased chance of cancer cannot yet be addressed. The message must be that lichen sclerosus has a small but significant association with carcinoma. Patients with lichen sclerosus, and probably those with lichen planus, squamous hyperplasia and even lichen simplex, need appropriate assessment when they present with symptoms; thickened hyperkeratotic or irregular areas must be biopsied. Patients should be reviewed yearly if lesions are quiescent, but more frequently if symptom control is poor. Although self-examination

is difficult or not always acceptable, patients must be encouraged to return if lesions change appearances. Not only do patients need appropriate instructions, but primary care physicians and gynaecologists, dermatologists and genitourinary medicine physicians must refer if lesions are altered or show untoward features. It is not appropriate to treat these premalignant lesions by vulvectomy, but adequate biopsy and an understanding of potent topical steroids use must be available to those gynaecologists who treat these lesions.

REFERENCES

1 Berkeley C, Bonney V. Leucoplakic vulvitis and its relation to kraurosis vulvae and carcinoma vulvae. *BMJ* 1909; **ii**: 1739–44.
2 Ridley CM. *The vulva*. London: Churchill Livingstone, 1988.
3 Janovski A, Douglas CP. *Diseases of the vulva*. London: Harper and Row, 1972.
4 Knight R van D. Bowen's disease of the vulva. *Am J Obstet Gynecol* 1943; **46**: 514–24.
5 Jeffcoate TNA, Davie TB, Harrison CV. Intra-epidermal carcinoma (Bowen's disease) of the vulva (a report of two cases). *J Obstet Gynaecol Br Empire* 1944; **51**: 377–85.
6 Jeffcoate TNA, Woodcock AS. Premalignant conditions of the vulva, with particular reference to chronic epithelial dystrophies. *BMJ* 1961; **ii**: 127–34.
7 Jeffcoate TNA. *Principles of gynaecology*. London: Butterworths, 1962.
8 Friedrich E. New nomenclature for vulvar disease. Report of the committee on terminology. *Obstet Gynecol* 1976; **47**: 122–4.
9 Walter JB, Israel MS. *General pathology*. London: Churchill, 1967.
10 MacLean AB. Vulval dystrophy – the passing of a term. *Curr Obstet Gynaecol* 1991; **1**: 97–102.
11 Ridley CM, Frankman O, Jones ISC et al. New nomenclature for vulvar disease . Report of the committee on terminology. *Am J Obstet Gynecol* 1989; **160**: 769.
12 Wallace HJ. Lichen sclerosus et atrophicus. *Trans St John's Dermatol Soc* 1971; **57**: 9–30.
13 Friedrich EG. Vulvar dystrophy. *Clin Obstet Gynecol* 1985; **28**: 178–87.
14 MacLean AB, Roberts DT, Reid WMN. Review of 1000 women seen at two specially designated vulval clinics. *Curr Obstet Gynaecol* 1998; **8**: 159–62.
15 Franck JM, Young AW. Squamous cell carcinoma in-situ

arising within lichen planus of the vulva. *Dermatol Surg* 1995; **21**: 890–4.

16 MacKie RM. *Clinical dermatology: an illustrated textbook*. Oxford: Oxford University Press, 1986.

17 Anderson MC. *Systemic pathology*, 3rd edn, Vol 6, *Female reproductive system*. Edinburgh: Churchill Livingstone, 1991.

18 Fox H, Buckley CH. Pathology for gynaecologists, 2nd edn. London: Arnold, 1991.

19 Taussig FJ. Cancer of the vulva. An analysis of 155 cases (1911–1940). *Am J Obstet Gynecol* 1940; **40**: 764–79.

20 Bibby AVG. Carcinoma of the vulva – a review of 71 cases. *J Obstet Gynaecol Br Empire* 1957; **64**: 253–66.

21 Langley II, Hertig AT, Smith G van S. Relation of leucoplakic vulvitis to squamous carcinoma of the vulva. *Am J Obstet Gynecol* 1951; **62**: 167–9.

22 McAdams AJ, Kistner RW. The relationship of chronic vulvar disease, leukoplakia, and carcinoma in-situ to carcinoma of the vulva. *Cancer* 1958; **11**: 740–57.

23 Woodruff JD, Baens JS. Interpretation of atrophic and hypertrophic alterations in the vulvar epithelium. *Am J Obstet Gynecol* 1963; **86**: 713–23.

24 Woodruff TJD, Borkowf HI, Holzman GB et al. Metabolic activity in normal and abnormal vulvar epithelia. An assessment by the use of tritiated nucleic acid precursors. *Am J Obstet Gynecol* 1965; **91**: 809–19.

25 Hart WR, Norris HJ, Helwig EB. Relation of lichen sclerosus et atrophicus of the vulva to development of carcinoma. *Obstet Gynecol* 1975; **45**: 369–77.

26 Rodke G, Friedrich EG, Wilkinson EJ. Malignant potential of mixed vulvar dystrophy (lichen sclerosis associated with squamous cell hyperplasia). *J Reprod Med* 1988; **33**: 545–50.

27 Meffert JJ, Davis BM, Grimwood RE. Lichen sclerosus. *J Am Acad Dermatol* 1995; **32**: 393–416.

28 Meyrick-Thomas RH, Ridley CM, McGibbon DH, Black MM. Lichen sclerosus et atrophicus and autoimmunity – a study of 350 women. *Br J Dermatol* 1988; **118**: 41–6.

29 Meyrick-Thomas RH, Ridley CM, McGibbon DH, Black MM. Anogenital lichen sclerosus in women. *J R Soc Med* 1996; **89**: 694–8.

30 Eng AM, Jacobs RA. Lichen sclerosus et atrophicus and squamous cell carcinoma. *J Cutan Pathol* 1980; **7**: 123–4.

31 August PJ, Milward TM. Cryosurgery in the treatment of lichen sclerosus et atrophicus of the vulva. *Br J Dermatol* 1980; **103**: 667–70.

32 Di Paola GR, Leverone NGR, Belardi MG. Recurrent vulvar malignancies in an 11 year prospectively

followed vulvar dystrophy: a gynaecologist's permanent concern. *Gynecol Oncol* 1983; **15**: 120–1.

33 Cario GM, House MJ, Paradinas FJ. Squamous cell carcinoma of the vulva in association with mixed vulvar dystrophy in an 18 year old girl: Case report. *Br J Obstet Gynaecol* 1984; **91**: 87–90.

34 Lindeque BG, Nel AE, Du Toit JP. Immune deficiency and invasive carcinoma of the vulva in a young woman: A case report. *Gynecol Oncol* 1987; **26**: 112–18.

35 Roman LD, Mitchell MF, Burke TW, Silva EG. Unsuspected invasive squamous cell carcinoma of the vulva in young women. *Gynecol Oncol* 1991; **41**: 182–5.

36 MacLean AB. Intraepithelial neoplasia of the lower genital tract: Its significance, detection, and management. In: Studd J (ed). *The yearbook of the Royal College of Obstetricians and Gynaecologists*. London: RCOG Press, 1995: 145–50.

37 MacLean AB, Buckley CH, Luesley D et al. Squamous cell carcinoma of the vulva: the importance of 'non-neoplastic epithelial disorders'. *Int J Gynecol Cancer* 1995; **5**: 70.

38 Buscema J, Stern J, Woodruff JD. The significance of the histologic alterations adjacent to invasive vulvar carcinoma. *Am J Obstet Gynecol* 1980; **137**: 902–8.

39 Choo YC. Invasive squamous carcinoma of the vulva in young patients. *Gynecol Oncol* 1982; **13**: 158–64.

40 Zaino RJ, Husseinzadeh N, Nahhas W, Mortel R. Epithelial alterations in proximity to invasive squamous carcinoma of the vulva. *Int J Gynecol Pathol* 1982; **1**: 173–84.

41 Podratz KC, Symmonds RE, Taylor WF, Williams WF. Carcinoma of the vulva: analysis of treatment and survival. *Obstet Gynecol* 1983; **64**: 63–74.

42 Hacker NF, Berek JS, Lagasse LD et al. Individualisation of treatment for stage 1 squamous cell vulvar carcinoma. *Obstet Gynecol* 1984; **63**: 155–62.

43 Hewitt H. Pre-neoplastic lesions of the vulva. *Eur J Gynaecol Oncol* 1988; **9**: 377–80.

44 Borgno G, Micheletti L, Barbero M et al. Epithelial alterations adjacent to 111 vulvar carcinomas. *J Reprod Med* 1988; **33**: 500–2.

45 Leibowitch M, Neill S, Pelisse M, Moyal-Baracco M. The epithelial changes associated with squamous cell carcinoma of the vulva: a review of the clinical, histological and viral findings in 78 women. *Br J Obstet Gynaecol* 1990; **97**: 1135–9.

46 Gomez-Rueda N, Garcia A, Vighi S et al. Epithelial alterations adjacent to invasive squamous carcinoma of the vulva. *J Reprod Med* 1994; **39**: 526–30.

47 Walkden V, Chia Y, Wojnarowska F. The association of squamous cell carcinoma of the vulva and lichen sclerosus: implications for management and follow-up. *J Obstet Gynaecol* 1997; **17**: 551–3.

48 Scurry J, Vanin K, Ostor A. Comparison of histological features of vulvar lichen sclerosis with and without adjacent squamous cell carcinoma. *Int J Gynecol Cancer* 1997; **7**: 392–9.

49 Clark DGC, Zumoff B, Brunschwig A, Hellman L. Preferential uptake of phosphate by premalignant and malignant lesions of the vulva. *Cancer* 1960; **13**: 775–9.

50 Karram M, Tarber B, Smotkin D et al. Detection of human papillomavirus deoxyribonucleic acid from vulvar dystrophies and vulval intraepithelial neoplastic lesions. *Am J Obstet Gynecol* 1988; **159**: 22–3.

51 Kim Y-T, Thomas NF, Kessis TD et al. p53 mutations and clonality in vulvar carcinomas and squamous hyperplasia: Evidence suggesting that squamous hyperplasias do not serve as direct precursors of human papillomavirus-negative vulvar carcinomas. *Hum Pathol* 1996; **27**: 389–95.

52 MacLean AB, Reid WMN, Perrett CW. Molecular and biophysical assessment of vulval lesions. *Int J Gynecol Cancer* 1997; **7**: 83.

53 Kohlberger PD, Kainz CH, Breitenecker G et al. Prognostic value of immunohistochemically detected p53 expression in vulvar carcinoma. *Cancer* 1995; **76**: 1786–9.

54 Kagie MJ, Kenter GG, Tollenaar RAEM et al. p53 protein overexpression, a frequent observation in squamous cell carcinoma of the vulva and in various synchronous vulvar epithelia, has no value as a prognostic parameter. *Int J Gynecol Pathol* 1997; **16**: 124–30.

55 Tan S-H, Derrick E, McKee PH et al. Altered p53 expression and epidermal cell proliferation is seen in vulval lichen sclerosus. *J Cutan Pathol* 1994; **21**: 316–23.

56 Soini Y, Kamel D, Paakko P et al. Aberrant accumulation of p53 associates with Ki67 and mitotic count in benign skin lesions. *Br J Dermatol* 1994; **131**: 514–20.

57 Zaki I, Dalziel KL, Solomonsz FA, Stevens A. The under reporting of skin disease in association with squamous cell carcinoma of the vulva. *Clin Exp Dermatol* 1996; **21**: 334–7.

58 Dwyer CM, Kerr RE, Millan DW. Squamous cell carcinoma following lichen planus of the vulva. *Clin Exp Dermatol* 1995; **20**: 171–2.

59 Duffey DC, Eversole LR, Abemayor E. Oral lichen planus and its association with squamous cell carcinoma: an update on pathogenesis and treatment implications. *Laryngoscope* 1996; **106**: 357–62.

60 Sigurgeirsson B, Lindelof B. Lichen planus and malignancy: an epidemiologic study of 2071 patients and a review of the literature. *Arch Dermatol* 1991; **127**: 1684–8.

61 Fulling H-J. Cancer development in oral lichen planus. *Arch Dermatol* 1973; **108**: 667–9.

62 Harland CC, Phipps AR, Marsden RA, Holden CA. Squamous cell carcinoma complicating lichen planus of the lip. *J R Soc Med* 1992; **85**: 235–6.

63 Cox NH. Squamous cell carcinoma arising in lichen planus of the penis during topical cyclosporin therapy. *Clin Exp Dermatol* 1996; **21**: 323–4.

64 Helm TN, Camisa C, Liu AY et al. Lichen planus associated with neoplasia: a cell mediated immune response to tumor antigens. *J Am Acad Dermatol* 1994; **30**: 219–24.

7

Vaginal intraepithelial neoplasia: presentation, diagnosis and management

MJ KAGIE, A ANSINK

The incidence of vulvar intraepithelial neoplasia (VIN) has increased considerably over the last two decades, particularly among women under the age of 40 years.[1–4] This increase parallels similar trends in cervical intraepithelial neoplasia (CIN) and is associated with changing sexual mores, human papillomavirus (HPV) infection and smoking. Women with VIN (and other vulvar lesions) may present to general practitioners, dermatologists, gynaecologists and urologists, and thus offer not only opportunities for interdisciplinary cooperation but also the potential for confusion and mismanagement.

In this chapter, an outline of the management of women with VIN is presented.

CLINICAL PRESENTATION AND EXAMINATION

Symptoms

The most common presenting symptom in VIN is pruritus (60 per cent).[1,5–14] Vulvar (burning) pain and dyspareunia are also common complaints.[15] Planner and Hobbs[16] reported that 15 per cent of patients had dyspareunia severe enough to result in avoidance of intercourse. Warts and/or discoloration occur less fre-

quently. Of patients with VIN, 10–60 per cent are assumed to be asymptomatic.[17–21] However, because of a probable selection bias, this is an imprecise estimate. The prevalence of VIN in a population of women aged 35 and over was reported by Broen and Ostergard,[22] who screened asymptomatic women. Of 1071 women screened there were four (0.4 per cent) women with VIN 3, and two (0.2 per cent) with VIN 1. Therefore, one in 200 women have VIN with no symptoms. Buscema and colleagues[5] reported 20 per cent of patients as asymptomatic, the lesions being discovered only by careful evaluation of the external genitalia. Most patients had neoplasia elsewhere in the lower genital tract, however, and the physician may have been alerted to the possibility of a new lesion in the area at risk.

A long duration of symptoms before presentation appears to be a feature of this condition. Bernstein and colleagues[6] reported that 40 per cent of the patients had complaints for more than 2 years whereas Shafi and colleagues[23] reported a median duration of symptoms of 22 months.

Examination

Ideally, women with vulvar lesions should be examined in a dedicated vulvar clinic, staffed by a gynaecologist and a dermatologist. Both gross examination and vulvoscopic examination are essential parts of the diagnostic procedure. Biopsies are usually taken under vulvoscopic guidance.

GROSS APPEARANCE

There is considerable variation in the clinical presentation of VIN, with patterns of varying colour and surface configuration[24] (Figs 7.1–7.4). There is no 'typical characteristic VIN lesion,'[8] so there are no pathognomonic features. In our experience, the most common finding is a raised lesion or hyperkeratosis,

which concurs with the observations of Herod and colleagues,[13] who found that 41 per cent of cases had these features.

Most VIN lesions are situated on the labia.[18] Crum and colleagues[9] reported that 81 per cent of the patients had gross involvement of the labia, 5 per cent of the clitoris and 14 per cent of the perineum.

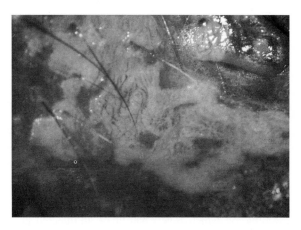

Figure 7.3 *VIN 3, after application of acetic acid. Note the mosaicism. (Reprinted with permission from M. van Beurden, Antonie van Leeuwenhoek hospital, Amsterdam, the Netherlands.) This figure also appears in the colour plate section.*

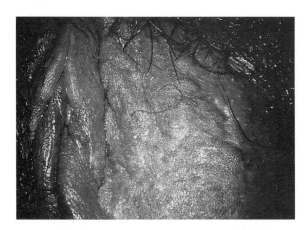

Figure 7.1 *VIN 3, with verrucous surface. (Reprinted with permission from M. van Beurden, Antonie van Leeuwenhoek hospital, Amsterdam, the Netherlands.) This figure also appears in the colour plate section.*

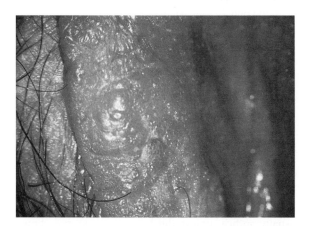

Figure 7.2 *VIN 3. Red lesions with erosion. (Reprinted with permission from M. van Beurden, Antonie van Leeuwenhoek hospital, Amsterdam, the Netherlands.) This figure also appears in the colour plate section.*

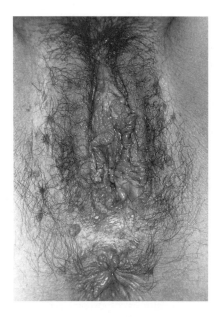

Figure 7.4 *VIN 3. Brown papules. (Reprinted with permission from M. van Beurden, Antonie van Leeuwenhoek hospital, Amsterdam, the Netherlands.) This figure also appears in the colour plate section.*

Multifocality is present in varying percentages (40–100 per cent),[14,18,25] depending on the population and the intensity of the search for lesions.

When examining the vulva, the following aspects should be described and documented:

- topography (uni- or multifocal)
- surface configuration (flat, raised, micropapillary, verrucous, ulcerative)
- colour (white, red, dark, no discoloration).

Examination can be extended when indicated to cover all the skin surfaces and other systems. Natural daylight is best for the appreciation of colour change, but artificial illumination will often be needed to illuminate the interstices of the anogenital area. It is of vital importance to record the exact morphology and location of the lesions. A routine order of examination of each part of the area is advisable. When there is a suggestion of an infective lesion it is mandatory to diagnose and treat the infection before vulvoscopic examination, this is because acetic acid is used in this examination, which is very painful on an infected surface. Notes should be supplemented by a drawing and/or photographs.

VULVOSCOPIC EXAMINATION

The use of the colposcope to perform vulvoscopy is, in our opinion, a helpful adjunct to inspection. Vulvoscopy is a safe, non-invasive and non-expensive technique for assessing the severity; it detects small areas of atypical epithelium, particularly on the inner aspects of the labia and in the vestibule. Biopsies can easily be taken under vulvoscopic control. The whole procedure can be carried out with the aid of local anaesthetics in an outpatient setting. Although vulvoscopic appearances do not predict histological outcome, vulvoscopy is helpful in finding the best place to take biopsies for two reasons. First, the lesions can be better demarcated and, second, with the aid of vulvoscopy, multifocality is recognized more frequently. In a recent study of VIN, all lesions were classified as multifocal in cases when vulvoscopy was used.[14]

Although the classification of vulvoscopically visible lesions is the same as that used for cervical colposcopy, it is uncertain whether vulvoscopy has the same predictive value as colposcopy in this classic context. So far, no attempt has been made to classify vulvoscopic findings.[26] The normal distribution of vulvoscopic findings has recently been reported by van Beurden and colleagues[27] who described them in 40 healthy volunteers; they found that vestibular erythema, vestibular papillomatosis and acetowhite lesions are common in healthy women who have no complaints, so the significance of acetowhitening on the vulva is questionable. Blood vessel patterns (punctation, mosaic or atypical vessels) in vulvar lesions can sometimes be seen after the application of acetic acid. The predictive value of these findings is, however, unknown. In a study by Kagie and colleagues[14] these vascular patterns were only found in VIN lesions and lesions of non-neoplastic epithelial disorders (NNEDs) and not in chronic non-specific infections of the vulva.

The use of toluidine blue as a superficial dye test is no longer recommended because of the high proportion of false-positive lesions associated with fissures and infection, and of false-negative lesions in thick keratinized epithelium.[28]

Vulvoscopy procedure

- An anaesthetic ointment such as Emla is applied 30–60 min before the procedure.
- Systematic gross inspection of the entire vulva including the perineal and anal region.
- Systematic microscopic inspection with low magnification without 3 per cent acetic acid.
- Systematic microscopic inspection with low magnification with 3 per cent acetic acid; waiting time after application is 5 min.
- Microscopic inspection with high magnification of the aberrant areas.
- Colourless disinfection.
- Local anaesthesia with lignocaine with adrenaline 1:200 000 or general anaesthesia.
- (Multiple) punch biopsies (Keyes).

DIAGNOSIS

It is essential to establish an initial diagnosis based on histology, because other methods such as gross appearance and cytology are unreliable. A pathologist specializing in gynaecological pathology is invaluable in this situation.

Where there is a single lesion, a single biopsy will usually suffice, unless the lesion is large and shows marked variance. However, in multifocal disease, particularly when not all of the lesions have the same appearance, multiple biopsies are indicated. If invasive disease is suspected, excision biopsy is recommended, provided that this is feasible without the excision of any essential midline structure. Where there are suspicious lesions close to the midline, a diagnostic rather than an excisional biopsy should be taken.

When VIN is diagnosed histologically, the vagina should be fully assessed for the possible coexistence of vaginal intraepithelial neoplasia (VaIN) and the cervix examined colposcopically for possible CIN. This is because of the high incidence of concurrence of these conditions. Concurrent or previous CIN, most commonly CIN 3, is reported in 30 per cent (range 12–48 per cent), and concurrent or previous VaIN in 10 per cent (2–40 per cent).[5,6,12,13,18,20,21,23,29–31]

In 1984, Buckley and colleagues[32] described two subtypes of VIN 3 on the basis of histological features. They described two basic patterns: the basaloid and bowenoid type. These are discussed in greater detail in Chapter 2. In 1991, Toki and colleagues[33] suggested a subdivision, based on the observation that there are two different clinical groups of women with VIN. They observed that one group consisted of relatively young women with HPV-positive VIN and another group of elderly women with HPV-negative VIN. They noted a correlation between the histological VIN type and the HPV distribution. These findings suggested that there were at least two different types of VIN with different clinical, pathological and virological features. The HPV-positive VIN was named warty VIN and the HPV-negative type basaloid VIN (see Chapter 4).

MANAGEMENT

Indications for the treatment of VIN

In patients with VIN, there are two problems that must be addressed: first, they often have severe symptoms such as pruritus and, second, they have a disorder that may have malignant potential (see Chapter 5). It is obvious that symptoms have to be treated. This can be done on a individual basis, depending on the preference of the patient and her doctor, and depending on the localization on the vulva.

Traditionally, VIN 3 has been considered to be a precursor of squamous cell carcinoma (SCC) of the vulva. However, the relationship between VIN and SCC is far from clear[26] and is the subject of Chapter 5.

There is considerable discussion about whether VIN 1 and VIN 2 are true precursors, and whether there is a sequential progression from VIN 1 to 2 and

3. The large spatial disparity between the mean peak incidence of VIN 3 (35 years) and SCC (68 years) leads to the conclusion that these two conditions may not always be directly related.

It has also been noted that VIN 3 is commonly multifocal, whereas SCC is usually unifocal.[24] The frequency and significance of the association of VIN with SCC are hard to assess, not least because many women with VIN are probably not seen by a doctor, because first women of advanced age with VIN often hesitate to visit a physician with a vulvar problem, and second approximately 0.6 per cent of the female population have asymptomatic VIN.[22]

Identification of vulvar epithelial changes and careful follow-up of women so identified to the time when they develop vulvar cancer would appear to be the only adequate method for evaluating which lesions are true precursors. Nevertheless, this sequence of events is rarely documented because most precursor lesions are destroyed in an effort to eliminate the potential for the development of cancer.

The overall percentage of malignant progression of VIN 3 varies from 2 per cent to 12 per cent for treated cases.[4,5,8–10,13,16,19,21,34–39] Barbero and colleagues[39] described malignant progression of VIN 1 and VIN 2 in 10 per cent and 11 per cent respectively. However, Herod and colleagues[13] found no malignant progression in patients with VIN 1 and VIN 2.

In the only study[4] of malignant progression in untreated patients (no treatment was defined as either biopsy alone, or grossly incomplete excision of VIN 3), there was a malignant progression in VIN 3 of 87.5 per cent. The authors found that the average time between the diagnosis of VIN 3 and invasion, in both treated and untreated patients, was 6.5 years.

Many authors have described risk factors for malignant progression of VIN. Advanced age,[5,9,40] immunosuppressed status[4,5,21] and perianal localization[5,9,34] have all been cited. However, these risk factors are all based on a small numbers of patients.

There is scant information available on spontaneous regression of VIN, because only a minority of patients are left untreated. Nevertheless, some have described spontaneous regression of VIN 3, such as Friedrich and colleagues,[21] who found that five of 50 patients with VIN 3 underwent regression without treatment. In addition, Jones and Rowan[4] described one untreated patient (of eight) with regression of VIN 3. Finally, Bernstein and colleagues[6] found that five of 13 untreated patients with VIN 3 underwent regression. However, all of these patients undergoing 'spontaneous' regression had biopsies taken from their lesions, which may have altered the natural history of the disease.

Options for the treatment of VIN

Treatment should not be undertaken before thorough gross and vulvoscopic examinations have been done with, if necessary, multiple biopsies to rule out (occult) invasive disease.

The optimal treatment for VIN has not been determined because the natural course of the disease in any individual patient remains uncertain. Various treatment options are discussed, and range from one extreme, such as radical vulvectomy, to observation alone (Table 7.1).

EXCISIONAL

Vulvectomy

The acceptance of vulvectomy as the proper treatment of VIN 3 was based on the tendency of VIN to be multicentric, the frequent association of other pathological vulvar conditions that may obscure the presence of additional foci, and the presumed high risk of progression to invasive cancer.

In the 1950s, some cases of radical vulvectomy for VIN were described. In 1992, Crawford and colleagues[41] described a patient with extensive intraepithelial neoplasia of the lower genital tract who was treated by radical exenterative surgery. The recurrence rates after radical vulvectomy in most (small) series is low. Collins and colleagues[8] reported 7.5 per cent (3 of 40) recurrence after radical vulvectomy for VIN. The

Table 7.1 *Treatment options*

1.	Excisional
	Radical vulvectomy
	Simple vulvectomy
	Wide local excision
	Local excision
	Skinning vulvectomy
2.	Local destructive
	Laser vaporization
	Cryosurgery
	5-Fluorouracil (5-FU)
	2,4-Dinitrochlorobenzene (DNCB)
3.	Medical therapy
	Interferon
	Topical corticosteroids
4.	Observation only

follow-up time was not specified. In the 1960s, simple vulvectomy became the standard management for VIN. Boutselis[7] advocated simple vulvectomy as the surgical procedure of choice. Recurrence was reported as 4 per cent (1 of 24) for follow-up of 1 to more than 10 years. In 1980, Buscema and colleagues,[5] in a rather large study of 106 patients with follow-up varying from 1 to 15 years, found no difference in recurrence rates between patients treated with simple vulvectomy and those treated with wide local excision. Recurrence rates were 30 per cent after wide local excision and 32 per cent after simple vulvectomy.

The trend has been set in favour of more conservative therapeutic modalities in managing VIN. Skinning vulvectomy using a split-thickness skin graft was introduced by Rutledge and Sinclair in 1968[42] and modified by Rettenmaier and colleagues in 1987.[43] They claimed that this procedure offered the opportunity to excise wide surgical margins, to provide an adequate specimen for pathological assessment, and to permit a satisfactory cosmetic and functional result by covering the defect with a graft. However, the method has the disadvantage of producing an additional scar at the donor site and because, after skin grafting, prolonged bedrest is necessary, there appeared to be an increased risk of thromboembolic phenomena. The skinning vulvectomy and skin graft procedure was indicated particularly for extensive, multifocal VIN. Rettenmaier and colleagues[43] reported a recurrence rate of 27 per cent (13 of 48) at intervals of 4–87 months after skinning vulvectomy for multifocal VIN. The risk of recurrence did not appear to be related to the status of the surgical margins.

As VIN appears to be increasing in frequency in younger women, the sequelae of vulvectomy are particularly undesirable; these include loss of perianal padding and protection, introital stenosis and dyspareunia, loss of secretion from vulvar glands, loss of sensation, loss of elasticity for vaginal delivery, urinary stream problems and a castration-like self-image.[44] Vulvectomy is associated with a high incidence of psychosexual problems. More than half of the patients reported psychosexual problems after vulvectomy[45] (see Chapter 16). Additionally, major postoperative complications such as pulmonary embolism can occur. Furthermore, wound breakdown and infection are not uncommon.

Local excision

As vulvectomy is a mutilating procedure and it does not significantly reduce the recurrence rates, wide local excision or even local excision would appear to be the surgical procedure of choice. Most localized lesions are managed effectively by wide local excision, allowing a disease-free border of at least 5–10 mm with primary approximation of the defect. However, for lesions that approach the midline, a disease-free border of 5–10 mm can be a problem. DiSaia and Rich[46] reported a 39 per cent recurrence after wide local excision (follow-up of 12–18 years). Leuchter and colleagues[47] described a 33 per cent recurrence after local excision. Wolcott and Gallup[48] found a 54 per cent recurrence (follow-up of 23 months to 10 years). This last high recurrence rate was attributed to the high frequency of involved margins; however, some patients without involved margins, no matter what type of operation, had recurrence of VIN.

On the basis of these data, we feel that there is no evidence for recommending radical excision for VIN, particularly if the justification is to minimize the risk of recurrence. All management options are associated with high recurrence rates, probably because the area at risk includes the entire lower genital tract. It is even possible that the status of the surgical margins is not related to the risk of recurrence. However, no randomized prospective studies have been carried out in this area. Thus, in our opinion, local excision can be used for most lesions that do not approach the midline. As has been discussed above, it is not necessary to aim for a complete excision of the abnormality, because there is no proof that this influences recurrence rates.

LOCAL DESTRUCTIVE TECHNIQUES

A major disadvantage of all destructive methods is the lack of a specimen for histopathological examination. For this reason, it is essential to rule out occult invasive disease by meticulous vulvoscopic examination and multiple biopsies.

Carbon dioxide laser

Carbon dioxide laser has become more widely used in the management of VIN, providing an effective and non-mutilating treatment. Laser vaporization, using a colposcope to determine the surgical plane, facilitates accurate control over the depth of destruction.[49,50] For lesions close to the anus, urethra or clitoris, laser vaporization is a good alternative to cold knife excision, because it offers the potential for avoiding damage to these structures.

The rationale for using the carbon dioxide laser to treat VIN is to destroy the entire area of abnormal epithelium to a shallow depth, so that rapid healing will occur from normal keratinocytes in the underlying pilosebaceous glands. After the first laser impact, anatomical landmarks in the crater are disguised by a layer of charred proteins, and any structure that is visible will already have suffered thermal necrosis. Accurate control of depth depends upon surgical strategies that correlate the level of the underlying zone of thermal necrosis with specific visual appearances within the zone of vaporization. A method for preserving anatomical orientation is wiping the surface char after the first impact of the laser, so that the visual characteristics of the different levels are recognized. Reid and colleagues[49] advise destruction until the third surgical plane, recognized by coarse collagen fibres for VIN, without involvement of the pilosebaceous glands. The healing of the wound is mostly cosmetic, although it may be hypertrophic. For VIN involving pilosebaceous glands, destruction to the fourth surgical plane is advised. The visual landmark of this plane is the 'sand grain' appearance. Healing is atrophic or hypertrophic and therefore requires grafting. For keratinized areas of the vulva and the perineum, power densities of 600–800 W/cm^2 are suggested, and for the non-keratinized vulvar mucosa, anus and urethra, 450–600 W/cm^2.

After laser vaporization, recurrence percentages range from 12 per cent to 88 per cent.[47,51–54] After laser vaporization combined with local excision, Bornstein and colleagues reported a 70 per cent recurrence.[55] Reid and colleagues[56] combined extended laser vaporization with topical 5-fluorouracil and reported a 3 per cent recurrence.

In conclusion, recurrence rates vary from 3 per cent to 88 per cent with an average of 30 per cent, regardless of treatment modality. An explanation for these observations is the possibility of the presence of an HPV reservoir, as HPV infection is present in approximately 75 per cent of the VIN lesions.[30,55,57–63] Furthermore, subclinical lesions that have not been treated may still be present in the remaining parts of the vulva, vagina and cervix. Finally, reinfection with HPV via sexual intercourse could also explain high recurrence rates.

Cryosurgery

As successful management of VIN requires careful microscopic control, cryosurgery is, in our opinion, not advisable for use on the vulva, because of the lack of precision associated with the technique.

5-Fluorouracil

In 1985, Sillman and colleagues[64] reviewed the use of topical 5-fluorouracil (5-FU) for the treatment of lower genital intraepithelial neoplasia. 5-FU is a pyrimidine analogue made by fluorination of uracil. The principal mechanism of action is to inhibit DNA synthesis. The most commonly used cream is a 5 per cent 5-FU concentrate. When 5-FU is applied directly to a neoplasm, erythema and oedema appear within 48 hours. If daily or twice-daily application continues, vesiculation, frequently accompanied by pain, occurs. The more advanced local effects of erosion, ulceration and necrosis commence after 2 weeks of treatment. When 5-FU is stopped, healing occurs within 2–6 weeks by granulation and re-epithelialization. After complete healing, scarring and hyperpigmentation may occur. Sillman and colleagues reviewed the results of 15 groups of investigators who had reported the use of 5-FU for the treatment of VIN. The overall outcome was a 59 per cent failure rate, 34 per cent remission and 7 per cent improvement in disease. There was a large spread of individual results (success rate from 0 to 100 per cent). This seems to be a reflection of the variables involved in the treatment of VIN with 5-FU. First, the size of the lesion plays a role: a large and widespread volume lesion is unfavourable. Second, the accessibility varies. Excessive keratinization and involvement of hair follicles and sebaceous glands might prevent penetration of 5-FU to sufficient depth. Furthermore, there was a great variance in how the 5-FU was used. The frequency of application varied from once to three times daily and the duration of treatment varied from 7 days to 4 months.

In attempting to compromise between sufficient therapy and patient discomfort, shorter, but more frequent, courses were used in some patients. This could be detrimental by allowing normal epithelium to grow over the ulcerated areas that had not yet been cleared of all neoplasia. Finally, pain and burning frequently limit the duration of 5-FU treatment. Most patients can tolerate 1 week of vulvar 5-FU (early erythema phase). With good patient–physician rapport and support and some discomfort tolerance, a 2-week course could be achieved. Supportive measures are advised and include good hygiene, sitzbaths, hydrogen peroxide treatment, topical lignocaine (Xylocaine) spray, analgesics, antipruritics, hypnotics and tranquillizers.

Beyond 2 weeks, when ulceration begins, heroic support and heroic patients are necessary to continue. Large, confluent lesions will develop wide, painful ulceration, which is particularly difficult to tolerate. The therapeutic end-point is often determined more by patient intolerance than by tumour clearance and, with 5-FU, response is hard to assess during therapy. Most authors agree that at least 6 weeks is required for a reasonable chance of remission. Many patients stop after 7–10 days.

We conclude that, because of the high failure rate and the excessive discomfort, there is no place for 5-FU treatment in the treatment of VIN.

2,4-Dinitrochlorobenzene

2,4-Dinitrochlorobenzene (DNCB) schedules have also been used to treat VIN. Weintraub and Lagasse[65] described six patients with VIN who were treated with DNCB. Cutaneous sensitization was achieved with 2 mg DNCB dissolved in 0.1 ml acetone applied to a 2 × 2 cm area on the right upper arm. Two weeks later a challenge dose of 100 μg DNCB was applied to the ipsilateral forearm. After 48 hours, the results were read. An indurated erythematous reaction was considered positive. Vulvar lesions were treated with a 0.1 per cent mixture of DNCB in a aqueous base. Erythema, oedema and tenderness were noted in the treated area. A daily application of DNCB was continued until bullous formation or superficial ulceration was noted. Medication was then stopped and healing allowed to begin. The question is whether the apparent destruction of the lesion is related to a specific immunological mechanism or is merely the result of the presence of a large number of mononuclear cells from an inflammatory stimulus. Only two of six patients responded in this study. Foster and Woodruff[66] described six patients treated with DNCB, of whom five demonstrated a reaction. As with 5-FU treatment, all patients suffered from extensive and sometimes apparently intolerable side effects.

We conclude that, because of the excessive discomfort, there is no place for DNCB in the treatment of VIN.

MEDICAL THERAPY

Interferon

De Palo and colleagues[67] reported a pilot study in 1985 of the results of human fibroblast interferon in the treatment of CIN and VIN. Interferon is a major component of the antiviral defence system. It also has complex immunomodulating activity that encompasses stimulation of the natural killer cells and monocyte system functions. It is assumed that interferon may be useful in the treatment of HPV-related

VIN. Interferon was administered topically with intra- and perilesional injections. The treatment schedule used was two to three applications/day for 5 days. One of two patients with VIN responded to this regimen with a complete remission. Fever, chills, fatigue and headache were common side effects; they were tolerable and did not lead to any change in treatment. Spirtos and colleagues[68] reported the results of topical interferon-α for the treatment of VIN. Interferon gel was applied three times daily, as long as a response of consistent diminution in lesion size was observed. Of the 18 patients, 14 (77 per cent) demonstrated some response to interferon.

As the results of interferon therapy on vulvar lesions are disappointing we do not advise this treatment for VIN.

Topical corticosteroids

No data are available on the effectiveness of topical steroids for the treatment of VIN. Data are available on the treatment of NNEDs of the vulva with topical steroids,[69–72] and they all report good clinical responses. However, VIN is felt, at least in some cases, to be an HPV-related problem, and it is not known how immunosuppression with steroids will interfere with the host–viral interface. Studies on this issue are warranted. Our clinical experience and that of others have shown that women with VIN lesions, who have an inflammatory reaction, experience considerable relief of symptoms when using topical steroids. In 1996, Tidy and colleagues[73] reported the results of a study on the management of lichen sclerosus and VIN by dermatologists and gynaecologists, in the UK. For both dermatologists and gynaecologists topical steroids were an unusual treatment method for VIN. We advise topical steroids twice daily for VIN lesions with inflammatory components.

OBSERVATION ONLY

On the basis of these data, we feel that there is no evidence to recommend radical excision for VIN in order to reduce the risk of progression to invasive disease. Furthermore, there is no evidence that asymptomatic VIN should be treated. Conservative management can be an excellent alternative in patients with and without symptoms, because excisional as well as ablative treatment modalities may cause severe cosmetic and functional disfigurement.

Follow-up of patients with VIN

After initial diagnosis and treatment, it is advisable to see patients in 6 weeks to assess their response to therapy. When a good result is achieved, patients should be seen in the vulvar clinic twice a year for gross examination and vulvoscopy. Biopsies are taken only if invasive disease is suspected or when the patient has persistent symptoms, i.e. does not respond to conservative treatment. When the lesions appear to be inactive, the patient can be seen once a year.

After diagnosis and treatment, all patients with VIN, including those who have no evidence of disease, may require lifelong follow-up because of previously reported high recurrence rates. In addition to examination of the vulva, cervical cytology and inspection of the cervix and vagina should be carried out because of the frequent multilocality of intraepithelial neoplasia of the female lower genital tract.

Summary of management

In summary, we advise 'wait and see' for cases of VIN 1, 2 and 3 provided that there are no symptoms and that invasive disease has been excluded by thorough vulvoscopic examination and biopsies. Conservative treatment, using corticosteroids, is advised when the patient has symptoms. If symptoms do not disappear with conservative treatment, destruction, using laser vaporization in combination with local excision, is advised. However, in cases of (even minimal) suspicion of invasive disease, excision is mandatory. Patients should be seen for follow-up once a year for the rest of their lives, or more often if indicated.

REFERENCES

1 Campion MJ, Singer A. Vulvar intraepithelial neoplasia: clinical review. *Genitourin Med* 1987; **63**: 147–52.

2 Jones RW, Baranyai J, Stables S. Trends in squamous cell carcinoma of the vulva: The influence of vulvar intraepithelial neoplasia. *Obstet Gynecol* 1997; **90**: 448–52.

3 Sturgeon SR, Brinton LA, Devesa SS, Kurman RJ. In situ and invasive vulvar cancer incidence trends. *Am J Obstet Gynecol* 1992; **166**: 1482–5.

4 Jones RW, Rowan DM. Vulvar intraepithelial neoplasia III: a clinical study of the outcome in 113 cases with

relation to the later development of invasive vulvar carcinoma. *Obstet Gynecol* 1994; **84**: 741–5.

5 Buscema J, Woodruff JD, Parmley TH, Genadry R. Carcinoma in situ of the vulva. *Obstet Gynecol* 1980; **55**: 225–30.

6 Bernstein SG, Kovacs BR, Townsend DE, Morrow CP. Vulvar carcinoma in situ. *Obstet Gynecol* 1983; **61**: 304–7.

7 Boutselis JG. Intraepithelial carcinoma of the vulva. *Am J Obstet Gynecol* 1972; **113**: 733–8.

8 Collins CG, Roman-Lopez JJ, Lee FYL. Intraepithelial carcinoma of the vulva. *Am J Obstet Gynecol* 1970; **108**: 1187–91.

9 Crum CP, Liskow A, Petras P, Keng WC, Frick II HC. Vulvar intraepithelial neoplasia (severe atypia and carcinoma in situ). A clinicopathologic analysis of 41 cases. *Cancer* 1984; **54**: 1429–34.

10 Iversen T, Abeler V, Kolstad P. Squamous cell carcinoma in situ of the vulva. A clinical and histopathological study. *Gynecol Oncol* 1981; **11**: 224–9.

11 DiPaola GR, Gomez-Rueda N, Belardi MG, Vighi S. Vulvar carcinoma in situ: A report of 28 cases. *Gynecol Oncol* 1982; **14**: 236–42.

12 Powell LC, Dihn TV, Rajaraman S et al. Carcinoma in situ of the vulva. A clinicopathologic study of 50 cases. *J Reprod Med* 1986; **31**: 808–13.

13 Herod JJO, Shafi MI, Rollason TP, Jordan JA, Luesley DM. Vulvar intraepithelial neoplasia: long term follow up of treated and untreated women. *Br J Obstet Gynaecol* 1996; **103**: 446–52.

14 Kagie MJ, Kenter GG, Fleuren GJ, Trimbos JB. Vulvoscopy in benign and premalignant vulvar lesions: results of seven year vulvoscopy clinic. *J Gynecol Techn* 1997; **3**: 21–6.

15 Buscema J, Stern J, Woodruff JD. The significance of the histologic alterations adjacent to invasive carcinoma. *Am J Obstet Gynecol* 1980; **137**: 902–9.

16 Planner RS, Hobbs JB. Intraepithelial and invasive neoplasia of the vulva in association with human papillomavirus infection. *J Reprod Med* 1988; **33**: 503–9.

17 Wright VC, Chapman WB. Colposcopy of intraepithelial neoplasia of the vulva and adjacent sites. *Obstet Gynecol Clin North Am* 1993; **20**: 231–55.

18 Husseinzadeh N, Newman NJ, Wesseler TA. Vulvar intraepithelial neoplasia: A clinicopathological study of carcinoma in situ of the vulva. *Gynecol Oncol* 1989; **33**: 157–63.

19 Ragnarsson B, Raabe N, Willems J, Pettersson F. Carcinoma in situ of the vulva. Long term prognosis. *Acta Oncol* 1987; **26**: 277–80.

20 Woodruff JD, Julian C, Puray T, Mermut S, Katayama P. The contemporary challenge of carcinoma in situ of the vulva. *Am J Obstet Gynecol* 1973; **115**: 677–86.

21 Friedrich EG, Wilkinson EJ, Fu YS. Carcinoma in situ of the vulva: A continuing challenge. *Am J Obstet Gynecol* 1980; **136**: 830–43.

22 Broen EM, Ostergard DR. Toluidine blue and colposcopy for screening and delineating vulvar neoplasia. *Obstet Gynecol* 1971; **38**: 775–8.

23 Shafi MI, Luesley DM, Byrne P et al. Vulvar intraepithelial neoplasia – management and outcome. *Br J Obstet Gynaecol* 1989; **96**: 1339–44.

24 Singer A, Monaghan JM. Vulvar intra-epithelial neoplasia. In: Singer A, Monaghan JM (eds). *Lower genital tract precancer*. Boston: Blackwell Scientific Publications, 1994: 177–226.

25 Kuppers V, Stiller M, Somville T, Bender HG. Risk actors for recurrent VIN. *J Reprod Med* 1997; **42**: 140–4.

26 Reid R. Preinvasive disease. In: Berek JS, Hacker NF (eds). *Practical gynecologic oncology*. Baltimore: Williams & Wilkins, 1994: 201–42.

27 Beurden M van, Vange N van der, Craen AJM de et al. Normal findings in vulvar examination and vulvoscopy. *Br J Obstet Gynaecol* 1997; **104**: 320–4.

28 Editorial. Clinical stains for cancer. Lancet 1982; **i**: 320–1.

29 Twiggs LB, Okagaki T, Clark BA, Fukushima M, Ostrow RS, Faras AJ. A clinical, histopathologic, and molecular biologic investigation of vulvar intraepithelial neoplasia. *Int J Gynecol Pathol* 1988; **7**: 48–55.

30 Barbero M, Micheletti L, Preti M et al. Vulvar intraepithelial neoplasia. A clinicopathologic study of 60 cases. *J Reprod Med* 1990; **35**: 1023–8.

31 Kagie MJ, Kenter GG, Hermans J, Trimbos JB, Fleuren GJ. The relevance of various vulvar epithelial changes in the early detection of squamous cell carcinoma of the vulva. *Int J Gynecol Cancer* 1997; **7**: 50–7.

32 Buckley CH, Butler EB, Fox H. Vulvar intraepithelial neoplasia and microinvasive carcinoma of the vulva. *J Clin Pathol* 1984; **37**: 1201–11.

33 Toki T, Kurman RJ, Park JS, Kessis T, Daniel RW, Shah KV. Probable nonpapillomavirus etiology of squamous cell carcinoma of the vulva in older women: A clinico-pathologic study using in situ hybridisation and poly-merase chain reaction. *Int J Gynecol Pathol* 1991; **10**: 107–25.

34 Japaze H, Garcia-Bunuel R, Woodruff JD. Primary vulvar neoplasia. A review of in situ and invasive carcinoma, 1935–1972. *Obstet Gynecol* 1977; **49**: 404–11.

35 Caglar H, Tamer S, Hreshchyshyn MM. Vulvar intraepithelial neoplasia. *Obstet Gynecol* 1982; **60**: 346–9.

36 Ulbright TM, Stehman FB, Roth LM, Ehrlich CE, Ransburg RC. Bowenoid dysplasia of the vulva. *Cancer* 1982; **50**: 2910–19.

37 Andreasson B, Bock JE. Intraepithelial neoplasia in the vulvar region. *Gynecol Oncol* 1985; **21**: 300–5.

38 Wilkinson EJ, Cook JC, Friedrich EG, Massey JK. Vulvar intraepithelial neoplasia: Association with cigarette smoking. *Colposcopy Gynecol Laser Surg* 1988; **4**: 153–9.

39 Barbero M, Micheletti L, Preti M et al. Biologic behaviour of vulvar intraepithelial neoplasia: histologic and clinical parameters. *J Reprod Med* 1993; **38**: 108.

40 Milde-Langosch K, Becker G, Loning T. Human papillomavirus and c-myc/c-erbB2 in uterine and vulvar lesions. *Virchows Arch A Pathol Anat Histopathol* 1991; **419**: 479–85.

41 Crawford RA, Shepherd JH, Jobling T, Woodhouse CR, Breach N. Radical exenterative surgery as the treatment for perineal intraepithelial neoplasia. *Br J Obstet Gynaecol* 1992; **99**: 158.

42 Rutledge F, Sinclair M. Treatment of intraepithelial carcinoma of the vulva by skin excision and graft. *Am J Obstet Gynecol* 1968; **102**: 806–18.

43 Rettenmaier MA, Berman ML, DiSaia PJ. Skinning vulvectomy for the treatment of multifocal vulvar intraepithelial neoplasia. *Obstet Gynecol* 1987; **69**: 247–50.

44 Bradley JJ, Buckley CH, Campion MJ et al. *The vulva*. Melbourne: Churchill Livingstone, 1988: 1–363.

45 Thuesen B, Andreasson B, Bock JE. Sexual function and somatopsychic reactions after local excision of vulvar intra-epithelial neoplasia. *Acta Obstet Gynecol Scand* 1992; **71**: 126–8.

46 DiSaia PJ, Rich WM. Surgical approach to multifocal carcinoma in situ of the vulva. *Am J Obstet Gynecol* 1981; **140**: 136–45.

47 Leuchter RS, Townsend DE, Hacker NF, Pretorius RG, Lagasse LD, Wade ME. Treatment of vulvar carcinoma in situ with the CO_2 laser. *Gynecol Oncol* 1984; **19**: 314–22.

48 Wolcott HD, Gallup DG. Wide local excision in the treatment of vulvar carcinoma in situ: A reappraisal. *Am J Obstet Gynecol* 1984; **150**: 695–8.

49 Reid R, Elfont EA, Zirkin RM, Fuller TA. Superficial laser vulvectomy. II. The anatomic and biophysical principles permitting accurate control over the depth of dermal destruction with the carbon dioxide laser. *Am J Obstet Gynecol* 1985; **152**: 261–71.

50 Reid R. Superficial laser vulvectomy III. A new surgical technique for appendage-conserving ablation of refractory condylomas and vulvar intraepithelial neoplasia. *Am J Obstet Gynecol* 1985; **152**: 504–9.

51 Townsend DE, Levine RU, Richart RM, Crum CP, Petrilli ES. Management of vulvar intraepithelial neoplasia by carbon dioxide laser. *Obstet Gynecol* 1982; **60**: 49–52.

52 Ferenczy A. Using the laser to treat vulvar condylomata acuminata and intraepithelial neoplasia. *Can Med Assoc J* 1983; **128**: 135–7.

53 Riva JM, Sedlacek TV, Cunnane MF, Mangan CE. Extended carbon dioxide laser vaporization in the treatment of subclinical papillomavirus infection of the lower genital tract. *Obstet Gynecol* 1989; **73**: 25–30.

54 Helmerhorst ThJM, Vaart CH, Dijkhuizen GH, Calame JJ, Stolk JG. CO_2–laser therapy in patients with vulvar intraepithelial neoplasia. *Eur J Obstet Gynecol Reprod Biol* 1990; **34**: 149–55.

55 Bornstein J, Kaufman RH, Adam E, Adler-Storthz K. Multicentric intraepithelial neoplasia involving the vulva. *Cancer* 1988; **62**: 1601–4.

56 Reid R, Greenberg MD, Lorincz AT, Daoud Y, Pizzuti D, Stoler M. Superficial laser vulvectomy. IV. Extended laser vaporisation and adjunctive 5–fluorouracil therapy of human papillomavirus-associated vulvar disease. *Obstet Gynecol* 1990; **76**: 439–48.

57 Kagie MJ. Aspects of maligant progression of vulvar epithelial disorders. Leiden, thesis, 1997.

58 Ferenczy A, Mitao M, Nagai N, Silverstein SJ, Crum CP. Latent papillomavirus and recurring genital warts. *N Engl J Med* 1985; **313**: 784–8.

59 Pilotti S, Donghi R, D'Amato L et al. Papillomavirus, p53 alteration and primary carcinoma of the vulva. *Eur J Cancer* 1993; **29A**: 924–5 (letter).

60 Park JS, Jones RW, McLean MR et al. Possible etiologic heterogeneity of vulvar intraepithelial neoplasia. *Cancer* 1991; **67**: 1599–607.

61 Hording U, Daugaard S, Iversen AKN. Human papillomavirus type 16 in vulvar carcinoma, vulvar intraepithelial neoplasia, and associated cervical neoplasia. *Gynecol Oncol* 1991; **42**: 22–6.

62 Beckmann AM, Acker R, Christiansen AE, Sherman KJ. Human papillomavirus infection in women with multicentric squamous cell neoplasia. *Am J Obstet Gynecol* 1991; **165**: 1431–7.

63 Kaufman RH, Bornstein J, Adam E, Burek J, Tessin B, Adler-Storthz K. Human papillomavirus and herpes simplex virus in vulvar squamous cell carcinoma in situ. *Am J Obstet Gynecol* 1988; **158**: 862–71.

64 Sillman FH, Sedlis A, Boyce JG. A review of lower genital intraepithelial neoplasia and the use of topical 5–fluorouracil. *Obstet Gynecol Surv* 1985; **40**: 190–220.

65 Weintraub I, Lagasse LD. Reversibility of vulvar atypia by DNCB-induced delayed hypersensitivity. *Obstet Gynecol* 1973; **41**: 195–9.

66 Foster DC, Woodruff JD. The use of dinitrochlorobenzene in the treatment of vulvar carcinoma in situ. *Gynecol Oncol* 1981; **11**: 330–9.

67 De Palo G, Stefanon B, Rilke F, Pilotti S, Ghione M. Human fibroblast interferon in cervical and vulvar intra-epithelial neoplasia associated with viral cytopathic effects. A pilot study. *J Reprod Med* 1985; **30**: 404–8.

68 Spirtos NM, Smith LH, Teng NNH. Prospective randomized trial of topical α-interferon (α-interferon gels) for the treatment of vulvar intraepithelial neoplasia III. *Gynecol Oncol* 1990; **37**: 34–8.

69 Mahmud N, Murakami T, Gyotoku Y, Nakazima H, Ishimaru T, Yamabe T. Vulvar dystrophy: A clinical follow-up. *Asia Oceania J Obstet Gynaecol* 1992; **18**: 231–8.

70 Bergman A, Karram M, Bhatia NN. Local steroid application for hyperplastic dystrophy of the vulva. *J Reprod Med* 1988; **33**: 542–4.

71 Kerns B-JM, Jordan PA, Moore M-BH et al. p53 overexpression in formalin-fixed, paraffin-embedded tissue detected by immunohistochemistry. *J Histochem Cytochem* 1992; **40**: 1047–51.

72 Bracco GL, Carli P, Sonni L et al. Clinical and histologic effects of topical treatments of vulval lichen sclerosus. *J Reprod Med* 1993; **38**: 37–40.

73 Tidy JA, Soutter WP, Luesley DM, MacLean AB, Buckley CH, Ridley CM. Management of lichen sclerosus and intraepithelial neoplasia of the vulva in the UK. *J R Soc Med* 1996; **89**: 699–701.

8

Clinical presentation and assessment of vulvar cancer

JB MURDOCH

A DISEASE OF DELAY

Vulvar cancer is a skin cancer affecting a specialized area of the body surface. As such, it should be easily identifiable at an early, curable stage. It is, however, characterized by neglect and delay by both patients and doctors. Approximately a third of vulvar cancers present late, with International Federation of Gynaecology Obstetrics (FIGO) stage III or IV disease. Reasons for this preventable delay include:

- reluctance by the patients to attend their doctor
- failure of the doctor to examine the patient adequately
- the rarity of the condition
- the heterogeneous appearance of vulvar skin conditions
- reluctance to biopsy suspicious lesions
- confusion over the malignant potential of precursor lesions.

Further difficulties arise when gynaecologists offer insufficiently radical treatment to often elderly patients. Such consideration is misplaced. All too often the disease returns as a result, leaving the patient with fewer therapeutic options and the prospect of an unpleasant demise.

The intimate nature of the disease, its associations with poor hygiene and the advanced age of many patients probably account for delays such as those cited by Monaghan[1] who found that 32 of 335 patients delayed more than 24 months and only 35 of 335 presented within 3 months in his series. Similar delays, ranging from 1 to 36 months with a mean of 10 months, were noted by Hacker and colleagues.[2] The problem is compounded by the symptoms associated with the condition. Typically, pruritus and irritation predominate, which are often long-standing problems that are ignored by patient and practitioner. They are non-specific, being common to all malignant and non-malignant vulvar conditions.

The rarity of the condition, particularly in young women, is one of several reasons for delay both in the patient seeking help and in the attending doctor's failure to refer promptly and appropriately. Vulvar cancer will present to the average general practitioner no more than once or twice in a professional lifetime and no more than once or twice a year in the case of the general gynaecologist. Traditionally, general gynaecologists cared for these occasional cases with no attempt at centralization.[3]

Increasingly clear guidance on the subject[4] is making an impact. A recent survey of Scottish gynaecologists confirmed that more than 90 per cent of gynaecologists referred cases to acknowledged subspecialists.[5]

It might be hoped that the combination of cervical screening with its attendant patient education and greater self-awareness and an increased willingness for patients to come forward for examination would shorten the delay in presentation. The Georgia study[6] failed to find this, with an average delay of 6 months for both young and old.

PRECURSOR LESIONS

Debate about the malignant potential of precursor lesions creates further confusion and delay. Non-neoplastic epithelial disorders (NNEDs) of the vulva include lichen sclerosus, squamous cell hyperplasia and other dermatoses. Lichen sclerosus is a common cause of prolonged bouts of itch and irritation. Surgery is unhelpful, biopsy is seldom used and the appearance of the skin can be deceptive. The potential for malignant progression of VIN and the so-called NNEDs is debated in Chapters 5 and 6.

The terminology may be falsely reassuring. In one study of synchronous epithelial changes in 63 women with vulvar cancer, the authors reported 39 cases of VIN (all grades), 31 cases of lichen sclerosus and 49 cases of squamous cell hyperplasia.[7] The authors noted that only a third of the patients had epithelial changes diagnosed before their cancer developed. It is estimated that 3–5 per cent of cases of lichen sclerosus will progress to invasive cancer.[8] The superficial response to this is to advocate more careful diagnosis, treatment and surveillance of such patients. This is unhelpful; for example, in a series of 211 women followed up for a mean of 20 months only two invasive cancers were identified.[9] This represents a relative risk of 3.17 compared with that for unaffected women. It also represents a large investment of resources for a low return and is inefficient. We need a clearer understanding of the natural history of the condition and the ability to identify the small number of women who will progress to cancer.

VIN 3 is now widely regarded as a premalignant condition and the terminology suggests parallels with cervical disease. This may be misleading because only about half of all cancer cases have known precursor or concomitant VIN. Furthermore, reports suggesting a potential for progression of less than 5 per cent were based on a follow-up of treated cases.[10,11] Jones and Rowan[12] produced data that confirmed a progression rate of 3.8 per cent in treated cases compared with seven of eight (87.5 per cent) cases of untreated VIN 3. They estimate that the progression rate for untreated VIN 3 is about 10 per cent per annum. This would suggest that complacency about the malignant potential of VIN 3 is misplaced and failure to treat detected VIN 3 actively is an important contributor to delay resulting in cancer in a proportion of cases.

Symptoms and signs

The most common symptom associated with vulvar cancer is pruritus, with a reported frequency ranging from 38.6 per cent[13] to 71 per cent.[1] Less frequent symptoms comprise swelling, ulceration, pain, burning and discharge. A similar profile of symptoms was found for VIN by Herod and colleagues[14] comprising pruritus (56 per cent), pain and soreness (29 per cent), swelling (16 per cent), discoloration (14 per cent), discharge (7 per cent), bleeding (2 per cent) and no symptoms (5 per cent). In a parallel study, the same investigators identified a subgroup of 26 patients with superficially invasive cancer in association with VIN; they found no pathognomonic clinical features of malignancy and diagnoses were made histologically.[15] It is clear that a history and clinical examination alone are not enough.

When presented with a mass or ulcer with the typical rolled edge and the consistency of malignancy, the diagnosis is straightforward (Fig. 8.1). Smaller lesions and superficially invasive foci in a field change of VIN can be more challenging. The use of a colposcope or magnifying glass with illumination can be helpful, if only to map a lesion and to identify the areas likely to yield the most severe histological abnormality. Detailed vulvoscopy is of debatable value (see Chapter 7) in the keratinized, squamous, hair-bearing tissues of much of the vulva, because most of the subtle changes are lost. In the non-keratinized skin of the labia minora and vestibule, suspicious findings similar to those on the cervix, such as mosaic, punctation, atypical vessels and superficial ulceration, may guide appropriate biopsy. Some authorities advocate the use of toluidine blue which stains dedifferentiated tissues.[8]

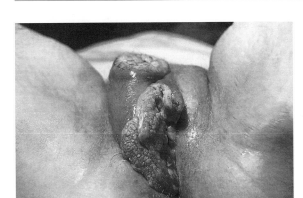

Figure 8.1 *Typical appearance of vulvar carcinoma showing an ulcerating mass with rolled edges. This figure also appears in the colour plate section.*

It is important to remember, however, that detailed vulvoscopy is not diagnostic and must be supplemented by appropriate biopsy. Vulvoscopically directed multiple biopsies can be very useful with mixed superficially invasive and preinvasive disease for accurate mapping of lesions. This allows the surgeon to tailor the radicality of the surgery to the patient's needs. The colposcope is also useful to identify multifocal disease. It is mandatory to inspect the cervix and vagina in such circumstances and some authorities recommend inspection of the anal canal as well.[16]

DIAGNOSIS

The diagnosis of vulvar cancer is histological. Inspection, with or without optical aids, is insufficient and only of value in defining optimal targets for biopsy. The diagnosis of superficially invasive disease can almost always be achieved as an outpatient procedure using 1 per cent lignocaine for local infiltration. Simple instruments such as a scalpel and forceps suffice, but can produce a distorted, crushed specimen. The Keyes punch is recommended to provide a good quality biopsy that is easy for the pathologist to handle.[17] Similarly, large ulcerating lesions can be diagnosed with local anaesthesia and wedge excision of part of the edge, including some of the adjacent normal skin. This simplifies the pathologist's task and ensures a diagnosis based on viable tumour rather than necrotic tissue from the centre of a lesion.

General anaesthesia is reserved for the following: anxious patients; patients with multifocal disease for which multiple biopsies are needed to map the disease

accurately; patients with extensive disease encroaching on the vagina, urethra, bladder, bone, anus or rectum, which is too uncomfortable to assess fully with the patient awake as part of treatment planning; or patients in whom excisional biopsy is appropriate. Excisional biopsy is not recommended for large or widespread, superficially invasive disease, which must be treated with radical excision. Such radical excision is not justified before a histological diagnosis is made. Excisional biopsy is appropriate in the case of small (< 1 cm) unifocal disease when a 1–1.5 cm margin can easily be achieved without undue morbidity or postoperative scarring. Much depends on the site of the lesion and the status of the patient. Excisional biopsy of a 1-cm lesion on the posterior vulva of a frail elderly patient, to plan therapy and avoid unnecessary anaesthesia, is appropriate, while it would be inappropriate if the lesion was less than 1 cm from the clitoris in a sexually active, younger woman.

NODAL ASSESSMENT

The sequential involvement of superficial inguinal, deep femoral and pelvic lymph nodes is sufficiently predictable to have a significant impact on management planning. Node status is the single most important prognostic factor for survival. Groin dissection has substantial morbidity comprising wound infection and wound breakdown, lymphocyst formation and lymphoedema. The development of an accurate predictive test of node status is urgently required.

Careful palpation of the groins is part of the assessment of women with vulvar carcinoma. It is low-tech, easy and free, but it is notoriously unreliable. False-negative rates of 23 per cent and false-positive rates of 60 per cent are typical when palpability of nodes is the criterion.[18] Radiology, including computed tomography (CT) and magnetic resonance imaging (MRI) appear to offer few advantages. Lymphangiography is uncomfortable for the patient, time-consuming and difficult to interpret. One review recorded a positive predictive value of only 54 per cent.[19]

As an alternative, intraoperative lymphatic mapping of vulvar cancer has been described.[20] This technique involves injection of isosulfan blue around the tumour. The dye is selectively taken up by lymphatics and travels to the sentinel node for that tumour, which is removed for frozen section. The authors reported on 21 patients, finding six with node metastases. In no cases was a false-negative sentinel node found. A recent multicentre attempt to repeat this study in Europe showed that sentinel node detection by this method was unreliable (A Ansink 1999, unpublished data).

Another approach using lymphoscintigraphy was described by DeCesare and colleagues.[21] Here technetium-99m (^{99m}Tc)-labelled sulphur colloid was injected at the tumour site and a gamma counter was used to find the sentinel nodes. None of 10 patients had a false-negative sentinel node. Ultrasonography has been explored in evaluation of the groins[22] with a reported sensitivity of 82 per cent and specificity of 87 per cent. Work in progress, combining real-time ultrasonography and ultrasonographically directed fine needle aspiration, is showing promising results (AQ Moskovic, unpublished data, 1997). The main problem with this technique is that it is highly dependent on operator skill, so there is a learning curve. The average UK cancer centre serves 1 million people, which should yield 10 new vulvar cancers per year. Three of these will be advanced tumours; of the remaining seven, one might be node positive. This is not sufficient to maintain quality assurance. The technique would have to have applications in other tumours to be reliable.

None of these techniques is in mainstream clinical use. The challenge is to devise a test that is easy, reproducible and safe; it also has to be very accurate. If we assume that 10 per cent of apparent stage T1 or T2 disease will be node positive, then simply omitting groin dissection will be safe in 90 per cent of cases. The test must therefore be more than 90 per cent accurate and, as salvage of recurrence away from the vulva is poor,[23] it must be virtually 100 per cent accurate.

It has been postulated that laparoscopically assisted surgical staging of pelvic lymph nodes may have a place in vulvar cancer (J Childers 1998, personal communication).

Although this is superficially attractive, it is essential that we do not lose sight of clinical reality. Of vulval cancers, 60 per cent are stage T1 or T2 at presentation; they do not need pelvic node dissection because they are groin node negative. Of the other 40 per cent, only 15 per cent[24] will be pelvic node positive; i.e. 6 per cent of new cases. Even if radiation offered a currently unattainable 50 per cent salvage rate for established pelvic disease, only 3 per cent of patients might gain a survival advantage. In the terms of 10 new cases being seen each year at a standard UK cancer centre, this equates to one patient every 4 years.

The alternative argument for laparoscopic surgical staging is to allow tailoring of radiotherapy to patient needs. Again this is superficially attractive, but the evidence suggests that groin and pelvic irradiation is effective by prevention of groin recurrence rather than by eradication of pelvic disease.[25] It could equally be argued that we should simply confine radiation fields to the groin alone in all cases to reduce treatment morbidity, a reasonable basis for a randomized trial of groin versus groin and pelvic radiotherapy. Laparoscopic pelvic lymphadenectomy is being advocated to identify, on the one hand, a small group of patients who have disease but for whom we have an inefficient therapeutic response and, on the other, a large group of patients who can be identified without the procedure.

STAGING

FIGO staging has evolved over years, taking into account the development of understanding of the natural history of the disease. Of greatest import is the change from clinical to surgical staging, which recognizes the limitations of node palpation. The latest version was agreed in 1994 (Table 8.1).[26]

Internationally agreed staging systems are important because they:

- allow broad comparison of results between centres
- inform clinical decision-making when linked to management protocols and survival data
- define similar risk patients for entry into clinical trials.

To achieve these ends, staging must separate patients into reasonably accurate risk groups without making the system so complex that it is not used. The old clinical staging was deficient in this respect, because it did not adequately define node status, which is overwhelmingly the most important risk factor in vulvar cancer.[27–29]

Shanbour and colleagues[30] who retrospectively confirmed a 35 per cent false-negative and a 36 per cent false-positive rate for clinical staging, explored the relative merits of clinical versus surgical staging. They showed that substantial staging shifts occurred (Table 8.2) and that better prognostic separation was achieved by surgical staging (Table 8.3). This shift results from reassigning clinically node-negative but surgically node-positive cases out of stage II.

The standard test of node status is complete

Table 8.1 *The FIGO staging of vulvar cancer after the Montréal Meeting in September 1994 (the TNM classification is included for comparison)*

Stage	Description	TNM
I	Lesions ≤2 cm confined to the vulva or perineum. No lymph node metastases	T1N0M0
Ia	Lesions ≤2 cm confined to the vulva or perineum with stromal invasion ≤1 mm.[a] No lymph node metastases	
Ib	Lesions ≤2 cm confined to the vulva or perineum with stromal invasion >1 mm.[a] No lymph node metastases	
II	Tumour confined to the vulva and/or perineum of >2 cm in the greatest dimension with no nodal metastases	T2N0M0
III	Tumour of any size arising on the vulva and/or perineum with (1) adjacent spread to the lower urethra and/or the vagina or anus and/or (2) unilateral regional lymph node metastases	T3N0M0 T3N1M0 T1N1M0 T2N1M0
IVa	Tumour invading any of the following: upper urethra, bladder mucosa, rectal mucosa, pelvic bone and/or bilateral regional nodal metastases	T1N2M0 T2N2M0 T3N2M0 T4anyNM0
IVb	Any distant metastasis including pelvic lymph nodes	AnyTanyNM1

[a] The depth of invasion is defined as measurement of the tumour from the epithelial stromal junction of the adjacent most superficial dermal papilla, to the deepest point of invasion.

inguinofemoral groin node dissection. This has a dual function both as a diagnostic and prognostic indicator and as part of therapy. Its appropriateness as a test will be considered here. Groin node dissection has considerable morbidity and is used on a population among whom there are subgroups with a chance as high as 95 per cent that the procedure will in retrospect prove to be unnecessary. DiSaia and colleagues[31] suggested an alternative strategy in a report on 20 patients for whom a superficial inguinal node dissection with

frozen section analysis was used as a screening test for node positivity. Full groin dissection was reserved for node-positive patients. This study, of course, proved little because the expected prevalence of node positivity in the study group was too low and the numbers too small to test the hypothesis. The Gynecologic Oncology Group (GOG), however, responded by studying the concept further. Unfortunately, the issue was prejudged and a formal randomized trial of superficial node dissection versus formal complete node dissection was eschewed in favour of an observational study with one arm. The study design was flawed further when no provision was made for recording data on the superficial node-positive patients (true positives), so preventing assessment of the performance of the screening test. Fortunately, the results were sufficiently

Table 8.2 *Staging shift when comparing clinical and surgical staging[30]*

Stage	Clinical stage	Surgical stage	% Change[a]
I	28	25	21 (6)
II	29	23	48 (14)
III	44	44	45 (20)
IV	5	a = 10 b = 4	60 (3)
Total	106	106	

[a] This means the percentage upstaged as a result of using surgical rather than clinical measurements. The figures in parentheses are the numbers.

Table 8.3 *Five-year survival rates according to clinical versus surgical staging in vulvar cancer[30]*

Stage	Clinical stage survival rate (%)	Surgical stage survival rate (%)
I	100	100
II	50	82
III	58	51
IV	40	a = 33 b = 0

robust to overcome these difficulties. There were nine groin recurrences with five related deaths.[32] Historical controls suggested that there should be no recurrences, so these results are compatible with failure of the strategy to achieve its aims. Furthermore, the evidence for reduced morbidity when there is no deep femoral dissection is weak. Alternatively, it has been argued that the frequency of poorly differentiated tumours in the study group was twice that of the control group,[33] six of the nine recurrences being in poorly differentiated tumours. Until publication of a proper randomized controlled trial with enough power to compare recurrence, mortality and morbidity rates between superficial and complete groin dissection, it seems clear that the value of superficial node dissection has not been proved. The case is similarly argued, although from a therapeutic perspective, in Chapter 9.

Despite this, the technique continues to be used. Burke and colleagues[34] offered superficial node dissection to the 76 patients who had radical wide excision of their T1 or T2 tumours. Seven true positives were identified but four false negatives subsequently appeared, i.e. a sensitivity of only 64 per cent. This is not acceptable given that one of seven true positives died compared with three of four false negatives.

The current staging system is less precise in the case of advanced disease. Stage III encompasses small volume T1N1 disease and large-volume T2N1 disease, despite the fact that the latter has significantly higher recurrence risks than the former.[35] The staging system performs rather better in considering node status in advanced disease, differentiating unilateral (stage III) and bilateral (stage IV) node positivity. Burger and colleagues[36] noted a 5-year survival rate of 51 per cent for patients with unilateral metastases versus 29 per cent for those with bilateral metastases. Finally, it should be remembered that it is the therapy, not the process of staging, that affects the outcome. There can be no justification outside clinical trials for performing staging procedures with no inherent clinical benefit. Thus, the evidence currently suggests that groin dissection for staging purposes in stage 1a is not justified[37] and that pelvic node dissection in stage 1b or greater is not justified.[25]

OTHER CHARACTERISTICS INFLUENCING RISK

The central role of groin node status in predicting survival is acknowledged in the FIGO staging system, and validated using multivariate analysis.[38] The standard response to this remains inguinofemoral node dissection, despite its morbidity. This prompted the study of the characteristics of the primary tumour in an attempt to define the risk of positive nodes.

Tumour size

The first characteristic to be studied was the size of the tumour. It is clear that increasing size of tumour has an impact on survival when assessed by univariate analysis[39] and that depth of invasion is the most useful measurement. Wharton and colleagues[40] reviewed their data and identified 10 patients who had primary tumours less than 2 cm in diameter with less than 5 mm invasion and no evidence of node metastases. Their suggestion that node dissection could be omitted in this group was met by a vigorous response from other workers, and the consensus view is that the node positivity rate in this group of patients ranges from 7 per cent to 34 per cent[41] and as such the size of the tumour is not sufficiently discriminating.

There would appear to be no acceptable watershed of depth of invasion more than 1 mm deep, below which node dissection can be abandoned (see Table 9.3). A GOG study found no incidence of node metastases in 63 such patients.[42] This study found a 20 per cent node-positive rate in disease that was less than 5 mm thick. Indeed, Podczaski and colleagues[43] recorded groin recurrence and death in two patients with maximum depth of disease of 1.5 mm and 2 mm. In addition, there are two case reports of metastatic disease in early invasive cancers that were less than 1 mm deep.[44]

Tumour grade

The histological grade of tumours has been suggested as an important prognostic variable.[33] There is support for this in the literature, with a statistical multivariate association between histological grade and node status.[45,46] Similarly, there is a highly significant correlation between vascular channel involvement and node status.

An alternative method of assessing tumour aggressiveness is suggested by Obermair and colleagues.[47] They measured microvessel density and expression of vascular permeability factor as tests of angiogenesis, which is well recognized as an important facet of tumour growth. There was a significant correlation

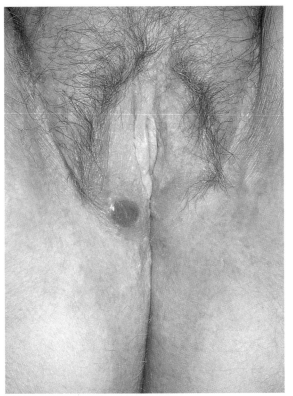

Fig. 6.1 *Early cancer in a field of lichen sclerosus.*

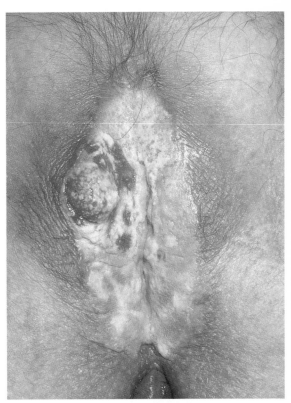

Fig. 6.2 *Larger cancer in a field of lichen sclerosus plus squamous hyperplasia.*

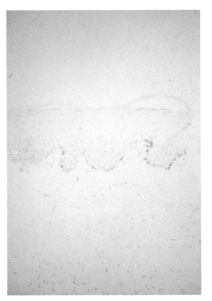

Fig. 6.3 *Overexpression of protein p53 in the basal cells of an area of lichen sclerosus; to the right p53 is seen immediately adjacent to invasive carcinoma while, on the left and away from the cancer, p53 expression is absent or reduced.*

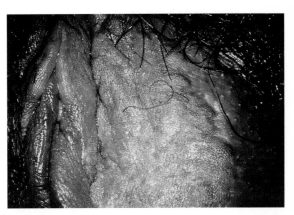

Fig. 7.1 *VIN 3, with verrucous surface. (Reprinted with permission from M. van Beurden, Antonie van Leeuwenhoek hospital, Amsterdam, the Netherlands.)*

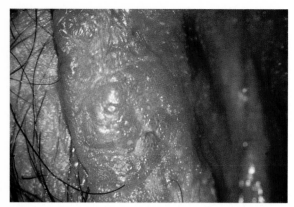

Fig. 7.2 *VIN 3. Red lesions with erosion. (Reprinted with permission from M. van Beurden, Antonie van Leeuwenhoek hospital, Amsterdam, the Netherlands.)*

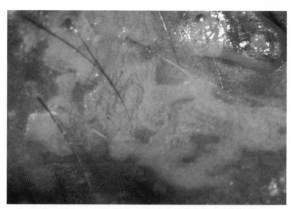

Fig. 7.3 *VIN 3, after application of acetic acid. Note the mosaicism. (Reprinted with permission from M. van Beurden, Antonie van Leeuwenhoek hospital, Amsterdam, the Netherlands.)*

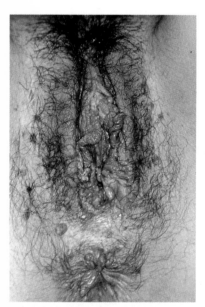

Fig. 7.4 *VIN 3. Brown papules. (Reprinted with permission from M. van Beurden, Antonie van Leeuwenhoek hospital, Amsterdam, the Netherlands.)*

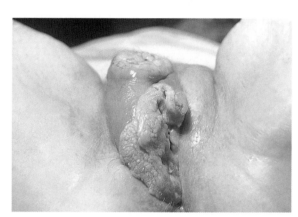

Fig. 8.1 *Typical appearance of vulvar carcinoma showing an ulcerating mass with rolled edges.*

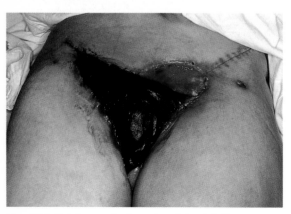

Fig. 12.1 *Total necrosis of a rectus abdominis flap.*

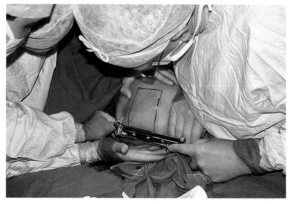

Fig. 12.2 *Use of a traditional Humby knife to take a split-thickness skin graft from the thigh.*

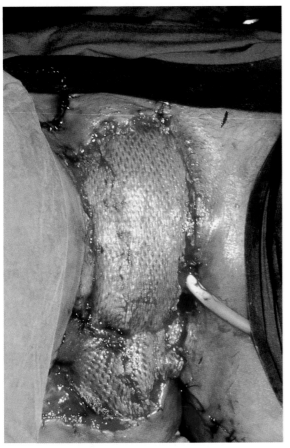

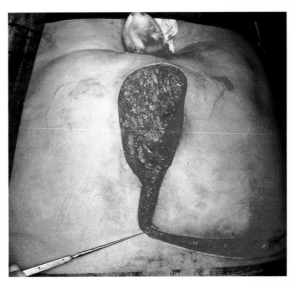

Fig. 12.4 *Large cutaneous advancement flap from above the right gluteus maximus used to fill a defect in the natal cleft.*

Fig. 12.3 *Split-thickness skin graft on vulva.*

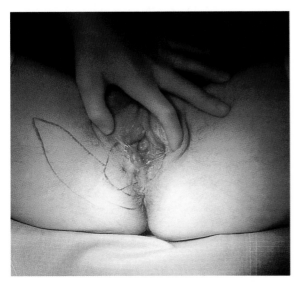

Fig. 12.5 *Preoperative marking for lateral transposition cutaneous flap from the right thigh.*

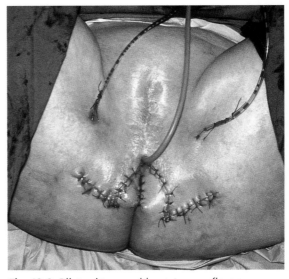

Fig. 12.6 *Bilateral transposition cutaneous flaps.*

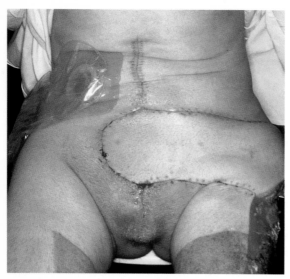

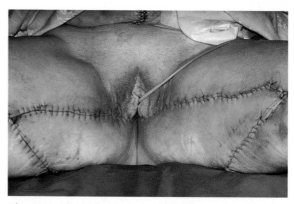

Fig. 12.8 *Bilateral gluteus maximus flaps.*

Fig. 12.7 *Large tensor fascia lata fasciocutaneous flap rotated from the left thigh.*

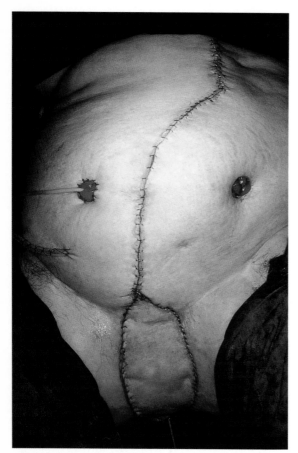

Fig. 12.9 *Rectus abdominis flap used to form pelvic floor after total pelvic exenteration.*

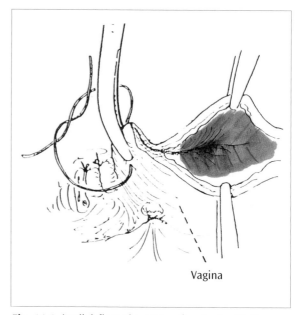

Vagina

Fig. 14.1 *'Red' defines about 1cm of vaginal epithelium that is buried when the vaginal cuff is sutured closed at hysterectomy. (Reproduced with permission from WB Saunders.[9])*

between these factors and survival in their small group of 25 patients. The authors acknowledge that larger multivariate studies are necessary. Finally, a regression analysis of 136 cases revealed not only the expected factors of node status and tumour size but also the novel observation that smoking is also an independent predictor for survival.[48]

It is important to assess each patient and each tumour to define the optimum management. All of the above-mentioned, independently significant characteristics can be considered in planning. It remains the case that tumour size and node status dominate the prognosis so much that they are pre-eminent. The others – differentiation, vascular channel involvement and smoking status – are not sufficiently discriminating clinically to have a major role in decision-making, although they influence choices in marginal cases.

Disease site and proximity to other structures

The management of all solid tumours can be considered in three parts, i.e. local disease, locoregional disease and systemic disease. Although many medical oncologists believe that cancer beyond its earliest stages is always a systemic disease, the surgical gynaecological oncologist finds that clinical experience does not support this concept. There is no effective systemic response to vulvar cancer, certainly not that beyond the pelvis and usually not that beyond the inguinal ligament where 5-year survival rates of 10 per cent are quoted.[49] The management of the groin nodes can be varied according to the size and the laterality of the tumour. The surgical management of the central tumour is where the skill and experience of the surgical oncologist have most impact in planning and executing therapy. The traditional Halsteadean approach to management[50–52] has given way to individualized care, most clearly seen in the treatment of the primary tumour.[18] Tumour size coupled with tumour site are the crucial elements to be considered and are discussed in detail in Chapter 9.

FORMULATING MANAGEMENT PLANS

Management planning must draw a series of considerations together to make an individualized whole. These considerations comprise:

Table 8.4 *The vulvar cancer team*

- Trained gynaecological oncologist
- Special interest radiation oncologist
- Special interest histopathologist
- High quality nursing
- Nurse/physiotherapist with interest in lymphoedema
- Stoma therapist
- Plastic surgeon
- Psychosexual support

- the site and size of the tumour
- involvement of other structures
- the extent of surgery required to extirpate the tumour
- the impact of treatment on bladder or bowel function
- the impact of the disease on the psychosexual and psychological well-being of the patient
- the impact of therapy on the psychosexual and psychological well-being of the patient
- the general health of the patient and her ability to withstand both the surgery and treatment-related sequelae
- the potential for reconstructive surgery.

The days of the generalist gynaecologist managing the odd case of vulvar cancer should be long gone. A team approach is essential to provide comprehensive care in this difficult area (Table 8.4). It is the function of the surgical gynaecological oncologist to coordinate the activity of the team, arriving at treatment plans by working through these eight considerations. This requires consultation with other team members. He or she must address the logistics of bringing together appropriate specialists as required. Improvements in vulvar cancer care in the last 20 years have not resulted in improved cure rates. They have, rather, maintained cure rates with reduced morbidity through selection of patients for less radical surgery, judicious use of chemotherapy and radiotherapy, and provision of comprehensive physical and psychological support for the patient.

CONCLUSION

The successful management of vulvar cancer depends on the patient having sufficient self-awareness of a problem to attend early for consultation. The general practitioner must be willing to examine the patient carefully, be aware of the possibility of the diagnosis, and be able to identify and refer to a relevant specialist. The specialist requires a detailed knowledge of the natural history of the disease and must be willing to biopsy appropriately at an early stage. The pathologist must be experienced in gynaecological cancer. The surgical gynaecological oncologist must be willing and able to select the right operation and ensure that it is sufficiently radical to extirpate the tumour. He or she must lead a multidisciplinary team to coordinate care and ensure that the appropriate expertise is brought to bear. It is only through these activities that the goal of optimum cure rates with minimum morbidity will be achieved.

REFERENCES

1 Monaghan JM. Management of vulval carcinoma. In: *Clinical gynaecological oncology*. Oxford: Blackwell Scientific Publications, 1990: 145.

2 Hacker NF, Leucher RS, Berek JS, Casaldo TW, Lagasse LD. Radical vulvectomy and inguinal lymphadenectomy through separate groin incisions. *Obstet Gynecol* 1981; **58**: 574–9.

3 Murdoch JB, Torbet TE. Carcinoma of the vulva. A ten year retrospective study in the West of Scotland (1972–1982). *Scot Med J* 1986; **31**: 166–9.

4 Scottish Office Home and Health Department. Report of the Study Group on the management of gynaecological services in Scotland. Edinburgh: HMSO, 1991.

5 Penny G, Kitchener HC, Templeton A. The management of carcinoma of the vulva: Current opinion and practice among consultant gynaecologists in Scotland. *Health Bull* 1995; **53**: 47–54

6 Messing MJ, Gallup DG. Carcinoma of the vulva in young women. *Obstet Gynecol* 1995; **86**: 51–4.

7 Kagie MJ, Kenter GG, Hermans J et al. The relevance of various vulvar epithelial changes in the early detection of squamous cell carcinoma of the vulva. *Int J Gynecol Cancer* 1997; **7**: 50–7.

8 Maclean AB, Reid WM. Benign and premalignant disease of the vulva. *Br J Obstet Gynaecol* 1995; **102**: 359–63.

9 Carli P, Cattaneo A, De Magnis A et al. Squamous cell carcinoma arising in vulval lichen sclerosus: a longitudinal cohort study. *Eur J Cancer Prev* 1995; **4**: 491–5.

10 Woodruff JD. Carcinoma in situ of the vulva. *Clin Obstet Gynecol* 1991; **34**: 669–76.

11 Singer A, Monaghan JM. Vulval intraepithelial neoplasia. In: *Lower genital tract precancer.* Boston: Blackwell Science, 1994: 177–226.

12 Jones RW, Rowan DM. Vulval intraepithelial neoplasia III: a clinical study of the outcome in 113 cases with relation to the later development of invasive vulvar carcinoma. *Obstet Gynecol* 1994; **84**: 741–5.

13 Kurzl R. Carcinoma of the vulva. In: *Surgical gynaecological oncology.* New York: Thième, 1993: **150**.

14 Herod JJO, Shafi MI, Rollason TP et al. Vulval intraepithelial neoplasia: long term follow up of treated and untreated women. *Br J Obstet Gynaecol* 1996; **103**: 446–52.

15 Herod JJO, Shafi MI, Rollason TP et al. Vulval intraepithelial neoplasia with superficially invasive carcinoma of the vulva. *Br J Obstet Gynaecol* 1996; **103**: 453–6.

16 Ogunbiyi OA, Scholefield JH, Robertson G et al. Anal human papillomavirus infection and squamous neoplasia in patients with vulvar cancer. *Obstet Gynecol* 1994; **83**: 212–16.

17 McCullough AM, Seywright M, Roberts DT, Maclean AB. Outpatient biopsy of the vulva. *J Obstet Gynaecol* 1987; **8**: 166–9.

18 Monaghan JM. Vulvar carcinoma: the case for individualization of treatment. *Baillieres Clin Obstet Gynaecol* 1987; **1**: 263–76.

19 Weiner SA, Lee JKT, Kao MS, Moon TE. The role of lymphangiography in vulvar carcinoma. *Am J Obstet Gynecol* 1986; **154**: 1073–5.

20 Levenback C, Burke TW, Morris M et al. Potential applications of intraoperative lymphatic mapping in vulvar cancer. *Gynecol Oncol* 1995; **59**: 216–20.

21 DeCesare SL, Fiorica JV, Roberts WS et al. A pilot study utilizing intraoperative lymphoscintigraphy for identification of the sentinel lymph nodes in vulvar cancer. *Gynecol Oncol* 1997; **66**: 425–8.

22 Makela PJ, Leminen A, Kaariainen, Lehtovirta P. Pretreatment sonographic evaluation of inguinal lymph nodes in patients with vulvar malignancy. *J Ultrasound Med* 1993; **5**: 255–8.

23 Piura B, Masotino A, Murdoch J et al. Recurrent squamous cell carcinoma of the vulva: a study of 73 cases. *Gynecol Oncol* 1993; **48**: 189–95.

24 Collins CG, Collins JH, Barclay DL, Nelson EW. Cancer involving the vulva. *Am J Obstet Gynecol* 1963; **87**: 762.

25 Homesley HD, Bundy BN, Sedlis A, Adcock L. Radiotherapy versus pelvic node resection for carcinoma of the vulva with positive groin nodes. *Obstet Gynecol* 1986; **68**: 733–40.

26 Shepherd JH. Cervical and vulva cancer: changes in

FIGO definitions of staging. *Br J Obstet Gynaecol* 1996; **103**: 405–6.

27 Morley GW. Infiltrative carcinoma of the vulva, results of surgical treatment. *Am J Obstet Gynecol* 1976; **124**: 874–88.

28 Way S. Surgery of vulval carcinoma: an appraisal. In: *Clinics in obstetrics and gynaecology*. London: WB Saunders, 1978: 623–8.

29 Benedet JL, Turko M Fairey RN, Boyes DA. Squamous carcinoma of the vulva: results of treatment, 1938 to 1976. *Am J Obstet Gynecol* 1979; **134**: 201–7.

30 Shanbour KA, Mannel RS, Morris PC et al. Comparison of clinical versus surgical staging systems in vulvar cancer. *Obstet Gynecol* 1992; **80**: 927–30.

31 DiSaia PJ, Creasman WT, Rich WM. An alternative approach to early cancer of the vulva. *Am J Obstet Gynecol* 1979; **133**: 825–30.

32 Stehman FB, Bundy BN, Dvoretsky PM, Creasman WT. Early stage 1 carcinoma of the vulva treated with ipsilateral superficial inguinal lymphadenectomy and modified radical hemivulvectomy: a prospective study of the Gynecological Oncology Group. *Obstet Gynecol* 1992; **79**: 490–7.

33 Cavanagh D. Vulvar cancer – continuing evolution in management. *Gynecol Oncol* 1997; **66**: 362–7.

34 Burke TW, Levenbach C, Coleman RL et al. Surgical therapy of T1 and T2 vulvar carcinoma: Further experience with radical wide excision and selective inguinal lymphadenectomy. *Gynecol Oncol* 1995; **57**: 215–20.

35 Ndubisi B, Kaminski PF, Olt G et al. Staging and recurrence of disease in squamous cell carcinoma of the vulva. *Gynecol Oncol* 1995; **59**: 34–7.

36 Burger MPM, Hollema H, Emanuels AG et al. The importance of the groin node status for the survival of T1 and T2 vulval carcinoma patients. *Gynecol Oncol* 1995; **57**: 327–34.

37 Murdoch JB. Management options in vulval cancer. *Contemp Rev Obstet Gynaecol* 1994; **6**: 142–6.

38 Rutledge FN, Mitchell MF, Munnsell MF et al. Prognostic indicators for invasive carcinoma of the vulva. *Gynecol Oncol* 1991; **42**: 239–44.

39 Boyce J, Fruchter RG, Kassambilides E et al. Prognostic factors in carcinoma of the vulva. *Gynecol Oncol* 1985; **20**: 364–77.

40 Wharton JT, Gallagher S, Rutledge FN. Microinvasive carcinoma of the vulva. *Am J Obstet Gynecol* 1974; **118**: 159–62.

41 Hacker NF, Van der Velden J. Conservative management of early vulvar cancer. *Cancer* 1993; **71**: 1673–7.

42 Sedlis A, Homesley H, Bundy BN et al. Positive groin lymph nodes in superficial squamous cell vulvar cancer. *Am J Obstet Gynecol* 1987; **156**: 1159–64.

43 Podczaski E, Sexton M, Kaminski P et al. Recurrent carcinoma of the vulva after conservative treatment for 'microinvasive' disease. *Gynecol Oncol* 1990; **39**: 65–8.

44 Van der Velden J, Kooyman CD, Van Lindert ACM, Heintz APM. A stage 1a vulvar carcinoma with an inguinal lymph node recurrence after local excision. A case report and literature review. *Int J Gynecol Cancer* 1992; **2**: 157–62.

45 Binder SW, Huang I, Fu YS et al. Risk factors for the development of lymph node metastasis in vulvar squamous cell carcinoma. *Gynecol Oncol* 1990; **37**: 9–16.

46 Rueda NG, Vighi S, Garcia A et al. Histologic predictive factors. Therapeutic impact in vulvar cancer. *J Reprod Med* 1994; **39**: 71–6.

47 Obermair A, Kohlberger P, Bancher-Todesca D et al. Influence of microvessel density and vascular permeability factor/vascular endothelial growth factor expression on prognosis in vulvar cancer. *Gynecol Oncol* 1996; **63**: 204–9.

48 Kirchner CV, Yordan EL, De Geest K, Wilbanks GD. Smoking, obesity, and survival in squamous cell carcinoma of the vulva. *Gynecol Oncol* 1995; **56**: 79–84.

49 Homesley HD. Management of vulvar cancer. *Cancer, Supplement* 1995; **76**: 2159–70.

50 Basset A. Traitment chiurgical operatoire de l'epithelioma primitif due clitoris indications-technique-resultats. *Rev Chir Orthop Reparatrice Appar Mort* 1912; **46**: 546.

51 Taussig FJ. Cancer of the vulva. An analysis of 155 cases (1911–1940). *Am J Obstet Gynecol* 1940; **40**: 764–79.

52 Way S. Carcinoma of the vulva. *Am J Obstet Gynecol* 1960; **79**: 692–8.

9

Surgery in the primary management of vulvar cancer

J VAN DER VELDEN

Although the role of surgery in the treatment of squamous cell cancer of the vulva has changed over the last 20 years, surgery still provides the basis for management. This role has evolved from a resection of the vulva *en bloc* with the groin lymph nodes in every patient, towards a more individualized approach, taking into account variables such as stage and other tumour characteristics. It is not just the high morbidity that has prompted many authors to question the need for a radical approach in every individual patient, it is also the realization that cosmesis and maintenance of sexual functions are important issues.

The results of clinical evaluations such as assessment of prognostic variables has made it possible to define low- and high- risk groups, providing the basis for less radical and thus less mutilating surgery in the group of patients with a low risk of recurrence.

The recent trend has been for less radical surgery, both for the primary tumour and for the groin nodes. This has been introduced as part of a multidisciplinary approach (i.e. together with radiotherapy), even in locoregionally more advanced tumours.

This chapter focuses on the various surgical techniques in the treatment of the primary tumour and the groin lymph nodes, and on the supporting evidence for their use. The results will be discussed in terms of both decreased morbidity and the impact the modifications have on survival.

TREATMENT OF THE PRIMARY TUMOUR

En bloc versus 'triple incision' technique

In the early years of the twentieth century, vulvar cancer was treated by local excision only. The lymph nodes in the groin were removed only for palliative reasons when they showed obvious metastases. Survival was not much better than 20 per cent.

From 1930 onwards, the primary tumour of the vulva has been removed by a radical vulvectomy *en bloc* with the lymph nodes in the groin. This procedure, using a single incision to excise the epidermis, dermis and fatty tissue overlying the vulvar and groin areas, ensured removal of the primary tumour and its draining lymph nodes, together with the afferent lymph channels that run from the primary tumour anteriorly and laterally to the inguinal and femoral lymph nodes in the groin. The removal of these lymph channels together with the primary tumour and the nodes was based on the theoretical concept of arrested migration of tumour emboli, which resulted in tumour nodules in the skin bridge between the vulva and its draining nodes. The *en bloc* procedure was first popularized by Way[1] and because of the high survival of 60 per cent it became the standard technique. However, at the same time, Taussig,[2] using a triple incision technique and not removing the skin bridge, obtained the same favourable results. Hacker and colleagues[3] were the first to show that, in a large set of patients with T1, T2 and T3 tumours, survival with this triple incision technique was equal to that in historical controls who had the *en bloc* removal of the tumour and the nodes. Moreover, they demonstrated that morbidity was very likely to decrease when this triple incision technique was used.[3] These data have subsequently been confirmed by others.

Morbidity has been shown to decrease substantially when separate groin incisions are used instead of the *en bloc* procedure. Most notably, the frequency of major wound breakdown is reduced by almost a half in the various series reported. The differences in absolute frequencies of, for example, wound breakdown in different papers is, however, striking. One study reports the frequency of all wound breakdowns decreasing from 34 per cent to 19 per cent when separate incisions are used[4] whereas another reports a decrease in wound breakdown from 64 per cent to 38 per cent after introduction of the triple incision technique.[5] It is tempting to speculate that these differences reflect a difference in technique, a difference in the definition of wound breakdown, patient selection or a combination of these factors.

Skin bridge recurrences are reported in 1–2 per cent of the patients treated by separate groin incisions (Table 9.1). It is important to note that these bridge recurrences are found in patients with positive nodes and, less frequently, in those with negative nodes. It is likely that, in patients with positive groin nodes, stasis of the lymph flow causes retrograde permeation and skin bridge recurrences.

One might therefore suggest that, when clinically suspicious groin nodes are present, the patient is better treated with a radical excision *en bloc* with the groin nodes. Some authors favour a nodal debulking of the groin followed by irradiation;[10] however, the intent of the latter strategy is to decrease early postoperative morbidity and possibly late lymphoedema. When a triple incision technique has been carried out and unsuspected micrometastases are found, the question posed is whether adjuvant radiotherapy is mandatory. It appears clear, from at least one controlled trial, that adjuvant radiotherapy in patients with a single microscopically positive node does not improve groin control.[11] There are no data on the efficacy of adjuvant radiotherapy in preventing bridge recurrences in these cases.

Separate groin incisions are considered to be the standard surgical technique for lateral and posterior T1, T2 and some T3 tumours with clinically non-suspicious groin lymph nodes. More anteriorly placed lesions are conveniently treated with an *en bloc* technique because of the close proximity of the primary to the skin bridge. Validation of the concept of nodal debulking of the groin, with the intention of lowering morbidity and to start postoperative radiotherapy as soon as possible, awaits further data.

Local excision versus total vulvectomy

There is one major factor to be considered when deciding whether to use either a radical vulvectomy or a radical local excision to treat the primary vulvar tumour: the status of the remainder of the vulva and/or the risk of multifocal invasive disease. If a unifocal lesion is present and the remainder of the vulva is healthy, a

Table 9.1 *The frequency of bridge recurrences in patients with vulvar cancer treated with the triple incision technique*

Reference	Bridge recurrence/ all patients	Bridge recurrence/ negative nodes	Bridge recurrence/ positive nodes
Hacker[3]	2/100 (2[a])	0/75	2/25
Helm[4]	0/32	0/28	0/4
Hopkins[5]	3/42 (1[a])	2/34	1/8
Hoffmann[6]	0/45	0/42	0/3
Grimshaw[7]	1/90 (1[a])	1/64	0/26
Siller[8]	0/27	0/21	0/6
Kohler[9]	3/105	0/52	3/53
Total	**9/441 (2%)**	**3/316 (1%)**	**6/125 (5%)**

[a] Patients dead of disease.

radical local excision is the treatment of choice. Obviously, the larger the lesion and the more of the vulva affected, the closer will local excision approximate to a radical vulvectomy. Multifocal lesions probably still justify a radical vulvectomy approach.

Although no randomized clinical trials have been carried out on this topic, it is clear from the collated retrospective literature that, in early stage vulvar cancer, the risk of local recurrence after a radical local excision is only slightly higher than that after a radical vulvectomy (7.2 per cent versus 6.3 per cent).[12] This does not, however, result in lower survival because local recurrences can be salvaged by re-excision in most cases.[13] In support of this, a prospective Gynecologiconcology Group (GOG) study, using historical controls for comparison, did not demonstrate reduced survival in relation to the extent of surgery, although local control with radical vulvectomy seemed slightly better (6.0 per cent versus 8.2 per cent local recurrences for radical vulvectomy and radical local excision respectively).[14]

When the remainder of the vulva is clinically normal, there is still a risk of occult multifocal disease and/or subepithelial growth of the primary tumour. Although vulvoscopy is recommended as a diagnostic aid in the detection of occult multifocal disease, no data are available to prove that vulvoscopy is better than careful clinical examination.

Occult microscopic invasive disease is most often restricted to the vicinity of the clinically apparent tumour.[15] This means that, when sufficient lateral clearance is obtained, the risk of local recurrence is minimized. A clinicopathological review of the data from one group indicated that local recurrence was unlikely with a tumour-free margin of at least 10 mm.[16]

When vulvar cancer arises in the presence of multifocal vulvar intraepithelial neoplasia (VIN) or maturation disorder, it may be difficult to diagnose occult invasive disease. The decision to use either a radical local excision or a radical vulvectomy, in this group of patients, should be based on the results of a biopsy mapping procedure and on the patient's age and wishes. Vulvoscopy may be of help in directing punch biopsies of the most abnormal areas.

When no multifocal invasive disease is found in the areas of VIN and/or maturation disorder, the primary tumour can be treated by a radical local excision, whereas the rest of the non-invasive abnormalities can be treated either by, for example, topical steroids in cases where the maturation disorder extends to the clitoral area or by superficial local excision, if required, in cases of VIN. In severely symptomatic elderly

women who have a long-standing history of pruritus, radical vulvectomy may be the most appropriate form of treatment. In younger patients, there may be reluctance to undergo this procedure and treatment should be individualized.

When necessary, the distal 10 mm of the urethra can be resected. It is a general belief, and also the author's personal experience, that urinary incontinence is not common after such a procedure. However, robust data are scant. Reid and colleagues[17] reported on four patients who all had more than 1 cm of the distal urethra removed as part of a radical vulvectomy. Two patients experienced total incontinence, whereas the other two developed stress incontinence. Others have reported that radical vulvectomy itself (without urethral compromise) gives rise to urinary incontinence in 15 per cent of patients, whereas this was seen in only 4 per cent after radical local excision.[6]

If it is accepted that the appropriate procedure for the primary lesion is largely determined by the status of the remaining vulva, the size of the lesion may seem of less importance. However, most of the data on the (low) risk of local recurrence after radical local excision compared with radical vulvectomy derive from studies on early vulvar cancer. Is the same true for vulvar tumours with diameters of more than 2 cm (T2 and most T3 tumours)?

In 1988, Burrell and colleagues[18] reported on 14 patients with International Federation of Gynaecology and Obstetrics (FIGO) stage II disease treated by less extensive surgery than radical vulvectomy. With various methods such as 'posterior or anterior bilateral vulvectomy', 'hemivulvectomy' or 'wide local excision', no recurrences were found after a follow-up ranging from 1 to 87 months.

The data presented in Table 9.2, indicate that the risk of local recurrence and/or death after radical local excision in patients with a T2/T3 tumour is very low (4 per cent of 115 cases), and is even lower than that reported for T1 tumours. One might initially conclude that, using the selection criteria employed by the various authors, radical local excision for T2 tumours is a safe procedure. However, it seems that there must have been a selection of favourable T2 cases, although two authors state that the tumour diameter exceeded 4 cm in more than 30 per cent of their patient material. As the selection criteria used by the various authors were imprecise and because randomized data are lacking, it is not possible to give firm recommendations with regard to the extent of radicality in T2/T3 tumours.

In general, radical local excision seems appropriate

Table 9.2 *Frequency of local recurrence after radical local excision for T2 and T3 squamous cell carcinoma of the vulva*

	Number of patients	Local recurrence		Died of disease
		No.	Percentage	
Burrel[18]	14	0	0	0
Hoffman[6]	18	1	6	0
Hacker[12]	8	0	0	0
Farias-Eisner[19]	23	2	9	2[a]
Andrews[20]	9	1	11	0
Burke[21]	43	1	2	0
Total	**115**	**5**	**4**	**2**

[a] The two patients who died of disease both died from distant metastases; it is not stated whether these patients also had a local recurrence.

for most T2 and T3 tumours, providing that the tumour is unifocal and the remainder of the vulva normal. As with T1 tumours, excision margins should clear the tumour by at least 10 mm and the dissection should extend down to the deep fascia (urogenital diaphragm). If the tumour encroaches on the urethral meatus, the same tumour-free margin of 10 mm must be taken into account.

TREATMENT OF THE REGIONAL LYMPH NODES

Bilateral inguinofemoral and pelvic lymph node dissection, carried out routinely on almost any patient some decades ago, has been replaced by a more individualized approach, taking into account size and localization of the tumour and the depth of infiltration. The status of the inguinofemoral nodes will usually determine the need for treatment of the pelvic lymph nodes.

This chapter addresses the issue of the extent of regional lymph node dissection.

Omission of the groin dissection

In the 1970s, several authors tried to define subsets of

patients who had T1 tumours with a depth of invasion of less than 5 mm and a very low risk of inguinal node metastases.[22–24] Omission of the inguinal lymphadenectomy was advised in such patients. However, cumulative experience has demonstrated a considerable risk of lymph node metastases in patients whose T1 tumour invaded more than 1 mm (Table 9.3). The occurrence of lymph node metastases in a unifocal T1 tumour with an infiltration depth of less than 1 mm is rare. Only two case reports have been published.[34,35]

Apparently the 1-mm cut-off point is important and determines the risk of the absence or possible presence of groin node metastases. Based on this observation, the nomenclature committee of the International Society for the Study of Vulvar Disease (ISSVD) has tried to reach consensus on how and what to measure. They recommend that the depth of invasion be measured from the most superficial dermal papilla adjacent to the tumour to the deepest focus of invasion.[36] Although many investigators have measured from the surface of the epithelium (tumour thickness), the average difference between tumour thickness and depth of invasion between these two methods was only 0.3 mm.[37] As a consequence, this means that a depth of invasion ranging from 0.7 mm to 1.3 mm is still a 'grey' area from which it is very difficult to calculate the risk of groin node metastases.

In a large GOG study presented by Sedlis and col-

Table 9.3 *Nodal status in T1 vulvar cancer in relation to depth of invasion (collated literature data[15, 25–33])*

Depth of invasion (mm)	Total number	Number of positive nodes	Percentage positive nodes
< 1	163	0	0
1.1–2	145	11	7.6
2.1–3	131	11	8.3
3.1–5	101	27	26.7
> 5	38	13	34.2
Total	**578**	**62**	**10.7**

leagues,[38] a low-risk group of patients was defined using multivariate analysis. Low-risk patients had N0 or N1 groin nodes, and tumours with no capillary-like space involvement. The tumour was either well or moderately differentiated with thickness of less than 2 mm. The observed frequency of positive nodes in this group was 0 (0 of 63) whereas the 95 per cent confidence limits were calculated to be between 0 and 3 per cent.

From these data, it is clear that, in patients with a tumour thickness of 1 mm or less, the groin dissection can be safely omitted. Omission of the groin dissection in other subgroups of patients with infiltration between 1 and 2 mm has to be balanced against a very small risk of groin node metastases.

A new development in the treatment of vulvar cancer is the identification of the sentinel lymph node in the groin. The concept is based on the fact that the first lymph node identified by, for example, technetium scanning is the sentinel lymph node. Mapping of the sentinel node is dealt with in more detail in Chapter 8.

Extent of groin dissection

The primary lymphatic drainage from the vulva is to two groups of lymph nodes in the groin. Efferent lymphatic channels drain mainly into the superficial (inguinal) lymph node group, situated along the medial half of the inguinal ligament and around the proximal long saphenous vein, particularly where it passes through the cribriform fascia. All of these nodes are situated above the superficial fascia. A second group of nodes, the deep (femoral) nodes, is situated below the level of the cribriform fascia along the femoral vein. This group consists of only two to four nodes.[39]

DiSaia and colleagues[40] suggested omission of the deep lymphadenectomy, with the intention of decreasing morbidity with no compromise in survival.[40] Recently, the same group reported on 50 patients, with a tumour of 2 cm diameter or less, no clinically suspicious groin nodes and negative superficial nodes on frozen section, in whom the deep groin node dissection had been omitted.[41] No groin recurrences were seen in this group, and the follow-up was longer than 12 months in 84 per cent of the patients.

In contrast, a prospective, uncontrolled GOG trial showed that a superficial inguinal node dissection in a very favourable subgroup of T1 patients resulted in a groin recurrence rate of 6 per cent.[14] Later, DiSaia explained their favourable results with the superficial

groin node dissection by the fact that, frequently, the medial part of the cribriform fascia and possibly deep lymph nodes were removed *en bloc* with the superficial node-containing fat pad.[42]

The GOG data are in line with those of Burke and colleagues, who found three groin recurrences (4 per cent) after a superficial groin dissection with negative nodes in 76 patients. Somewhat surprisingly, they concluded that 'any degree of groin failure is undesirable but a small percentage of node negative T1/T2 patients treated with superficial and deep lymphadenectomy also develop groin recurrences'.[21] When the collated literature was reviewed, only two of 236 T1 patients (<1 per cent) with negative groin nodes after superficial and deep groin dissection experienced a groin recurrence (Table 9.4). Moreover, in large individual series of early stage or locally advanced vulvar cancer, the risk of groin recurrence after an inguinal and femoral groin dissection was less than 1 per cent in node-negative cases.[13,44]

Although inguinal dissection with omission of the femoral dissection was introduced to decrease morbidity, even this potential benefit seems unproven. Lin and colleagues[45] (1992) showed (in a non-randomized study) that the frequency of complications related to the groin dissection, including lymphoedema, lymphocysts and wound dehiscence or infections, did not decrease with the omission of the deep groin dissection. They found lymphoedema in two of 16 patients (13 per cent) and five of 30 patients (17 per cent) after superficial and deep dissection versus superficial dissection alone. The same figures were found for the incidence of lymphocysts.

One can conclude only that a superficial groin dissection, as performed in the GOG study, results in an unacceptably high groin recurrence rate with no improvement in morbidity. At present, when a groin dissection is indicated, superficial inguinal and deep femoral groups of nodes should be removed.

This may seem straightforward, but there is still controversy regarding the extent of this dissection.

Table 9.4 *The influence of omission of the groin dissection on groin recurrence in T1N0–1 vulvar cancer*

Surgery	Groin recurrence/total (%)
No groin dissection	10/107 (9.3)
Groin dissection (positive nodes)	3/28 (10.7)
Groin dissection (negative nodes)	2/236 (0.8)

From the literature.[15,26,27,31,43]

What does superficial and deep groin dissection mean? How much lymph node-bearing fat must be removed in a cranial and caudal direction, in a medial and lateral direction and last, but not least, what should be the deep margin of dissection?

Unfortunately, few clinical data are available to clarify this issue, and it can be addressed only by combining the scant clinical data with topographical anatomical data.

Recently, an interesting paper was published by Levenback and colleagues[46] regarding a survey of the current surgical practices of gynaecological oncologists treating patients with early vulvar cancer. Three different drawings of a groin dissection, each showing a different deep margin of dissection, were presented (Figs 9.1–9.3), and respondents were asked to give a name to the procedure. Figure 9.2 presents Scarpa's triangle after removal of superficial inguinal and lymph nodes medial to the femoral vein, with meticulous conservation of the fascia lata but removal of the medial part of the cribriform fascia, skeletonizing only a minimal part of the femoral vein. This was termed 'superficial inguinal lymphadenectomy' by 24 per cent of respondents.

With these results in mind, the high groin recurrence rate in the GOG study on 'superficial groin dissection' is even more worrisome. It must be suspected that some patients with groin recurrences have been treated by a method depicted in Fig. 9.2. Therefore the safest procedure regarding the deep margin of dissection seems to be that depicted in Fig. 9.3.

A modification of the lateral and medial extent of the groin dissection was presented by Nicklin and colleagues.[47] In a retrospective study, they analysed lymphangiograms of patients with vulvar and cervical cancer, with the intention of defining the most lateral inguinal node relative to the anterosuperior iliac spine. They calculated that by leaving 15 per cent of the fatty tissue overlying the lateral part of the inguinal ligament and 20 per cent over the medial part, the chance of complete nodal clearance was 99.8 per cent. Theoretically, this approach of conserving possible lymph channel-bearing fatty tissue should decrease morbidity, but this has not been evaluated prospectively.

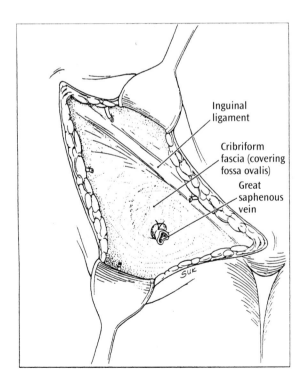

Figure 9.1 *Appearance of Scarpa's triangle after removal of superficial inguinal lymph nodes. (Reprinted with permission from Levenback et al.[46])*

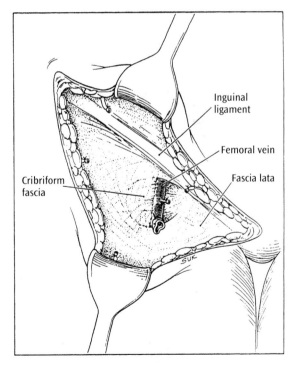

Figure 9.2 *Appearance of Scarpa's triangle after removal of superficial inguinal and medial femoral lymph nodes. (Reprinted with permission from Levenback et al.[46])*

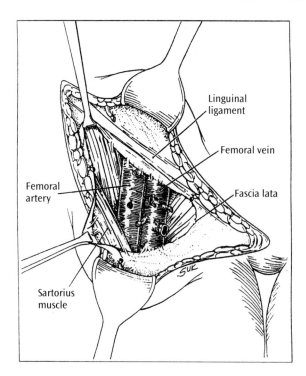

Figure 9.3 *Appearance of Scarpa's triangle after removal of superficial inguinal and femoral lymph nodes. (Reprinted with permission from Levenback et al.[46])*

Preservation of the saphenous vein may be of importance in patients with no varicose veins in order to prevent venous stasis. The few papers addressing this issue do not, however, provide evidence of benefit. Lin and colleagues[45] reported that leg oedema occurred in six of 36 patients (17 per cent) who had preservation of the long saphenous vein versus five of 40 (13 per cent) in whom the vein was sacrificed.[45] This was confirmed by Hopkins and colleagues,[48] who presented data on 17 patients in whom the saphenous vein was preserved. Paley and colleagues[49] recently presented data showing that lymphoedema occurred in 36 per cent of patients who had preservation of the saphenous vein, compared with 21 per cent in whom the vessel was removed. These data suggest that sacrificing the saphenous vein does not increase morbidity, so the vein should be removed *en bloc* with the lymph node-bearing, surrounding fatty tissue.

Other means of reducing morbidity after a groin dissection includes the so-called sartorius muscle transposition or covering the vessels with dura film. The latter method has not been proved to reduce groin morbidity.[50] Sartorius muscle transposition was popularized by vascular surgeons, creating a protective barrier against infection after arterial reconstructive surgery. Transposition of the sartorius muscle to cover the inguinal vessels has been widely used to protect the vessels from erosion and even rupture of the artery, in the event of wound dehiscence after infection. Total wound dehiscence and infection were common after *en bloc* resection, so the introduction of the separate incision technique, with a resultant reduction in wound dehiscence and infections, reduced the need for this technique. Way[51] published a paper on five patients with vessel rupture (three patients died) before he started to perform sartorius muscle transposition. No further vessel ruptures occurred after adopting the transposition procedure.[51]

Evidence for a negative or positive impact of this procedure on groin infections has only recently become available. Paley and colleagues[49] reported on the effect of this procedure on wound morbidity after the triple incision technique. Surprisingly, they reported an increase in wound breakdown and/or cellulitis in the group of patients in whom the sartorius muscle transposition was omitted, compared with historical controls in whom the procedure had been carried out (66 per cent versus 41 per cent). Moreover, in a multivariate analysis, only weight (< 68 kg) and sartorius muscle transposition were independently associated with a reduction in groin morbidity.

The conclusion must be that, although the sartorius muscle transposition has waned in popularity over the last decade, the available data suggest possible advantages and its re-introduction should be considered.

Omission of contralateral groin dissection in unilateral tumours

The work of Iversen and Aas[52] has indicated that the lymph flow from the vulva is predominantly ipsilateral for unilateral lesions, whereas midline lesions drain bilaterally. However, they also showed that significant bilateral flow occurred from the anterior labium minus. The observation by Magrina and colleagues is in agreement with this;[26] they found contralateral groin node metastases in two of 77 patients who had unilateral T1 tumours and negative ipsilateral nodes. Both patients had a unilateral tumour on the labium minus. A collection of retrospective data shows that the risk of contralateral groin metastases in unilateral T1 tumours with negative ipsilateral nodes is very low (Table 9.5).

One should, however, remember that all these patients had a bilateral groin dissection. Way[51] showed

Table 9.5 *Incidence of positive contralateral nodes in patients with lateral T1 squamous cell cancer of the vulva, who all had a bilateral inguinal node dissection with negative ipsilateral nodes*

Reference	Unilateral lesions	Contralateral nodes positive (%)[a]
Wharton[23]	25	0 (0)
Parker[25]	41	0 (0)
Magrina[26]	77	2 (2.6)
Iversen[27]	112	0 (0)
Hoffman[29]	70	0 (0)
Hacker[31]	60	0 (0)
Struijk[33]	53	0 (0)
Buscema[43]	38	0 (0)
Total	**476**	**2 (0.4)**

[a] Numbers in parentheses are the percentage.

Table 9.6 *Contralateral groin node metastases in patients with lateral T1 squamous cell cancer of the vulva, who had omission of the contralateral inguinal node dissection with negative ipsilateral nodes*

Reference	Unilateral lesions	Contralateral groin metastases (%)[a]
Lin[45]	14	1
Stehman[14]	107	3
Hoffman[6]	6	0
Tham[53]	7	0
Andrews[20]	19	0
Farias-Eisner[19]	6	0
Burke[21]	33	1
Total	**192**	**5 (2.6)**

[a] The number in parentheses is the percentage.

that, in doing more sections of blocks of tissue originating from the groin, previously unrecognized micrometastases were occasionally found. This suggests that evidence for the true safety of omission of the contralateral groin dissection can derive only from prospective data, when the contralateral groin dissection is really omitted. Only 192 patients with a unilateral T1 tumour, all treated by an ipsilateral groin dissection only, have been described in seven different papers (Table 9.6). Most of these patients had favourable tumour characteristics such as invasion of less than 5 mm and/or absence of vascular space invasion and/or well-differentiated tumours. Five patients (2.6 per cent) developed a metastasis in the undissected contralateral groin. Importantly 'only' two of the five patients in this small series died from their recurrence. In other larger collated series, a groin recurrence in an undissected groin carries a mortality rate of 90 per cent.[10]

Unfortunately, the exact location of the tumours in the five patients was not reported. It would be of interest to know whether these tumours were situated at the labia minora because both the imaging studies and the retrospective data suggest that tumours on the anterior aspect of the labia minora show contralateral lymph flow. One might therefore advise, at least until more data become available, that all tumours within 1 cm of the introitus be regarded as midline tumours.

The less favourable results of prospective data compared with retrospective data (2.6 per cent versus 0.4 per cent contralateral groin metastases), together with the patient groups from the prospective studies representing favourable subgroups, indicate a possibly greater risk of contralateral groin metastases in the group of patients with unilateral T1 tumours not selected on favourable prognostic variables. There is definitely a need for another prospective study including all patients with T1 tumours.

The risk of dying from a contralateral groin recurrence in small (T1) unilateral vulvar cancers is very low. This means that the benefit of omitting a groin dissection on one side seems to outweigh the 'costs'. Frequent follow-up and careful examination of the undissected groin remain mandatory in these patients.

ROLE FOR PELVIC NODE DISSECTION

In the past, pelvic lymphadenectomy was an integral part of the treatment of vulvar cancer. However, a review of published experiences reveals that only 2 per cent of patients with the old FIGO stage I and II[54] had pelvic lymph node metastases. In stages III and IV, 29 per cent and 75 per cent of patients, respectively, have positive pelvic nodes (Table 9.7).

Even in advanced disease, pelvic node dissection should not be recommended as routine because pelvic nodal involvement is seen only in the presence of positive inguinal nodes. Controversy exists regarding the correlation between the number of positive inguinal nodes and the risk of subsequent positive pelvic nodes. Curry and colleagues[56] did not find positive pelvic nodes unless four or more positive inguinal nodes were found, whereas Hacker and colleagues[57] and Podratz and colleagues[58] reported positive pelvic nodes only when three or more inguinal nodes were involved. Homesley and colleagues,[59] however, in the only available prospective study on this subject, report

Table 9.7 *Pelvic lymph node involvement in relation to old FIGO stage*

Stage	Number/total (%)[a]	Range (%)
I	3/158 (2)	0–8
II	1/60 (2)	0–8
III	15/52 (29)	22–39
IV	9/12 (75)	50–100

[a] Numbers in parentheses are the percentages.
From the literature.[15, 25–27,55,57]

a frequency of 14 per cent (two of 14) positive pelvic nodes with only one (N0–N1) positive groin node and a frequency of 45 per cent (10 of 22 patients) with two or more N2–N3 positive inguinal nodes. The risk of positive pelvic nodes is thus clearly related to the number of positive inguinal nodes and the clinical status of these nodes.

Recently several papers have been published on capsular breakthrough of the inguinal nodes as an adverse prognostic variable.[60–63] As shown in Fig. 9.4, this phenomenon is associated with a dramatic decrease in survival.

The results were strikingly similar in all of these studies. In a multivariate analysis, capsule breakthrough of the inguinal nodes proved to be the strongest independent prognostic variable for survival, in two of three studies. This means that, even in patients with a single microscopically positive node and capsule breakthrough, survival is compromised. Whether pelvic failures are a substantial part of the failures remains unclear. None of the forementioned papers addresses the issue of pelvic node metastases in relation to extracapsular growth.

The current consensus, based on the available data, is that treatment for the pelvic nodes is required when:

- two or more inguinofemoral nodes are found to be positive
- capsular breakthrough has occurred in any groin node
- there is cytological or histological confirmation of malignancy in a clinically suspicious groin node.

A randomized GOG study concluded that the addition of adjunctive groin and pelvic radiotherapy after radical vulvectomy and inguinal lymphadenectomy proved superior to pelvic node resection in patients with positive groin nodes.[59] On the basis of the recurrence pattern in both treatment arms, it was clear that the survival benefit was not caused by better pelvic control in the group of patients who received adjunctive radiotherapy (6.8 per cent pelvic recurrences after radiotherapy versus 1.8 per cent pelvic recurrences after pelvic node dissection). This was largely as a result of better inguinal control in the group of patients who had a radical vulvectomy, inguinal node dissection and adjuvant groin radiation with adjunctive pelvic radiation.

One can conclude from this randomized study that pelvic radiation does not seem to result in better pelvic control compared with pelvic node dissection. Taking into account the slightly higher frequency of pelvic recurrences after radiotherapy alone, probably caused by bulky nodes that could not be sterilized by this treatment, pelvic node debulking should be considered when enlarged pelvic nodes are found on computed tomography (CT) scan. When enlarged groin nodes are found and confirmed as malignant by frozen section, the horizontal groin incision can be extended above the inguinal ligament, allowing an extraperitoneal pelvic node resection to be performed which removes only enlarged nodes. Adjuvant radiation to the groin and pelvis is then warranted.

The validity of such a proposal can be tested only in a randomized study. This study should randomize patients with enlarged pelvic nodes on CT scan or patients with multiple positive inguinal nodes into either a group in which only adjuvant inguinal and adjunctive pelvic radiation is administered or a group in which pelvic nodal debulking is followed by adjuvant inguinal and pelvic irradiation.

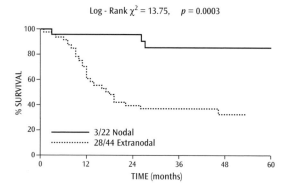

Log - Rank $\chi^2 = 13.75$, $p = 0.0003$

— 3/22 Nodal
········· 28/44 Extranodal

Figure 9.4 *Survival estimate according to extranodal spread in patients with vulvar cancer (numbers on the figure mean patients dead from disease versus total number of patients). (Reprinted with permission from van der Velden et al.[62])*

SURGERY AS A PLANNED PART OF MULTIDISCIPLINARY MANAGEMENT

The treatment of locally advanced vulvar cancer with a combination of radiotherapy, chemotherapy or both with surgery should ideally result in less radical surgery, less morbidity and uncompromised survival. As yet there are no results of controlled studies indicating that this combined modality treatment offers advantages over surgery alone. However, there is evidence from uncontrolled retrospective studies that combination treatment does decrease morbidity and indeed results in 'acceptable' survival. In Table 9.8, the results of seven studies on the combination of radiotherapy and surgery are summarized.

In these seven studies, the radiation dose varies from 36 Gy to 55 Gy and the type of surgery varies from local excision to radical vulvectomy with inguinal and pelvic node dissection. The problem in interpreting the data is that there is no definition of 'locally advanced vulvar cancer', which means that patient groups in the different studies are very heterogeneous. This is best reflected by the differences in survival rates of from 25 per cent[67] to 89 per cent.[69]

The lack of definition of locally advanced vulvar cancer also makes it difficult to interpret the possible benefits of the combined modality treatment. Does 'locally advanced' mean involvement of the proximal urethra or anal mucosa, necessitating colostomy formation, or does it mean large tumours encroaching on to the urethra, the anus or the vagina? Or does it mean

'large tumour'? Only Hacker and colleagues[65] and Rotmensch and colleagues[68] attempt a classification. They defined locally advanced as those cases that would have required a colostomy in order to achieve surgical clearance. Using this definition, Hacker and colleagues[65] avoided colostomies in all seven patients and Rotmensch and colleagues[68] in 10 of 16. Moore and colleagues treated 71 patients with T3/T4 vulvar cancers with preoperative chemoradition and surgery. They stated that initially 50 of the 71 patients required exenterative surgery. After preoperative chemoradiation only 1 of 50 patients required an exenteration and another 2 patients required a colostomy.[71]

In most studies, radiotherapy was administered before surgery. This seems logical where the intention is to avoid stoma formation. However, this then poses the question of appropriate management of the locoregional nodes. There are several possibilities. Primary radiotherapy to the vulvar tumour can be extended with an inguinal and pelvic field, and surgery entails a radical local excision and an inguinofemoral lymph node dissection. Assuming that half of the patients will not have lymph node metastases, this will result in considerable overtreatment (and extra morbidity) for this group of patients. This was the policy adopted in most retrospective studies.

To avoid overtreatment, one can elect to give radiotherapy to the primary tumour first and then perform an inguinal node dissection (with or without a pelvic node dissection) after radiotherapy. Adjuvant inguinal and pelvic radiotherapy can be administered in node-positive cases. The disadvantage of such a

Table 9.8 *Results of combined radiotherapy and surgery for locally advanced vulvar cancer*

Reference	Number	Radiotherapy field	Radiotherapy dose (GY)	Surgery	Residual tumour (%)	Survival rate (%)	Local recurrence (%)	Colostomy
Acosta[64]	14	P + N	36–55	RV + N	70	62	NK	2
Hacker[65]	7	P + N	44–54	RLE + (N)	40	62	14	0
Boronow[66]	37	NK	45–50	RLE + (N)	57	76	14	4
Carson[67]	8	P + N	45–50[a]	RLE[b]	25	25	NK	0
Rotmensch[68]	16	P + N	45	RV + N	85	45	25	6
Wahlen[69]	19	P + N	45–50[a]	RLE	47	89	37	2
Lupi[70]	24	P + N	36[a]	RV + N	67	55	21	0
Moore[71]	71	P + M[c]	47	RLE + N	69	55	16	3

[a] Chemoradiotherapy.
[b] Five out of eight patients had an inguinofemoral lymphadenectomy before radiotherapy.
P, radiotherapy towards primary; N, radiotherapy towards regional lymph nodes; NK, no data available; in the surgery column: RV, radical vulvectomy; N, lymph node dissection; (N), some patients also without lymph node dissection; RLE, radical local excision.
[c] Only patients with N2/N3 nodes received radiotherapy in the groin and pelvis.

policy is the 6- to 8-week delay in treating the regional nodes. This may result in the development of clinically suspicious nodes.[65]

A third possibility is to perform the groin, and if necessary the pelvic, node dissection first followed by radiotherapy to the primary tumour. The advantage is that, depending on the status of the lymph nodes, primary radiotherapy to the tumour can be combined with adjuvant radiotherapy to the groin and pelvis in selected patients. The delay in treating the primary is only 3–4 weeks. Although this seems a very logical sequence of treatments, only one author mentions such a policy.[67]

Another option is treating the primary tumour and the lymph nodes with radiotherapy, followed by a local excision only. The lymph nodes are not surgically treated in these cases. This policy could be criticized based on two studies. First, a randomized study of the treatment of groin nodes with either radiotherapy or surgery (GOG 88) was closed prematurely because of an excessive number of groin recurrences in the radiotherapy arm.[72] A weakness of this study was that the radiation was focused at a fixed depth of 3 cm[73] (femoral nodes) whereas Koh and colleagues[74] demonstrated by CT scan that the mean depth of the femoral nodes was 6.1 cm dependent upon the body mass index (BMI). This suggests that the depth of radiation may well have been insufficient to sterilize deeper groin nodes in obese patients. In a second, but uncontrolled, study, Manavi and colleagues[75] reported that even with proper primary radiotherapy to the inguinal region (45 Gy at a depth of 5 cm), a 5 per cent inguinal recurrence rate was seen in patients with T1N0–1 tumours (including 17 very low-risk patients with less than 2 mm of invasion). In a large individual series, this risk was about 1 per cent after inguinal lymph node dissection in similar patients.[44]

For these reasons, lymphadenectomy still remains the standard treatment for the groin nodes, even in patients whose primary tumour is treated by radiotherapy. The use of radiotherapy as sole treatment for the groins must be limited to patients who are medically unfit to withstand surgery.

In contrast to neoadjuvant radiotherapy, neadjuvant chemotherapy has not been seriously investigated until recently. In 1990, study by the EORTC (European Organization for Research and Treatment of Cancer) demonstrated that a combination of bleomycin, methotrexate and lomustine given to patients with 'advanced inoperable squamous cell cancer of the vulva' resulted in a reponse rate of 64 per cent.[76] Of the 35 inoperable patients, seven became operable. Severe mucositis was, however, seen in 21 per cent of patients, whereas severe infections occurred in 15 per cent of patients. Haematological toxicity was also severe. One patient died from pulmonary fibrosis (bleomycin related) and one patient from myelosuppression. The severe toxicity of this combination resulted in a waning popularity for neoadjuvant chemotherapy. More recently, experience with a combination of 5-fluorouracil and mitomycin C as neoadjuvant chemotherapy was published in a small number of patients (n = 10) with advanced vulvar cancer.[77] Seven patients (70 per cent) responded, with two patients demonstrating a complete response. No complications as a result of this regimen were seen. These preliminary data are promising and warrant further investigation, particularly as a neoadjuvant with surgery.

REFERENCESS

1 Way S. The anatomy of the lymphatic drainage of the vulva and its influence on the radical operation. *Ann R Coll Surg Engl* 1948; **3**: 1159–64.

2 Taussig FJ. Cancer of the vulva: An analysis of 155 cases (1911–1940). *Am J Obstet Gynecol* 1949; **40**: 764–79.

3 Hacker NF, Leuchter RS, Berek JS, Castaldo TW, Lagasse LD. Radical vulvectomy and bilateral inguinal lymphadenectomy through separate groin incisions. *Obstet Gynecol* 1981; **58**: 574–9.

4 Helm CW, Hatch K, Austin JM et al. A matched comparison of single and triple incision techniques for the surgical treatment of carcinoma of the vulva. *Gynecol Oncol* 1992; **46**: 150–6.

5 Hopkins MP, Reid GC, Morley GW. Radical vulvectomy, The decision for the incision. *Cancer* 1993; **72**: 799–803.

6 Hoffman MS, Roberts WS, Finan MA et al. A comparative study of radical vulvectomy and modified radical vulvectomy for the treatment of invasive squamous cell carcinoma of the vulva. *Gynecol Oncol* 1992; **45**: 192–7.

7 Grimshaw RN, Murdoch JB, Monaghan JM. Radical vulvectomy and bilateral inguinal-femoral lymphadenectomy through separate incisions – experience with 100 cases. *Int J Gynecol Cancer* 1993; **3**: 18–23.

8 Siller BS, Alvarez RD, Conner WD et al. T2/T3 vulva cancer: a case control study of triple incision versus en bloc radical vulvectomy and inguinal lymphadenectomy. *Gynecol Oncol* 1995; **57**: 335–9.

9 Kohler U, Schone M, Pawlowitsch T. Ergebnisse einer individualizierten operatieven therapie des vulvakarzinoms von 1973 bis 1993. *Z Gynakol* 1997; **119**: 8–16.

10 Hacker NF. Vulvar cancer. In: Berek JS, Hacker NF (eds). *Practical gynecologic oncology*. Baltimore: Williams and Wilkins, 1989.

11 Homesley HD, Bundy BN, Sedlis A, Adcock L. Radiation therapy versus pelvic node resection for carcinoma of the vulva with positive groin nodes. *Obstet Gynecol* 1986; **68**: 733–40.

12 Hacker NF, van der Velden J. Conservative management of early vulvar cancer. *Cancer* 1993; **71**: 1673–7.

13 Podratz KC, Symmonds RE, Taylor WF. Carcinoma of the vulva: analysis of treatment failures. *Am J Obstet Gynecol* 1982; **143**: 340–7.

14 Stehman FB, Bundy BN, Dvoretsky PM, Creasman WT. Early stage 1 carcinoma of the vulva treated with ipsilateral superficial inguinal lymphadenectomy and modified radical hemivulvectomy: A prospective study of the Gynaecologic Oncology Group. *Obstet Gynecol* 1992; **79**: 490–7.

15 Ross M, Ehrmann RL. Histologic prognosticators in stage I squamous cell carcinoma of the vulva. *Obstet Gynecol* 1987; **70**: 774–84.

16 Heaps JM, Fu YS, Montz FJ, Hacker NF, Berek JS. Surgical pathological variables predictive of local recurrence in squamous cell carcinoma of the vulva. *Gynecol Oncol* 1990; **38**: 309–14.

17 Reid GC, Delancy JO, Hopkins MP, Roberts JA, Morley GW. Urinary incontinence following radical vulvectomy. *Obstet Gynecol* 1990; **75**: 852–8.

18 Burrell MO, Franklin EW, Campion MJ, Crozier MA, Stacy DW. The modified radical vulvectomy with groin dissection: an eight year experience. *Am J Obstet Gynecol* 1988; **159**: 715–22.

19 Farias-Eisner R, Cirisano FD, Grouse D et al. Conservative and individualized surgery for early squamous carcinoma of the vulva: the treatment of choice for stage I and II (T1–2N0–1M0) disease. *Gynecol Oncol* 1994; **53**: 55–8.

20 Andrews SJ, Williams BT, DePriest PD et al. Therapeutic implications of lymph nodal spread in lateral T1 and T2 squamous cell carcinoma of the vulva. *Gynecol Oncol* 1994; **55**: 41–6.

21 Burke TW, Levenback C, Coleman RL, Morris M, Silva EG, Gershenson DM. Surgical therapy of T1 and T2 vulvar carcinoma; further experience with radical wide excision and selective inguinal lymphadenectomy. *Gynecol Oncol* 1995; **57**: 215–20.

22 Rutledge F, Smith PJ, Franklin EW. Carcinoma of the vulva. *Am J Obstet Gynecol* 1970; **106**: 1117–30.

23 Wharton JT, Gallager S, Rutledge FN. Microinvasive carcinoma of the vulva. *Am J Obstet Gynecol* 1974; **118**: 159–62.

24 Kunschner A, Kanbour AL, David B. Early vulvar carcinoma. *Am J Obstet Gynecol* 1978; **132**: 599–606.

25 Parker RT, Duncan I, Rampone J, Creasman W. Operative management of early epidermoid carcinoma of the vulva. *Am J Obstet Gynecol* 1975; **123**: 349–55.

26 Magrina JF, Webb MJ, Gaffey TA, Symmonds RE. Stage I squamous cell cancer of the vulva. *Am J Obstet Gynecol* 1979; **134**: 453–9.

27 Iversen T, Abeler V, Aalders J. Individualized treatment of stage I carcinoma of the vulva. *Obstet Gynecol* 1981; **57**: 85–9.

28 Wilkinson EJ, Rico MJ, Pierson KK. Microinvasive carcinoma of the vulva. *Int J Gynecol Pathol* 1982; **1**: 29–39.

29 Hoffman JS, Kumar NB, Morley GW. Microinvasive squamous carcinoma of the vulva: search for a definition. *Obstet Gynecol* 1983; **61**: 615–18.

30 Boice CR, Seraj IM, Thrasher T, King A. Microinvasive squamous carcinoma of the vulva: present status and reassessment. *Gynecol Oncol* 1984; **18**: 71–6.

31 Hacker NF, Berek JS, Lagasse LD, Nieberg RK, Leuchter RS. Individualization of treatment for stage I squamous cell vulvar carcinoma. *Obstet Gynecol* 1984; **63**: 155–62.

32 Rowley K, Gallion HH, Donaldson ES et al. Prognostic factors in early vulvar cancer. *Gynecol Oncol* 1988; **31**: 43–9.

33 Struijk APHB, Bouma JJ, van Lindert ACM et al. Early stage cancer of the vulva. A pilot investigation on cancer of the vulva in gynecologic oncology centers in the Netherlands. In: *Book of abstracts, second meeting of the International Gynecologic Cancer Society*. Toronto: Blackwell Science, 1989: 303.

34 Atamtede F, Hoogerland D. Regional lymph node recurrence following local excision for microinvasive vulvar carcinoma. *Gynecol Oncol* 1989; **34**: 128–9.

35 Van der Velden J, Kooyman CD, van Lindert ACM, Heintz APM. A stage IA vulvar carcinoma with an inguinal lymph node recurrence after local excision. A case report and literature review. *Int J Gynecol Cancer* 1992; **2**: 157–9.

36 Kneale BL. Announcement. *Gynecol Oncol* 1984; **18**: 134.

37 Fu YS, Reagan JW. Benign and malignant epithelial tumours of the vulva. In: Fu YS, Reagan JW (eds). *Pathology of the uterine cervix, vagina and vulva*. Philadelphia: WB Saunders, 1989: 138–92.

38 Sedlis A, Homesley H, Bundy BN et al. Positive groin lymph nodes in superficial squamous cell vulvar cancer. A Gynecologic Oncology Group study. *Am J Obstet Gynecol* 1987; **156**: 1159–64.

39 Borgno G, Micheletti L, Barbero M et al. Topographic distribution of groin lymph nodes. A study of 50 female cadavers. *J Reprod Med* 1990; **35**: 1127–9.

40 DiSaia PJ, Creasman WT, Rich WM. An alternative approach to early cancer of the vulva. *Am J Obstet Gynecol* 1979; **133**: 825–32.

41 Berman ML, Soper JT, Creasman WT, Olt GT, DiSaia PJ. Conservative surgical management of superficially invasive stage I vulvar carcinoma. *Gynecol Oncol* 1989; **35**: 352–7.

42 DiSaia PJ, Hacker NF. Is superficial inguinal lymphadenectomy sufficient for treatment of early vulvar cancer? In: *Proceedings*, Annual Meeting of the Society of Gynecologic Oncologists, San Francisco, USA, 1995: 17.

43 Buscema J, Stern JL, Woodruff JD. Early invasive carcinoma of the vulva. *Am J Obstet Gynecol* 1981; **140**: 563–9.

44 Iversen T, Aalders JG, Christensen A, Kolstad P. Squamous cell carcinoma of the vulva: a review of 424 patients, 1956–1974. *Gynecol Oncol* 1980; **9**: 271–9.

45 Lin JY, DuBeshter B, Angel C, Dvoretsky PM. Morbidity and recurrence with modifications of radical vulvectomy and groin dissection. *Gynecol Oncol* 1992; **47**: 80–6.

46 Levenback C, Morris M, Burke TW, Gershenson DM, Wolf JK, Wharton JT. Groin dissection practices among gynecologic oncologists treating early vulvar cancer. *Gynecol Oncol* 1996; **62**: 73–7.

47 Nicklin JL, Hacker NF, Heintze SW, van Eijkeren M, Durham NJ. An anatomical study of inguinal lymph node topography and clinical implications for the surgical managment of vulval cancer. *Int J Gynecol Cancer* 1995; **5**: 128–33.

48 Hopkins MP, Reid CC, Vettrano I, Morley GW. Squamous cell carcinoma of the vulva: prognostic factors influencing survival. *Gynecol Oncol* 1990; **43**: 113–17.

49 Paley PJ, Johnson PR, Adcock LL et al. The effect of sartorius transposition on wound morbidity following inguinal femoral lymphadenectomy. *Gynecol Oncol* 1997; **64**: 237–41.

50 Finan MA, Fiorica JV, Roberts WS et al. Artificial dura film for femoral vessel coverage after inguinofemoral lymphadenectomy. *Gynecol Oncol* 1994; **55**: 333–5.

51 Way S. *Malignant disease of the vulva*. Edinburgh: Churchill Livingstone, 1982.

52 Iversen T, Aas M. Lymph drainage from the vulva. *Gynecol Oncol* 1983; **16**: 179–89.

53 Tham KF, Shepherd JH, Lowe DG, Hudson CN, van Dam PA. Early vulvar cancer: the place of conservative management. *Eur J Surg Oncol* 1993; **19**: 361–7.

54 Classification and staging of malignant tumours in the female pelvis. *Acta Obstet Gynecol Scand* 1971; **50**: 1–7.

55 Boyce J, Fruchter RG, Kasambilides E, Nicastri AD, Sedlis A, Remy JC. Prognostic factors in carcinoma of the vulva. *Gynecol Oncol* 1985; **20**: 364–77.

56 Curry SL, Wharton JT, Rutledge F. Positive lymph nodes in vulvar squamous carcinoma. *Gynecol Oncol* 1980; **9**: 63–7.

57 Hacker NF, Berek JS, Lagasse LD, Leuchter RS, Moore JG. Management of regional lymph nodes and their prognostic influence in vulvar cancer. *Obstet Gynecol* 1983; **61**: 408–12.

58 Podratz KC, Symmonds RE, Taylor WF, Williams TJ. Carcinoma of the vulva: analysis of treatment and survival. *Obstet Gynecol* 1983; **61**: 63–74.

59 Homesley H, Bundy BN, Sedlis A, Adcock L. Radiation therapy versus pelvic node resection for carcinoma of the vulva with positive groin nodes. *Obstet Gynecol* 1986; **68**: 733–40.

60 Origoni M, Sideri M, Garsia S, Carinelli SG, Ferrari AG. Prognostic value of pathological patterns of lymph node positivity in squamous cell carcinoma of the vulva stage III and IVA FIGO. *Gynecol Oncol* 1992; **45**: 313–16.

61 Paladini D, Cross P, Lopes A, Monaghan JM. Prognostic significance of lymph node variables in squamous cell cancer of the vulva. *Cancer* 1994; **74**: 2491–6.

62 van der Velden J, van Lindert ACM, Lammes FB et al. Extracapsular growth of lymph node metastases in squamous cell cancer of the vulva, the impact on recurrence and survival. *Cancer* 1995; **75**: 2885–90.

63 Burger MPM, Hollema H, Emanuels AG, Krans M, Pras E, Bouma J. The importance of the groin node status for the survival of T1 and T2 vulvar carcinoma patients. *Gynecol Oncol* 1995; **57**: 327–34.

64 Acosta AA, Given FT, Frazier AB, Cordoba RB, Luninari A. Preoperative radiation therapy in the management of squamous cell carcinoma of the vulva: preliminary report. *Am J Obstet Gynecol* 1978; **132**: 198–206.

65 Hacker NF, Berek JS, Juillard JF, Lagasse LD. Preoperative radiotherapy for locally advanced vulvar cancer. *Cancer* 1984; **54**: 2056–61.

66 Boronow RC, Hickman BT, Reagan MT, Smith A, Steadman RE. Combined therapy as an alternative to exenteration for locally advanced vulvovaginal cancer. *Am J Clin Oncol* 1987; **10**: 171–81.

67 Carson LF, Twiggs LB, Adcock LL, Prem KA, Potish RA. Multimodality therapy for advanced and recurrent vulvar squamous cell carcinoma: a pilot project. *J Reprod Med* 1990; **35**: 1029–32.

68 Rotmensch J, Rubin SJ, Sutton HG et al. Preoperative radiotherapy followed by radical vulvectomy with inguinal lymphadenectomy for advanced vulvar carcinomas. *Gynecol Oncol* 1990; **36**: 181–4.

69 Wahlen SA, Slater JD, Wagner RJ et al. Concurrent radiation therapy and chemotherapy in the treatment of primary squamous cell carcinoma of the vulva. *Cancer* 1995; **75**; 2289–94.

70 Lupi G, Raspagliesi F, Zucali R et al. Combined preoperative chemoradiotherapy followed by radical surgery in locally advanced vulvar carcinoma. *Cancer* 1996; **77**: 1472–8.

71 Moore DH, Thomas GM, Mantana GS, Saxer A, Gallup DG, OH G. Preoperative chemoradiation for advanced vulvar cancer: a phase II study of the Gynecologic Oncology Group. *Int J Radation Biol Phys* 1998; **42**: 79–85.

72 Stehman F, Bundy B, Thomas G et al. Groin dissection versus groin radiation in carcinoma of the vulva: a Gynecologic Oncology Group Study. *Int J Radiat Oncol Biol Phys* 1992; **24**: 389–96.

73 Lanciano RM, Corn BW. Groin irradiation for vulvar cancer: treatment planning must do more than scratching the surface. *Int J Radiat Oncol Biol Phys* 1993; **27**: 987–9.

74 Koh WJ, Chiu M, Stelzer KJ et al. Femoral vessel depth and the implications for groin node radiation. *Int J Radiat Oncol Biol Phys* 1993; **27**: 969–74.

75 Manavi M, Berger A, Kucera E, Vavra N, Kucera H. Does T1, N0–1 vulvar cancer treated by vulvectomy but not lymphadenectomy need inguinofemoral radiation? *Int J Radiat Oncol Biol Phys* 1997; **38**: 749–53.

76 Durrant KR, Mangioni C, Lacave AJ et al. Bleomycin, methotrexate, and CCNU in advanced inoperable squamous cell carcinoma of the vulva: a phase II study of the EORTC Gynecological Cancer Cooperative Group (GCCG). *Gynecol Oncol* 1990; **37**: 359–62.

77 Abdulhaya G, Sobel RM. Neoadjuvant chemotherapy and surgery for the treatment of advanced vulvar carcinoma (abstract). *Gynecol Oncol* 1998; **68**: 124.

10

Role of radiotherapy in the management of vulvar cancer

A JHINGRAN, P EIFEL

BACKGROUND

The traditional operative approach to invasive carcinoma of the vulva – radical *en bloc* resection of the vulva and inguinofemoral nodes – was developed at the beginning of the twentieth century and was popularized during subsequent decades. This procedure remained the standard of care until the early 1980s.[1,2] Radiotherapy was thought to have little role in the treatment of vulvar cancer because of early reports of severe local reactions and poor survival rates with primary radiotherapy.[3,4] Although this operative approach achieved gratifying 5-year survival rates of 60–70 per cent, the surgery caused significant physical and psychological complications. In 1981, Hacker and colleagues[5] demonstrated a less morbid surgical approach, which involved separate incisions in the vulva and groin and resulted in cure rates that were comparable with those of the traditional radical vulvectomy. Since then, there has been a continuing trend towards less radical surgery for early stage disease. In

addition, recent prospective and retrospective studies have clearly demonstrated that relatively high doses of radiation can be delivered safely and that, in carefully selected patients, treatment of the vulva or regional lymphatics can improve locoregional control rates, survival rates and even overall treatment morbidity.

RADIOTHERAPY ALONE

Results of radiotherapy in the treatment of carcinoma of the vulva are scarce and difficult to evaluate critically because of the various methods of treatment, doses of radiation and criteria used for patient selection; however, a significant improvement in results has been observed over the years with the use of modern equipment and adequate doses of radiation.[6] In 1930, Stoeckel[7] reported a 12 per cent 5-year survival rate in patients treated with X-rays or radium. Later, Backstrom and colleagues[8] reported a 21 per cent 5-year survival rate in patients with T4 tumours. Frischbier and Thomsen[9] reported a 47.5 per cent 5-year survival rate in 118 patients treated with higher-energy electrons; however, ulcers developed in 24 per cent of the patients, and extensive tissue necrosis was found in 5 per cent, which probably resulted from the use of a relatively large daily dose of 3 Gy. Nobler[10] addressed the issue of normal tissue tolerance to irradiation in the vulvar area in six patients treated with perineal portals of 50–70 Gy over 6–9 weeks at 2 Gy per day. No evidence of local recurrence was seen in five of these six patients for a period of 10–24 months, and tolerance of perineal and vulvar tissue was judged to be good. Pirtoli and Rottoli[11] described a 5-year survival rate of 42 per cent in 19 patients treated with radiation doses of 45–85 Gy to the primary tumour and 45–50 Gy to inguinal lymph nodes. However, all these survival rates are lower than those routinely mentioned with surgery: 80–90 per cent in patients with stages I and II disease, 60 per cent for stage III disease and 15 per cent for stage IV disease (based on the stage of the International Federation of Gynaecology and Obstetrics, FIGO). It is, however, very important to remember that all the studies mentioned above are old and selective for very advanced or medically inoperable cases, and so it is very hard to compare local control or survival against surgery. Radiotherapy alone should probably be reserved for patients who are not medically able to have any type of surgery, for palliation of very advanced tumours and maybe for patients with early T1 or T2 disease.[6] Nevertheless, radiotherapy has a definite role in combination with surgery, because it can reduce the extent of surgery needed in patients with locally advanced tumours and in the treatment of regional disease.

SURGERY COMBINED WITH RADIOTHERAPY

A number of authors have advocated the use of combined surgery and irradiation to improve local control of vulvar cancers that display features associated with a high rate of local recurrence, and to reduce the need for exenterative surgery in patients with tumours that are close to or involve the urethra or anus. In one of the larger reviews of the results of surgery alone, Podratz and colleagues[12] reported a 24 per cent incidence of vulvar recurrence in 71 patients with stage III carcinoma. Recurrence correlated with tumour size and nodal status. Heaps and colleagues[13] reported that

a close surgical margin was the most powerful predictor of local recurrence in their patients. They observed 21 vulvar recurrences in 44 patients with tumour margins that were less than 8 mm (deep or at the skin surface), compared with no local recurrences in 91 patients with margins of 8 mm or more. Invasion of the lymph vascular space and deep tumour penetration are also associated with a greater likelihood of recurrence.[13–15] Although many local recurrences are controlled with additional surgery or irradiation, salvage surgery is associated with some morbidity, and local recurrences may provide additional opportunity for regional and distant tumour spread.

Faul and colleagues[16] studied retrospectively patients with invasive vulvar cancer and either positive or close (<8 mm) surgical margins, who were either treated with radiotherapy or observed. Adjuvant radiotherapy significantly reduced local recurrence rates in both patients with close margins ($p = 0.036$) and those with positive margins ($p = 0.0048$). Univariate and multivariate analyses showed that adjuvant irradiation and surgical margins were significant prognostic predictors for local control. The patients observed with positive margins had a significantly poorer actuarial 5-year survival rate than other patients ($p = 0.0016$), and adjuvant irradiation significantly improved survival for this group (Fig. 10.1).

Perez and colleagues[6] studied retrospectively 50 patients with primary invasive vulvar carcinoma and 17 with histologically confirmed recurrent vulvar carcinoma, who were treated with radiotherapy for locoregional disease. Primary tumour control was 90

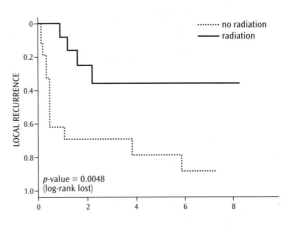

Figure 10.1 *Actuarial local control rates for the positive margin radiated group and observed group. Adjuvant radiation significantly improved survival in this group. (Reproduced with permission from Faul et al.[16])*

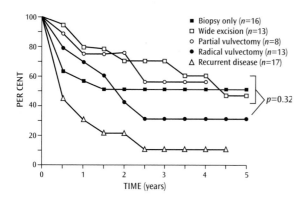

Figure 10.2 *Carcinoma of the vulva: disease-free survival correlated with type of surgical procedure. There was no statistical difference in the extent of surgery. (Reproduced with permission from Faul et al.[16])*

per cent in patients treated with partial or radical vulvectomy and radiotherapy for T1–3 tumours and any nodal stage, 33 per cent in patients with T-stage tumours and N3 lymph nodes, and 66 per cent in patients with recurrent tumours. The actuarial 5-year disease-free survival rates were 87 per cent for patients with T1N0 disease, 62 per cent for those with T2–3N0 disease, 30 per cent for those with T1–3N1 disease, and 11 per cent for patients with recurrent tumours. There were no long-term survivors with T4 or N2–3 disease, and there was no significant difference in the type of resection that was done (Fig. 10.2). The authors concluded that wide local excision and radiotherapy or irradiation alone was an alternative treatment with significantly less morbidity for controlling T1–2 vulvar carcinoma, and that irradiation after excision of locally advanced tumours improved tumour control at the primary site and regional lymphatics.

Postoperative irradiation may be helpful in preventing the need for radical surgery and preserving organs in cases where less radical surgery may leave close or microscopic positive margins. It may also prevent local recurrences in patients with high-risk factors such as close margins, invasion of the lymph vascular space and deep tumour penetration.

PREOPERATIVE RADIOTHERAPY

Some radiation oncologists advocate the use of preoperative irradiation for locally advanced vulvar cancer, based on the theory that it may sterilize microscopic

disease so that less radical resection is required to achieve local control. It may cause sufficient tumour regression to obtain adequate surgical margins without sacrificing important structures such as the urethra, anus and clitoris, and, if aimed at the inguinal nodes, it may obviate the need for radical dissection of the inguinal lymph nodes in patients with clinically uninvolved groins and mobilize fixed and matted nodes, facilitating subsequent surgical excision.[17]

Although not much has been published on preoperative radiotherapy, several investigators have reported excellent responses and high local control rates for advanced tumours after relatively modest doses of radiation (45–55 Gy). This has permitted organ-sparing surgery without sacrificing tumour control (Table 10.1).[17–22] Acosta and colleagues[18] found no macroscopic residual tumour in 10 of 13 patients (seven with stage II and six with stage III disease) who underwent surgery after receiving 35–55 Gy of radiation preoperatively. In a series of nine cases, Boronow[23] reported only one local recurrence. Operative morbidity was minimal, and five patients remained disease free for from 11 months to 4.5 years. When this experience was updated,[19] most of the 37 patients treated with this technique had advanced primary tumours of the vulva. The 5-year survival rate for patients with primary tumours was 75.6 per cent. For patients with recurrent disease, the 5-year survival rate was 62.6 per cent. In most patients (94.8 per cent), the bladder and rectum were preserved. In seven of eight patients (87.5 per cent) reported on by Hacker and colleagues,[20] significant tumour regression enabled conservative surgery. Four patients had no viable tumour in the surgical excision. Five of eight patients (62.5 per cent) were alive without evidence of disease at intervals ranging from 15 months to 10 years. Bilateral hip necrosis and fracture developed in one patient.

CHEMOTHERAPY COMBINED WITH RADIOTHERAPY

To reduce the need for morbid ultra-radical surgery, and to improve locoregional control rates, a number of investigators have explored combinations of chemotherapy with radiotherapy and surgery in patients with locally advanced vulvar carcinoma[21–33] (Table 10.2). Most studies have used combinations of cisplatin, 5-fluorouracil (5-FU) and mitomycin C, as a

Table 10.1 *Preoperative radiotherapy for locally advanced vulvar cancer*

	No. of patients	Radiotherapy dose (Gy)	Tumours in specimen (%)	Local recurrence[a]
Fairey (1985)	7	55	Uncertain	1 (14)
Hacker[20]	8	44–54	50	1 (12)
Boronow[19]	20	Uncertain	Uncertain	1 (5)
Jafari (1981)	4	30–42	100	0
Acosta[18]	14	36–55	36	1 (7)

[a] Numbers in parentheses are the percentage.

Table 10.2 *Chemoradiotherapy in the management of locally advanced or recurrent carcinoma of the vulva*

	Number	Chemotherapy	Dose (Gy)	NED (%)[a]
Cunningham (1997)	14	FM	50–65	57 (1–81 m)
Landoni (1996)	41	FM	54 (split)	36 (24 m)
Wahlen[33]	19	FM	45–50	79 (med 34 m)
Thomas[32]	24	FM	44–60	78 (med 20 m)
Eifel (1995)	12	FP	40–50	50 (17–30 m)
Russell[30]	18	FP	47–72	83 (med 24 m)
Koh[27]	20	F	40–54	49 (60 m)
Scheiströen[31]	20	B	30–43	5 (60 m)
Iverson[25]	15	B	15–40	7 (48 m)

NED, no evidence of disease; F, 5-fluorouracil; M, mitomycin C; P, platinum; B, bleomycin

result of the extrapolation of the high response rates observed when these drugs were used to treat locally advanced carcinomas of the cervix and head and neck, and of the results from studies that have demonstrated the efficacy of these drugs as radiosensitizers in the treatment of carcinomas of the anus.

The most impressive results of combined modality therapy for vulvar carcinoma are those reported by Thomas and colleagues.[32] A total of 33 patients with stage II, III or IV disease were treated: nine with irradiation and chemotherapy as preoperative adjuvant treatments, nine with definitive radiotherapy and chemotherapy, and 15 with radiotherapy and chemotherapy upon local recurrence after surgery. Chemotherapy consisted of infusional 5-FU given over 4–5 days at a dose of 1000 mg/m^2 daily; six patients received low-dose mitomycin C. Various radiation doses and delivery techniques were used. Seven of nine patients treated with neoadjuvant therapy remained free of disease for 5–45 months, one after local excision of a vulvar recurrence. Of the nine patients with primary disease who received chemotherapy and radiotherapy as definitive management, six were alive without evidence of disease for 5–45 months. Of the 15 patients treated after recurrence, seven were alive without evidence of disease for 5–45 months. Combined therapy was well tolerated, except for the expected oropharyngeal mucositis and haematological toxicity of 5-FU. Severe proctitis developed in one patient after receiving 55 Gy in 35 fractions with electrons to the vulva, and vascular hip necrosis developed in another patient after a dose of 47 Gy in 27 fractions. It is impossible to determine the role of chemotherapy in these patients, but it appears that combined modality therapy offers the potential for long-term disease control without the need for surgery, which would lead to significant functional morbidity.

Levin and colleagues[28] used preoperative chemotherapy with mitomycin C and 5-FU, followed by pelvic irradiation before surgery for advanced carcinoma of the vulva. They observed marked local tumour shrinkage in six patients, which allowed for more conservative surgery after the chemotherapy. Iverson[25] treated 15 patients with inoperable vulvar carcinoma with a combination of radiation (36–40 Gy) and bleomycin (30 mg every 2 days for total doses of 90–180 mg). Only two patients had complete tumour regression and survived 2.5 and 4 years. Recurrences in 11 of 15 patients developed a few weeks after the completion of therapy.

Koh and colleagues[27] described results in 20 patients with locally extensive recurrent carcinoma of the vulva treated with combined radiotherapy and chemotherapy (seven patients with FIGO stage III disease, 10 with stage IV disease, and three with recurrent disease). Median doses for microscopic disease and gross tumour were 40 Gy (range 30–54 Gy) and 54 Gy (range 34–70.4 Gy), respectively. All patients received two or three cycles of 5-FU together with the radiation; in addition, five patients received cisplatin and one mitomycin C. Ten patients (50 per cent) had complete resolution of tumour after initial chemoradiotherapy, and eight of these remained disease free (median follow-up of 37 months). Eight other patients had partial responses, with tumour bulk reduced by 60 per cent or more, and the remaining two patients had locoregional progression of disease. Six patients with partial responses had residual tumour successfully resected, but disease later recurred in a few of them (median follow-up of 37 months). For the 20 patients, the actuarial 5-year local tumour control rate was 48 per cent, and the disease-specific survival rate was 59 per cent. There was a suggestion that better local control was obtained in patients who received 50 Gy or more for gross tumour. Skin reaction was the major acute toxic effect and it responded well to conservative management.

Eifel[22] reported on 12 patients with locoregionally advanced vulvar carcinoma treated with a combination of radiation and continuous infusions of 5-FU and cisplatin. Eleven patients had advanced vulvar disease with tumours that were 5–18 cm in maximum diameter, eight had palpable inguinal nodes with biopsy-proven metastatic carcinoma, and five had fixed nodes. Patients received weekly 96-hour infusions of cisplatin (4 mg/m^2 per day) and 5-FU (250 mg/m^2 per day) for a total of 64 mg/m^2 of cisplatin and 4 g/m^2 of 5-FU in 4 weeks. Chemoradiotherapy was well tolerated with virtually no haematological toxicity and no unscheduled breaks in treatment. Of eight patients who underwent vulvar resection 6 weeks after treatment, four had no residual disease in the vulvar specimen and were disease free 17, 20, 25 and 37 months after surgery. Another patient was disease free 28 months after a complete clinical response without vulvar resection. However, of four patients who had residual disease in the vulvar surgical specimen, disease recurred within the radia-

tion field in three. Overall, six of 12 patients who had this chemoradiotherapy remained disease free 17–30 months after treatment.

Russell and colleagues[30] observed 16 complete responses in 25 women with locally advanced or recurrent squamous cell carcinoma of the vulva treated with a 96-hour continuous infusion of 5-FU (combined in 11 patients with three doses of cisplatin at 100 mg/m^2) and pelvic irradiation (median dose of 54 Gy). Of 18 previously untreated patients, 12 were cancer free 2–52 months after treatment. Intermittent urinary incontinence developed in three patients and leg oedema in four.

Wahlen and colleagues[33] described 19 patients with locally advanced vulvar cancer (four with stage II disease and 15 with stage III disease); 17 had clinically negative inguinal lymph nodes and the remaining two had had their ipsilateral inguinal nodes removed before treatment. The patients received 45–50 Gy of radiation to the pelvis and inguinal nodes with concurrent chemotherapy (96-hour continuous infusion of 5-FU at 1000 mg/m^2 per day during weeks 1 and 5 of radiotherapy). Ten patients received boosts with implants or electrons and six underwent local excision. After a median follow-up of 34 months, combination therapy resulted in a local tumour control rate of 74 per cent (14 of 19); all five failures occurred within 6 months of treatment. Four of these patients were rendered disease free by radical vulvectomy and/or exenteration, for an overall local control rate of 95 per cent (18 of 19).

Only one study has investigated the role of neoadjuvant chemotherapy. Benedetti-Panici and colleagues[34] treated 21 patients who had stage IVA vulvar cancer with two to three cycles of cisplatin, bleomycin and methotrexate, followed by radical surgery. Two patients (10 per cent) had partial responses, and 14 (67 per cent) had partial responses of regional nodes to chemotherapy; 90 per cent were considered to have operable tumours, but the 3-year survival rate was only 24 per cent.

These studies include small numbers of patients who usually had very advanced local or regional disease. Although the data are insufficient to determine whether concurrent chemotherapy adds to the efficacy of radiotherapy, most investigators have described impressive local responses of some very advanced lesions, suggesting that responses may be better than those achievable without concurrent chemotherapy. Well-controlled multi-institutional trials are necessary to clarify the role of chemotherapy as a radiosensitizer in this relatively rare disease.

Caution is warranted in designing aggressive treatment protocols for vulvar cancer in patients who, typically, are elderly and often have concurrent medical problems. Serious pulmonary toxicity has been observed in a number of patients whose treatment included bleomycin.[25,29,31] In the largest published series of patients treated with mitomycin C and 5-FU, haematological tolerance was acceptable, but the administered dose of mitomycin C was somewhat lower than that generally used in the treatment of anal cancers.[32]

TREATMENT OF REGIONAL DISEASE

The primary lymphatic drainage of the vulva and distal vagina is to the superficial femoral (or inguinal) nodes that lie along the femoral vein[35] (Fig. 10.3). Metastases are rarely found in the deep inguinal or pelvic nodes without evidence of spread to the superficial inguinal nodes. Various authors report the incidence of positive nodes in operable vulvar cancer to be between 20 per cent and 35 per cent. A number of factors have been correlated with the incidence of regional node metastasis at a significance of less than 0.01 (Table 10.3): clinical stage, depth of invasion, tumour diameter, tumour thickness, invasion of lymph vascular space, keratin level, mitotic activity, histological grade and cell type.[13] Effective regional treatment is the single most important factor in the curative management of early vulvar cancer. Survival correlates strongly with the presence, number and location of regional metastases. The survival rate for patients with more than two positive femoral nodes is less than 30 per cent.[36–38] Bilateral node involvement is associated with a particularly poor prognosis, as is pelvic node involvement. In a Gynecologic Oncology Group (GOG) study involving pelvic node dissection, Homesley and colleagues[39] reported a 23 per cent survival rate (at 2 years) in patients with positive pelvic nodes compared with 73 per cent in patients without pelvic node involvement (Fig. 10.4). In combination, information about tumour size and nodal status is

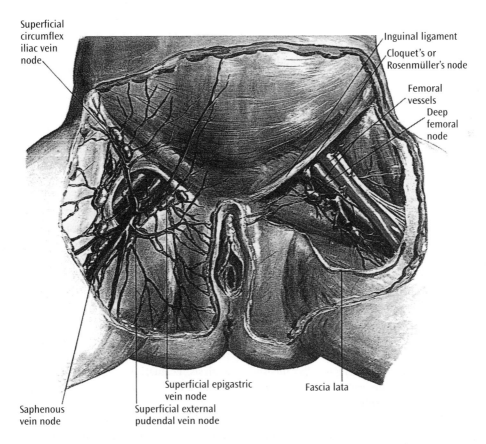

Figure 10.3 *Shows the lymphatic drainage of the vulva. (Reproduced with permission from Netter.[35])*

Table 10.3 *Predictors of node involvement*[14]

Predictor	Significance
Clinical stage	<0.01
Depth of invasion	<0.01
Tumour diameter	<0.01
Tumour thickness	<0.01
Vascular invasion	<0.01
Amount of keratin	<0.01
Mitotic activity	<0.01
Histological grade	<0.01
Cell type	<0.01

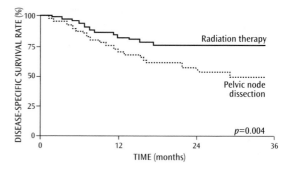

Figure 10.5 *Homesley and colleagues showed that radiotherapy significantly benefited patients with positive nodes. For patients with positive nodes, the 2-year survival rates were 59 and 31 percent for the radiotherapy and pelvic resection only, respectively. (Reproduced with permission from Holmesley et al.[39])*

highly predictive of prognosis[39] (Fig. 10.5). Although patients with vulvar recurrences can often be treated curatively with additional local therapy, patients whose disease recurs in the inguinal nodes are rarely cured.

All patients with primary tumours that invade more than 1 mm should have their inguinal nodes treated. Traditional management includes a bilateral radical dissection of the inguinal lymph nodes. Currently, this is usually carried out through separate groin incisions for most T1 and selected T2 tumours. At one time, pelvic node resection was also performed in all patients with invasive vulvar cancer. When subsequent studies demonstrated that pelvic node metastases were found only in patients with clinically suspicious or multiple positive inguinal nodes, the procedure was limited to patients determined intraoperatively to have positive inguinal nodes.[36,40,41]

Retrospective studies suggest that patients with multiple positive nodes and extranodal tumour spread

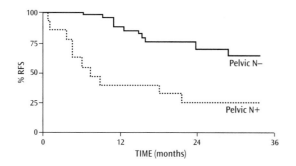

Figure 10.4 *Homesley and colleagues[39] showed that survival significantly decreased with positive nodes. The survival rate was 23 per cent in 2 years in patients with positive nodes, compared with 73 per cent in patients with negative nodes. RFS, relapse-free survival. (Reproduced with permission from Holmesley et al.[39])*

are at increased risk for recurrence in inguinal nodes after radical inguinal lymphadenectomy.[42]

In 1986, the GOG published the results of a prospective randomized trial that documented the important role of postoperative radiotherapy in the treatment of regionally advanced vulvar carcinoma.[39] All patients were initially treated with radical vulvectomy and inguinal lymphadenectomy. Patients were randomized intraoperatively, after frozen tissue from the inguinal nodes was evaluated, either to receive radiation at 45–50 Gy over 5–6 weeks to the pelvic and inguinal regions or to undergo pelvic lymph node dissection. No radiation was delivered to the central vulvar area. This trial was closed prematurely, after 114 eligible patients had been entered, when interim analysis revealed a survival advantage for the radiation treatment arm ($p=0.03$) (see Fig. 10.5). The difference was most marked for patients with clinically positive or multiple histologically positive groin nodes. For patients with clinically positive nodes, the 2-year survival rates were 59 per cent for those treated with radiation and 31 per cent for those who underwent pelvic node resection. There was no significant difference in survival between the treatment groups for patients with clinically negative nodes or microscopically positive nodes, but the authors commented that the patient numbers were insufficient for adequate subset analysis. Evaluation of the failure patterns revealed a significantly lower incidence of inguinal recurrences in patients who received radiation to the groin (Fig. 10.6). Patients in whom tumours recurred in the groin usually died from the disease. At the time of the analysis, disease had recurred in the primary site in approximately 9 per cent of patients in both treatment arms. We therefore concur with van der Velden (see Chapter 9) that irradiation appears to exert its influence by the reduction of groin recurrences and, as yet, we cannot confirm any benefit in terms of pelvic control.

Most of the serious acute and subacute complications of radical vulvectomy are related to lymph node dissection, although these risks have decreased somewhat with the use of separate groin incisions.[41,43–45] Complications include wound disruption or infection in 50–75 per cent of cases and chronic lymphoedema in 20–50 per cent. The perioperative mortality rate is between 2 per cent and 5 per cent. Patients who undergo vulvectomy without inguinal node dissection have significantly shorter hospital stays and fewer complications.[41,43,45]

Although radical inguinal lymphadenectomy has historically been considered the treatment of choice for regional management of invasive vulvar carcinoma, several retrospective studies have suggested that regional radiotherapy may be an effective and less morbid way of preventing recurrence in patients with clinically negative groins. In a review of 91 patients treated electively with radiation to the inguinal nodes for cancers with primary drainage to these nodes, Henderson and colleagues[46] observed only two failures after treatment with 45–50 Gy over 5 weeks, and both of these occurred outside the treatment fields. Complications were rare, with only one case of mild leg oedema, which may not have been treatment related.

The GOG attempted to define the optimal approach to clinically negative inguinal nodes in a trial that randomized patients between inguinal node irradiation and radical lymphadenectomy (followed by inguinopelvic irradiation in patients with positive nodes) after resection of the primary tumour. The study was closed after entry of only 58 patients when an interim analysis demonstrated a significantly higher rate of inguinal recurrence and death in the irradiated group[1] (Fig. 10.7). The authors concluded that lymphadenectomy was the superior treatment, although the morbidity was higher than that in patients who had groin irradiation. Radiotherapy consisted of 50 Gy given in daily 2-Gy fractions to a depth of 3 cm below the anterior skin surface. These results seem to raise serious questions about the efficacy of radiation in this setting. This study was criticized because the protocol prescription suggested that 50 per cent of the tumour dose be delivered with 9 to 12-MeV electrons, which are inadequate to treat the deep inguinal lymph nodes in most cases (a 90 per cent depth dose at 3.1 cm).

In point of fact, McCall and colleagues[47] evaluated the depth of inguinal lymph nodes with computed tomography (CT) in 100 women without palpable inguinal adenopathy or before inguinal surgery. The tumour doses that the patients would have received were determined using isodose curves, constructed according to the guidelines in GOG protocol 88. In only 18 per cent of women were all inguinal lymph nodes measured at a depth of 3 cm or less. More than

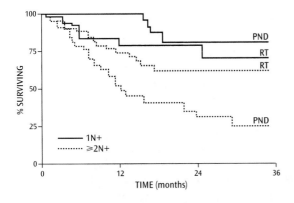

Figure 10.6 *Sites of recurrence in 114 patients with invasive squamous cell carcinoma of the vulva who were entered on a Gynecologic Oncology Group (GOG) protocol randomizing patients with positive groin nodes after radical vulvectomy and bilateral inguinal lymphadenectomies to receive pelvic lymph node dissection or postoperative irradiation to the pelvis and inguinal nodes. (Reproduced with permission from Holmesley et al.[39])*

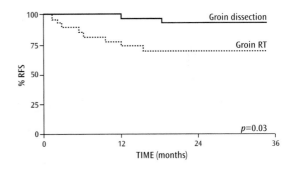

Figure 10.7 *Relapse-free survival from a GOG randomized trial comparing groin dissection and groin radiation in clinically node-negative patients. The trial was stopped early because of the significant advantage of the groin dissection over the radiation. (Reproduced with permission from Stehman et al.[45])*

half of all women would have received less than 60 per cent of the prescribed irradiation dose because their inguinal lymph nodes were deeper than 5 cm.

Koh and colleagues[48] quantified inguinofemoral node depths using pre-treatment computed tomography (CT) scans in 50 patients with gynaecological cancer. The distance of each femoral vessel beneath the overlying skin surface was determined as an indicator of the depth of the inguinofemoral nodes. Correlative data regarding height and weight were used to calculate Quetelet index or the body mass index (BMI), defined as the weight in kilograms divided by the square of the height in meters:

$$\text{Quetelet's index, } Q = \frac{\text{Weight (kg)}}{\text{Height}^2 \text{ (m}^2)}.$$

Individual femoral vessel depths ranged from 2.0 cm to 18.5 cm. When the depths of all four femoral vessels were averaged in each patient, the mean four-vessel average nodal depth was 6.1 cm. Recalculation of doses provided to five patients, in whom prophylactic groin irradiation failed in the GOG study, showed that all had received nodal tumour doses of less than 47 Gy, with three patients being underdosed by more than 30 per cent.

An example of this can be seen in Fig. 10.8, which shows a single CT slice from a relatively slender patient with a left vulvar lesion metastatic to superficial and deep left inguinal nodes. On the contralateral uninvolved side, the corresponding deep inguinal node is 5.5 cm from the surface of the patient. If this patient was treated with a 50:50 mix of 12-MeV electrons and 6-MV photons prescribed to a point 3 cm from the surface, the deep inguinal nodes would receive approximately 50 per cent of the prescribed dose. The superficial inguinal nodes, which were 4.2 cm from the surface, would also be underdosed. In very obese patients, the inguinal nodes may be located 8 cm or more beneath the surface of the patient. The convention of prescribing inguinal node fields at a depth of 3 cm was developed many years ago, before the advent of computed tomography and the widespread use of electron beam fields.

Another prospective GOG study published in 1992 by Stehman and colleagues[49] hints at the importance of the deep femoral nodes in vulvar carcinoma. In the study, 122 patients with early vulvar carcinomas (all < 2 cm in diameter) were observed after treatment with hemivulvectomy and superficial node dissection. All patients who had tumour invasion of more than 5 mm invasion, positive lymph nodes or lymph invasion of the vascular space were excluded. Despite the favourable characteristics of this group of patients, the investigators observed nine groin recurrences in 122 patients. Six of these recurrences were in the ipsilateral dissected groin. The authors speculated that, contrary

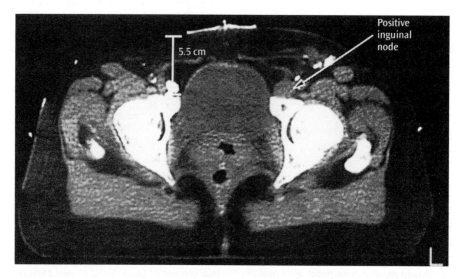

Figure 10.8 *A transverse CT slice through the deep femoral nodes of a 48-year-old woman with squamous carcinoma of the left labium metastatic to superficial and deep inguinal nodes. The patient was 1.7 m tall and weighed 77 kg (Quetelet's index = 26). Brightly opacified nodes are from a lymphangiogram done before the CT scan. On the uninvolved side, the node corresponding to the positive node on the left is 5.5 cm beneath the skin surface. (Reproduced with permission from Eifel.[22])*

to conventional wisdom, the deep femoral nodes sometimes harbour disease even when the superficial inguinal nodes are negative.

In a more recent retrospective review that attempted to address the confusion generated by these studies, Petereit and colleagues[43] found no difference in the groin recurrence rate for clinically negative inguinal nodes treated with radical lymphadenectomy or radiotherapy; 24 patients treated with radical vulvectomy and bilateral node dissection were compared with 18 patients who underwent radical vulvectomy and inguinofemoral node irradiation. Patients were treated with anterior and posterior opposed photon fields weighted to favour the anterior one. Although the patients treated with radiation had included a larger percentage of unfavourable T3 and T4 lesions (33 per cent versus 4 per cent), there was no significant difference in the incidence of inguinal node failures (one in the surgery group and two in the radiation group; $p=0.56$). The morbidity of lymphadenectomy included lymphoedema (16 per cent), seroma (16 per cent), infection (44 per cent), and wound separation (68 per cent). In the irradiated patients, lymphoedema developed in 16 per cent, and only 9 per cent had a significant skin reaction. The authors concluded that patients with clinically negative inguinal nodes were effectively treated with radiation alone, if radiation techniques were used that adequately encompassed the inguinofemoral nodes.

Some surgeons have tried to reduce surgical complications by reducing the extent of lymph node dissections. Burke and colleagues[50] reported four (5 per cent) groin recurrences in 74 patients with T1–2 tumours treated with wide local excision and superficial inguinal lymphadenectomy (unilateral or bilateral depending on the location of the tumour). More recently, this group has added intraoperative lymphatic mapping to the procedure to improve identification of the sentinel node, and they have reported an 11 per cent incidence of major perioperative complications.[51]

We can conclude that patients with multiple positive nodes or gross inguinal nodal disease at node dissection benefit from postoperative inguinal irradiation. Doses of radiation should range from 50 Gy to 65 Gy depending on the extent of disease. A less radical dissection, in which all gross disease is removed and then radiotherapy is given, may be less morbid. For fixed nodes, chemoradiotherapy may be helpful, with lymph node dissection reserved for after treatment if the nodes become mobile.

We can also conclude that occult inguinal metastases can probably be controlled with radiotherapy. The standard approach for clinical N0 or N1 disease is radical lymph node dissection plus irradiation for positive nodes, but irradiation alone may be equally effective and less morbid in experienced hands. If radiation is the treatment of choice, CT-based planning is a must, and a CT or magnetic resonance imaging (MRI) scan should be done first to rule out enlarged nodes. An alternative to irradiation may be superficial node dissection or lymphatic mapping plus irradiation for positive nodes. Relative indications for radiation treatment of a clinically negative groin would be medical problems that might complicate a prolonged surgical procedure, severe obesity or diabetes, and extensive primary disease that requires radiotherapy.

RADIOTHERAPY TECHNIQUES

Techniques commonly used for treatment of vulvar carcinoma reflect the need to encompass the lower pelvic and inguinal nodes, as well as the vulva, while minimizing the dose to the femoral heads.

Treatment of regional lymphatics

In patients with primary lesions smaller than 2 cm in diameter, the probability of nodal involvement is low, and irradiation of the pelvic lymph nodes may be omitted if only the inguinofemoral nodes are being treated (Fig. 10.9a).

In patients with primary tumours larger than 2 cm in diameter and no clinical evidence of regional lymphatic involvement, the inguinal and pelvic lymph nodes may be treated electively to a dose of 45–50 Gy in 1.8- to 2-Gy fractions per day instead of lymph node dissection. If palpable inguinal lymph nodes are present, the dose to the inguinofemoral lymph nodes needs to be 65–70 Gy (with reduced fields after 50 Gy), depending on the size of the involved nodes. If there is evidence of spread to the pelvic nodes, the dose must be increased to 60 Gy. As some patients with involved pelvic nodes can potentially be cured, irradiation of the lower periaortic chain in the presence of pelvic lymph node involvement may be appropriate. In patients in whom the pelvic nodes must be treated, anterior and posterior portals covering the vulvar and regional lymphatic volumes are required (Fig. 10.10).

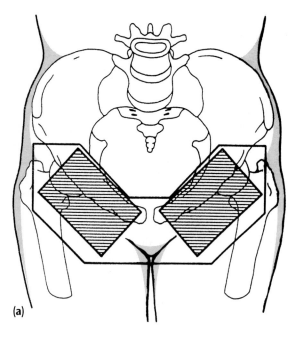

(a)

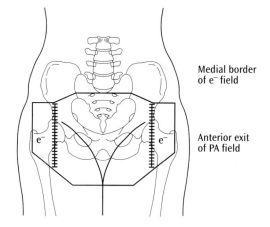

Medial border of e⁻ field

Anterior exit of PA field

e⁻   e⁻

Figure 10.10 *Portal for elective irradiation of regional lymphatics in patients with no clinical evidence of inguinal lymph node involvement.*

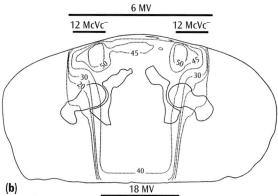

6 MV

12 McVc⁻   12 McVc⁻

(b)   18 MV

Figure 10.9 *Delivering part of the dose to inguinal nodes with appropriate energy electron fields can reduce the radiation dose to the femoral heads. In this example, a wide anterior 6-MV field encompasses the primary site and the inguinal and pelvic nodes. Electron fields are placed anteriorly to overlap slightly with the exit of a narrower posterior 18-MV field that encompasses the primary and pelvic nodes. (Reproduced with permission from Perez and Brady.[52])*

Radiation alone

One approach for radiotherapy alone is to use an anterior field that encompasses the inguinal regions, lower pelvic nodes and vulva, and a narrower posterior field

that encompasses the lower pelvic nodes and vulva, but excludes most of the femoral heads (Figs 10.9b and 10.10). The anterior field is treated with a 6-MV photon beam, whereas the posterior field is treated with an 18-MV photon beam. If an 18-MV photon beam is used for both fields, the bolus may need to be placed on the groins to avoid underdosing the nodes. If the fields are evenly weighted to the mid-plane of the pelvis using 6-MV photons, the contribution of the anterior field to the groin nodes at a depth of 3–5 cm will generally be 60–70 per cent of the dose to the mid-pelvis. The difference may be made up by supplementing the dose to the lateral groins with anterior electron fields of appropriate energy. Computed tomography is very helpful in treatment planning because it identifies the electron beam energy needed to cover the inguinal nodes and helps to exclude gross disease that may not be appreciated on clinical examination. Thermal luminescent dosimetry (TLD) may be used to determine the perineal dose. If an open leg position is used, a bolus on the vulva may be needed and an immobilization device for reproducibility would be helpful. After a dose of 45–50 Gy is delivered to the mid-pelvis, an *en face* electron field or a low-energy photon beam (4–6 MV) aimed directly at the vulva is used to deliver an additional 10–20 Gy to gross or microscopic tumour volumes. An interstitial implant may also be considered to deliver the boost dose to the primary tumour.

Palpable metastatic inguinofemoral lymph nodes receive an additional dose (15–20 Gy), preferably with electrons, to decrease the dose to the underlying

Preoperative radiotherapy

Patients with advanced primary lesions involving surrounding structures that are either of questionable resectability or clearly unresectable should receive preoperative irradiation. Moderate doses of 45–50 Gy over 5–6 weeks may increase the resectability rate and also avoid mutilating procedures such as exenteration. Treatment fields should encompass the pelvis, inguinal region and vulva.

Postoperative radiotherapy

Postoperative irradiation to the vulva alone is occasionally indicated when the margins of surgical resection are less than 8 mm and the inguinal lymph nodes are pathologically negative. This occurs most often with lesions that are very close to the urethra or anus. The close or positive margin may be treated to a dose of 50–70 Gy, depending on the proximity of disease to the surgical margin, with an appositional perineal electron-beam field or occasionally with an interstitial implant.[6]

Patients found, at node dissection, to have metastasis in inguinofemoral nodes benefit from postoperative irradiation, including radiation to at least the lower pelvic lymphatics of 40–50 Gy at the mid-plane of the pelvis, followed by a boost to the inguinal nodes, depending on the pathological findings. We recommend a total dose of 50 Gy for minimal microscopic disease, 55–60 Gy for large or multiple positive nodes, 60 Gy for extracapsular extension and 65–70 Gy for gross residual disease.

Treatment of recurrent lesions

Some recurrent lesions may be treated surgically. Recurrences after surgical resection remain potentially curable and must be treated aggressively, in the manner described previously, to deliver tumour doses of 65–70 Gy with reducing fields.

Brachytherapy

A few reports have described outcomes after interstitial irradiation. Pohar and colleagues[53] reported on 34 patients treated with iridium-92 (^{192}Ir) brachytherapy for vulvar cancer (21 at first presentation when surgery was contraindicated or declined); 12 patients had stage III or IV disease, eight had stage II, one had stage I and one had stage 0; 13 patients were treated for recurrent disease. Paris system brachytherapy rules were followed and the median reference dose was 60 Gy (range 53–88 Gy). Ten (29 per cent) of 34 patients were alive after a median follow-up of 31 months. Actuarial 5-year local tumour control was 47 per cent, and locoregional tumour control was 45 per cent; the 5-year disease-specific survival rate was 56 per cent, and the overall survival rate was 29 per cent. Subset analysis disclosed higher actuarial 5-year locoregional tumour control in patients treated at first presentation (80 per cent versus 16 per cent; $p = 0.01$).

At Washington University,[54] 20 patients had an interstitial implant as part of their therapy, usually as a boost at the primary tumour site, but occasionally for positive lymph nodes. The rate of locoregional tumour control was 100 per cent for T1 or T2 disease (four patients), 80 per cent for T3 disease (10 patients), and 50 per cent for T4 or recurrent disease (six patients). None of the five patients who received a total dose of 60 Gy or less had significant sequelae, in contrast to eight (53 per cent) of 15 patients treated with higher doses. Patients treated with external-beam radiation had only 11–26 per cent moderate or severe sequelae ($p = 0.16$).

Brachytherapy should be done carefully; it needs experience because the risk of necrosis is very high.

ACUTE SIDE EFFECTS OF RADIOTHERAPY

Acute radiation reactions are brisk, and doses of 40 Gy and higher routinely induce confluent moist desquamation. However, with adequate local care, this acute reaction usually heals within 2–3 weeks. Patients should be warned about side effects before treatment and told that the discomfort usually resolves after completion of treatment. Domobero's sitz baths, aquaphor ointment and oral treatment of possible superimposed candidal infection help to minimize discomfort. We believe that breaks during treatment should be avoided because the acute reaction usually takes more than 1 week to improve, allowing tumour cells time to repopulate.

LATE COMPLICATIONS

Numerous factors may add to the late morbidity of radiation treatment in patients with vulvar carcinoma. Patients with advanced vulvar carcinoma are often treated with radiation after radical surgery, which may include extensive dissection of the inguinal, and possibly pelvic, nodes. Large ulcerative cutaneous lesions frequently have superimposed infection. Patients are often elderly and may have complicating medical conditions such as diabetes, multiple prior operations and osteoporosis. The contribution of concurrent chemotherapy to local morbidity is not yet clearly defined.

The incidence of lower extremity oedema after inguinal radiation alone is negligible. Although radiotherapy probably contributes to the incidence of peripheral oedema after radical node dissection, no difference was noted in the GOG randomized study.[39] However, the authors admit that evaluation of lymphoedema was not a major consideration of the study and that the complication may have been underreported. Femoral head fractures have occasionally been reported in patients treated with radiation to the inguinal nodes. This risk is probably negligible when techniques are used that limit the dose to the femoral heads to less than 35–40 Gy. It is not known whether severe osteoporosis contributes to complications in the femoral head.

The long-term cosmesis and function of the irradiated vulva are poorly understood. Although treatment with radiation and wide excision is becoming a more accepted alternative to radical vulvectomy for selected patients, and major complication rates appear to be acceptable, very little has been reported about more subtle late effects of such treatment in the vulva. Late effects are dose related. Although Frischbier and Thomsen[9] reported a 24 per cent incidence of late ulceration in a large number of patients treated primarily with electron-beam radiation to the vulva, the relatively large dose per fraction used (3 Gy/day) probably contributed to this high incidence. Better information will become available only as treating physicians record and report the late cosmetic and functional results in patients treated in conjunction with surgery, chemotherapy or radiation alone.

CONCLUSION

The treatment of vulvar carcinoma, and particularly our understanding of the role of radiotherapy, have improved substantially over the past two decades and will continue to evolve as current investigations mature. Postoperative radiotherapy improves regional control and survival of patients with positive inguinal lymph nodes. The efficacy of radiotherapy alone in the management of clinically N0–1 disease remains controversial. Careful attention to radiotherapy technique is very important in achieving good local control. The combination of radiotherapy with organ-conserving surgery is being explored as a way of increasing the functional results of treatment. The role of chemotherapy in combination with surgery and radiotherapy is another area under active investigation.

REFERENCES

1 Taussig FJ. Cancer of the vulva: an analysis of 155 cases. *Am J Obstet Gynecol* 1940; **40**: 764.

2 Way S. Carcinoma of the vulva. *Am J Obstet Gynecol* 1960; **79**: 692.

3 Helgason NM, Hass AC, Latourette HB. Radiation therapy in carcinoma of the vulva. *Cancer* 1972; **30**: 997.

4 Tod MC. Radium implantation treatment of carcinoma vulva. *Br J Radiol* 1949; **22**: 508.

5 Hacker NF, Leuchter RS, Berek JS, Castaldo TW, Lagasse LD. Radical vulvectomy and bilateral inguinal lymphadenectomy through separate groin incisions. *Obstet Gynecol* 1981; **58**: 574.

6 Perez CA, Grigsby PW, Galakatos A et al. Radiation therapy in management of carcinoma of the vulva with emphasis on conservation therapy. *Cancer* 1993; **71**: 3703.

7 Stoeckel W. Zur Therapie des Vulvacarzinoms. *Z Gynaekologie* 1930; **54**: 47.

8 Backstrom A, Edsmyr R, Wicklund H. Radiotherapy of carcinoma of the vulva. *Acta Obstet Gynecol Scand* 1972; **51**: 109.

9 Frischbier HJ, Thomsen K. Treatment of cancer of the vulva with high-energy electrons. *Am J Obstet Gynecol* 1971; **111**: 431.

10 Nobler MP. Efficacy of a perineal teletherapy portal in the management of vulvar and vaginal cancer. *Radiology* 1972; **103**: 393.

11 Pirtoli L, Rottoli ML. Results of radiation therapy for vulvar carcinoma. *Acta Radiol Oncol* 1982; **21**: 45.

12 Podratz KC, Symmonds RE, Taylor WF et al. Carcinoma of the vulva analysis of treatment and survival. *Obstet Gynecol* 1983; **61**: 63.

13 Heaps JM, Fu YS, Montz FJ et al. Surgical–pathologic variables predictive of local recurrence in squamous cell carcinoma of the vulva. *Gynecol Oncol* 1990; **38**: 309.

14 Binder SW, Huang I, Fu YS et al. Risk factors for the development of lymph node metastasis in vulvar squamous carcinoma. *Gynecol Oncol* 1990; **37**: 9.

15 Boyce J, Fruchter RG, Kasambilides E et al. Prognostic factors in carcinoma of the vulva. *Gynecol Oncol* 1985; **20**: 364.

16 Faul CM, Mirmow D, Huang Q et al. Adjuvant radiation for vulvar carcinoma: improved local control. *Int J Radiat Oncol Biol Phys* 1997; **38**: 381.

17 Burke TW, Eifel PJ, McGuire W, Wilkinson EJ. Vulva. In: Hoskins WJ, Perez CA, Young RC (eds). *Principles and practice of gynecologic oncology*, 2nd edn. Philadelphia: Lippincott-Raven, 1997:.

18 Acosta AA, Given FT, Frazier AB et al. Preoperative radiation therapy in the management of squamous cell carcinoma of the vulva: preliminary report. *Am J Obstet Gynecol* 1978; **132**: 198.

19 Boronow RC. Combined therapy as an alternative to exenteration for locally advanced vulvo-vaginal cancer: rationale and results. *Cancer* 1982; **49**: 1085.

20 Hacker NF, Berek JS, Julliard GJF, Lagasse LD. Preoperative radiation therapy for locally advanced vulvar cancer. *Cancer* 1984; **54**: 2056.

21 Berek JS, Heaps JM, Fu YS et al. Concurrent cisplatin and 5-fluorouracil chemotherapy and radiation therapy for advanced-stage squamous carcinoma of the vulva. *Gynecol Oncol* 1991; **42**: 197.

22 Eifel PJ. Vulvar carcinoma: radiotherapy or surgery for the lymphatics? *Front Radiat Ther Oncol* 1994; **28**: 218.

23 Boronow RC. Therapeutic alternative to primary exenteration for advanced vulvo-vaginal cancer. *Gynecol Oncol* 1973; **1**: 223.

24 Evans LS, Kersh CR, Constable WC, Taylor PT. Concomitant 5-fluorouracil, mitomycin C, and radiotherapy for advanced gynecologic malignancies. *Int J Radiat Oncol Biol Phys* 1998; **15**: 901.

25 Iverson T. Irradiation and bleomycin in the treatment of inoperable vulva carcinoma. *Acta Obstet Gynecol Scand* 1982; **61**: 195.

26 Kalra JK, Grossman AM, Krumholz BA et al. Preoperative chemoradiotherapy for carcinoma of the vulva. *Gynecol Oncol* 1981; **12**: 256.

27 Koh WJ, Wallace HJ, Greer BE et al. Combined radiotherapy and chemotherapy in management of local-regionally advanced vulvar cancer. *Int J Radiat Oncol Biol Phys* 1993; **26**: 809.

28 Levin W, Goldberg G, Altaras M et al. The use of concomitant chemotherapy and radiotherapy prior to surgery in advanced stage carcinoma of the vulva. *Gynecol Oncol* 1986; **25**: 20.

29 Makinen J, Salmi T, Gronroos M. Individually modified treatment of invasive squamous cell vulvar cancer: 10-year experience. *Ann Chir Gynaecol* 1987; **76**: 68.

30 Russell AH, Mesic JB, Scudder SA et al. Synchronous radiation and cytotoxic chemotherapy for locally advanced or recurrent squamous cancer of the vulva. *Gynecol Oncol* 1992; **47**: 14.

31 Scheiströen M, Trope C. Combined bleomycin and irradiation in preoperative treatment of advanced squamous cell carcinoma of the vulva. *Acta Oncol* 1992; **32**: 657.

32 Thomas G, Dembo A, DePetrillo A et al. Concurrent radiation and chemotherapy in vulvar carcinoma. *Gynecol Oncol* 1989; 34: 263.

33 Wahlen SA, Slater JD, Wagner RJ et al. Concurrent radiation therapy and chemotherapy in the treatment of primary squamous cell carcinoma of vulva. *Cancer* 1995; **75**: 2289.

34 Benedetti-Panci, Greggi S, Scambia G, Salero G, Mancuso S. Cisplatin, bleomycin, and methotrexate preoperative chemotherapy in locally advanced vulvar carcinoma. *Gynecol Oncol* 1993; **50**: 49.

35 Netter F. *The Ciba collection of medical illustration*, Vol 2. *Reproductive system*. Summit, NJ: Ciba Pharmaceutical Products, Inc., 1988.

36 Hacker NF, Berek JS, Lagasse L et al. Management of regional lymph nodes and their prognostic influence in vulvar cancer. *Obstet Gynecol* 1983; **61**: 408.

37 Sedlis A, Homesley H, Bundy BN et al. Positive groin lymph nodes in superficial squamous cell vulvar cancer. *Am J Obstet Gynecol* 1987; **156**: 1159.

38 Homesley H, Bundy B, Sedlis A et al. Assessment of current International Federation of Gynecology and Obstetrics staging of vulvar carcinoma relative to prognostic factors for survival (ACOG Study). *Am J Obstet Gynecol* 1991; **164**: 997.

39 Homesley HD, Bundy BN, Sedlis A, Adcock L. Radiation therapy versus pelvic node resection for carcinoma of the vulva with positive groin nodes. *Obstet Gynecol* 1986; **68**: 733.

40 Figge CD, Gaudenz R. Invasive carcinoma of the vulva. *Am J Obstet Gynecol* 1974; **119**: 382.

41 Morley GW. Infiltrative carcinoma of the vulva: results of surgical treatment. *Am J Obstet Gynecol* 1976; **124**: 874.

42 Simonsen E, Nordberg UB, Johnsson JE et al. Radiation therapy and surgery in the treatment of regional lymph nodes in squamous cell carcinoma of the vulva. *Acta Radiol Oncol* 1984; **23**: 433.

43 Petereit D, Mehta M, Buchler D, Kinsella T. A retrospective review of nodal treatment for vulvar cancer. *Am J Clin Oncol* 1993; **16**: 38.

44 Podratz KC, Symmonds RE, Taylor WF. Carcinoma of the vulva: analysis of treatment failures. *Am J Obstet Gynecol* 1982; **143**: 340.

45 Stehman F, Bundy B, Thomas G et al. Groin dissection versus groin radiation in carcinoma of the vulva: a Gynecologic Oncology Group study. *Int J Radiat Oncol Biol Phys* 1992; **24**: 39.

46 Henderson RH, Parsons JT, Morgan L, Million R. Elective ileoinguinal lymph node irradiation. *Int J Radiat Oncol Biol Phys* 1984; **10**: 811.

47 McCall AR, Olsen MC, Potkul RK. The variation of inguinal lymph node depth in adult women and its importance in planning elective irradiation for vulvar cancer. *Cancer* 1995; **75**: 2286.

48 Koh WJ, Chiu M, Stelzer KJ et al. Femoral vessel depth and the implications for groin node radi-ation. *Int J Radiat Oncol Biol Phys* 1992; **27**: 969.

49 Stehman FB, Bundy BN, Dvoretsky PM, Creasman T. Early stage I carcinoma of the vulva treated with ipsilateral superficial inguinal lymphadenectomy and modified radical hemivulvectomy: a prospective study of the Gynecologic Oncology Group. *Obstet Gynecol* 1992; **79**: 490.

50 Burke TW, Levenback C, Coleman RC et al. Surgical therapy of T1 and T2 vulvar carcinoma: further experience with radical wide excision and selective inguinal lymphadenectomy. *Gynecol Oncol* 1995; **57**: 215.

51 Levenback C, Burke TW, Gershenson DM et al. Intraoperative lymphatic mapping for vulvar cancer. *Obstet Gynecol* 1994; **84**: 163.

52 Perez CA, Brady L. Carcinoma of the vulva. In: Perez CA, Grisby PW, Chao KSC, Garipagaoglu M (eds). *Principles and practice of radiation oncology*, 3rd edn. Philadelphia: Lippincott-Raven, 1997: 1036.

53 Pohar S, Hoffstetter S, Peiffert O et al. Effectiveness of brachytherapy in treating carcinoma of the vulva. *Int J Radiat Oncol Biol Phys* 1995; **32**: 1455.

54 Perez CA, Grisby PW, Chao KSC, Garipagaoglu M. *Principles and practice of radiation oncology*, 3rd edn. Philadelphia: Lippincott-Raven, 1997.

11

Management of relapsed vulvar cancer

FG LAWTON

Diagnosis and hence treatment at an earlier stage, accompanied by advances in the understanding of prognostic factors that influence regional lymph node involvement and local recurrence, have encouraged an individualized approach to the treatment of vulvar cancer. Traditionally, *en bloc* radical vulvectomy with bilateral inguinofemoral nodal excision was considered the treatment of choice for all cases of vulvar cancer, but several studies have shown that more limited vulvar surgery – radical local excision – combined with selective inguinofemoral node dissection gives results equivalent to those achieved with more extensive surgery with much reduced morbidity.[1]

Initially, critics of a less radical approach argued that such surgery might lead to a reduction in cure rates, but it is apparent, from a number of studies, that recurrent disease is a function of characteristics of the primary tumour, such as lesion size and position, tumour stage and nodal status.[2,3] However, recurrences in the undissected 'bridge' that results from the three-incision technique have been reported in both node-positive and node-negative tumours.[4]

FACTORS THAT MAY PREDISPOSE TO RECURRENT DISEASE

Suboptimal vulvar surgery

Provided that all surgical margins of the resected specimen are tumour free, the incidence of local, i.e. vulvar, recurrence should be the same after radical vulvectomy or radical local excision. In this context, radical local excision needs definition. It should not be seen as a procedure in which, merely, a lesser surface area of vulvar skin is removed. The aim is to carry out an excision that is wide and deep enough to obtain at least a 1-cm tumour-free margin at all surfaces. This requires that the incision be carried down to the inferior fascia of the urogenital diaphragm. A 'skinning' procedure, regardless of the area of vulvar skin removed, is inadequate.

It may be very difficult to obtain suitable negative margins for lesions on the perineum close to the anal margin, but periurethral lesions present less of a surgical problem because the distal 1 cm of the urethra can be excised without affecting continence.

Suboptimal groin surgery

It was thought that, for most patients with clinical stage I disease (based on the classification of the International Federation of Gynaecology and Obstetrics, FIGO), with depth of invasion of 5 mm or less, groin dissection was an unnecessary procedure. Numerous reports have, however, concluded that groin surgery can be omitted only in patients who have invasion of less than 1 mm, where the risk of nodal disease is, effectively, zero. Invasion of between 1 mm and 2 mm carries an almost 8 per cent risk of nodal spread, whereas deeper lesions, of between 3.1 mm and 5 mm, carry a risk of almost 27 per cent.[5]

A bilateral groin dissection is not indicated if the vulvar lesion is unilateral, posterior or medial in position and less than 2 cm in diameter, because less than 1 per cent of such patients will have disease in the contralateral groin.[5] Lymphatic drainage of more anterior lesions is frequently to the contralateral groin, so both groins should be dissected.[6]

A reduction in the extent of groin dissection, to reduce morbidity, may increase regional recurrence rates and hence mortality, because, essentially, recurrence in an undissected or inadequately dissected groin is not compatible with cure. Two studies undertaken by the Gynecologic Oncology Group (GOG) in the USA bear testimony to this. In both, all patients were previously untreated, and had clinical stage I–III disease that was resectable without excision of the urethra, bladder, rectum or anus, and had impalpable or clinically non-suspicious groin nodes. In GOG protocol 74, patients with stage I disease were treated with a modified radical hemivulvectomy and superficial groin node dissection. In protocol 88, patients were randomized to either groin dissection or radiotherapy of the surgically unexplored groin nodes. Of the patients in protocol 74, 120 had superficial groin surgery and 23 patients in protocol 88 had groin irradiation. These 143 patients formed the basis of the report.[7]

The vulva was the site of recurrence in 21 patients overall, comprising 15 per cent of patients in protocol 74 and 13 per cent in protocol 88. The groin recurrence rate was 5.8 per cent in protocol 74 and 21.7 per cent in protocol 88. The median time to groin recurrence was 7 months with a median survival after recurrence of only 9.4 months. The median time to vulvar relapse was 35.9 months with a median survival after recurrence at this site of 52.4 months.

Other studies have shown that most groin recurrences develop within a year of surgery; Iversen and colleagues[8] reported a 72.8 per cent rate within 12 months. Tilmans and colleagues[9] reported on recurrence pattern and interval in 40 patients: local recurrence alone was seen in 43 per cent of patients compared with 30 per cent who had recurrent groin disease. Interval to recurrence was a function of tumour grade and FIGO stage. Of the recurrences, 63 per cent were seen within 2 years. The median time to groin recurrence was 9 months, to pelvic recurrence 12 months, to distant recurrence 7 months and to vulvar recurrence 33 months. In Hopkins' study of 34 patients, 56 per cent recurred within the first 2 years of initial treatment.[10]

Tumour variables

Several studies have indicated a large number of surgicopathological variables that predict risk of recurrent disease. For local recurrence, these include initial stage, positive margins in the resected specimen, depth of invasion and tumour thickness, a pushing or infiltrative pattern of tumour growth and the presence of invasion of the lymph vascular (LVI). Heaps and colleagues[3] reported a statistically increased risk of local recurrence for patients with a tumour-free margin of less than 8 mm (21 of 44 compared with 0 of 91 for patients > 8 mm; $p < 0.0001$), no recurrences in 52 patients with tumour invasion to a depth of less than 2.5 mm, compared with 20 per cent of patients with 2.5–5 mm invasion and 45 per cent of patients with invasion of 5.1–7.5 mm ($p < 0.0001$), and a 39 per cent vulvar recurrence rate for patients with LVI compared with a 12 per cent rate without ($p = 0.003$). None of 44 patients with a 'pushing' type of tumour had a recurrence compared with 28 per cent who had an infiltrative type ($p = 0.0002$). These data underline the need for an adequate biopsy of a vulvar lesion because many of these variables are then known before planning definitive surgery.

Risk factors for predicting lymph node status are similar and include tumour grade and patient age.[11] Nodal relapse and hence survival are associated with intracapsular nodal size; 5-year survival rates approach 90 per cent for patients with nodal deposits of less than 5 mm compared with 20 per cent for those with larger nodal metastases or extracapsular spread.[12] Patients at high risk of recurrent groin disease may include those with positive inguinal nodes, bilaterally involved groins or large nodal deposits, and those with extranodal extension.

Second primaries

It has been suggested that some vulvar recurrences may actually be the result of the development of a second primary lesion, particularly in cases of more limited initial vulvar surgery.[5,7] In the latter report, only three of 18 patients with initial limited vulvar surgery had an ipsilateral vulvar recurrence. Further support to this hypothesis is given by the observation that appreciable long-term survival after recurrence is limited to those patients who recur following an interval of more than 2 years after initial surgery.[13]

Patient characteristics

Vulvar cancer tends to be a disease of elderly women with the mean age at diagnosis of about 65 years. Old age itself may be seen by some to preclude radical surgery, particularly in encouraging gynaecologists to omit groin surgery on the grounds of increased associated morbidity, but this is an erroneous assumption. Clearly, age and coexistent morbidity cannot be ignored, but, when scheduling vulvar surgery for an elderly patient, two important factors must be taken into consideration. The first is that the average life expectancy of a healthy 65-year-old woman is an additional 18 years, whereas for a fit 75 year old it is another 12 years.[14] Recurrent disease in an undissected groin is not compatible with cure; the consequence of suboptimal primary surgery is that an otherwise healthy patient will die a painful and undignified death.

The second factor to be considered is that radiotherapy, rather than radical surgery, should not be considered an 'easier' option for such patients. Up to 30 per cent of elderly patients may not be able to complete a course of radiotherapy for gynaecological cancer, and although inpatient stay after radical vulvectomy may be longer in the over-65s, compared with younger women (mean 18.2 days compared with 12.3 days, $p < 0.05$), surgical complication rates are similar.[15]

Surgeon-associated variables

Clearly, differences in the extent to which an individual clinician will undertake a planned surgical endeavour are associated with factors other than patient age and apparent fitness for surgery. A recent, retrospective, population based study from a single region in the UK has shown marked differences in the management of vulvar cancer. The study contained details of 411 patients with squamous cell carcinoma of the vulva treated over two 3-year periods, 1980–82 and 1986–88, in 35 hospitals.[16] Out of the hospitals, 46 per cent saw, on average, only one case per year, only 65 per cent of the 411 patients had a biopsy of the vulvar lesion, and 15 different surgical procedures were performed on the 344 woman who actually had an operation! Only 46 per cent of the patients underwent lymphadenectomy. The overall recurrence rate was 30 per cent, whereas 5-year survival rates were 78 per cent for FIGO stage I, 54 per cent for stage II, 27 per cent for stage III and 13 per cent for stage IV. These figures should be compared with recurrence rates of less than 20 per cent and survival rates of 89 per cent, 65 per cent and 40 per cent for stages I–III in reports from single institutions.[9,13,17] Population-based studies are more likely to reveal the true picture of the management of a particular disease compared with reports from single centres or specialist multicentre groups and, as such, it would be difficult to deny the adverse prognostic impact of inadequate surgery on the results of Rhodes'[16] study.

Multifocal preinvasive disease

Around 30 per cent of patients with vulvar intraepithelial neoplasia (VIN) have had a previous intercurrent diagnosis of other lower genital tract intraepithelial or anorectal disease, or will have intercurrent or future disease.[18] The risk of subsequent malignant change in patients with VIN 3 has been estimated at 5 per cent.[19] Jones and Rowan[20] reported a similar progression rate with 3.8 per cent of 113 women developing invasive disease 7–18 years after treatment. Recurrence, and hence progression to invasive disease, were more common in patients with multifocal disease. Determination of the limits of associated multifocal preinvasive disease at the time of surgery for vulvar cancer will be essentially impossible, particularly if there are 'skip lesions' anatomically separate from the area of macroscopic cancer.

An interesting study from the Netherlands[21] has shown a marked difference in the proportion of patients who had a diagnosis of abnormal vulvar epithelium (VIN, lichen sclerosus or squamous cell hyperplasia) made before the diagnosis of vulvar cancer – 30 per cent compared with 95 per cent who had synchronous epithelial changes after reviewing the vulvar cancer specimen.

RECURRENT VULVAR CANCER

The 5-year survival rate for operable, node-negative patients after primary surgery is about 90 per cent, but this falls to about 50 per cent for patients with nodal metastases. Around a quarter of patients will develop recurrence after treatment.[3,7,9,10,13,16,22] An isolated vulvar recurrence is seen in about 55 per cent of patients (Table 11.1). Recurrent groin or more distant disease tends to be a rapid event with a median interval of only about 9 months, whereas the median time to recurrent vulvar disease is about 34 months.[7,9] The interval between primary surgery and relapse is a strong predictor of the outcome of further treatment. Tilmans and colleagues[9] reported that patients who relapsed more than 16 months after primary treatment had a median survival of 13 months, compared with 5 months for those patients with a more rapid relapse. Podratz and colleagues[13] reported 94 per cent and 70 per cent 1- and 5-year survival rates for patients who relapsed after 2 years, compared with rates of 50 per cent and 14 per cent for those who recurred within 2 years of primary therapy.[13]

MANAGEMENT OPTIONS

As relapse beyond the pelvis is uncommon, a large number of patients with recurrent disease are candidates for further surgery. Factors that influence the type of surgery, which are common to both untreated patients and those with recurrent disease, include age,

general health and willingness to undergo treatment. Previous therapy is an important influence in planning treatment for recurrent disease.

Patients with an apparent isolated vulvar recurrence should be investigated thoroughly to document evidence of spread beyond the vulva and groins. Evidence of pelvic or distant recurrence (by computed tomography, magnetic resonance, radiograph or fine needle aspiration) should preclude a surgical attempt at cure, but surgical palliation of recurrent vulvar disease in such cases should be considered, particularly for patients with large, fungating, vulvar lesions.

Surgery for recurrent disease should, like that for primary disease, be individualized and may include excision of the recurrent vulvar tumour alone, by either simple vulvectomy or a more radical procedure. In patients who have not undergone previous groin surgery, inguinofemoral lymphadenectomy may be considered.

Factors that predict survival after secondary surgery have not been addressed much in the literature. In one of the largest series of 34 cases of recurrent vulvar cancer, all of whom were treated by surgery at recurrence, Hopkins and colleagues[10] reported a 74 per cent 2-year and a 61 per cent 5-year survival rate from the time of recurrence. Lymph node status at the time of secondary surgery had a major impact on further recurrence and survival, with none of 10 node-positive patients remaining disease free over a 5-year follow-up, compared with 19 of 24 node-negative patients ($p < 0.00001$). Of the node-negative patients, 80 per cent were alive at 10 years, compared with a median survival of around 2 years for node-positive patients.

In Tilmans' study,[9] 17 of 40 patients had recurrent disease confined to the vulva. Surgery consisted of simple vulvectomy in eight patients, modified radical vulvectomy in four and radical vulvectomy in one. A superficial lymph node dissection was, in addition, undertaken in four of these patients. A further vulvar recurrence was seen in 35 per cent of these 17 patients after salvage therapy, with half of them having evidence of additional groin or pelvic recurrence.

Treatment for the 12 patients with groin recurrences was either with curative or palliative intent. In the former group, treatment included surgery and radiotherapy ($n = 3$), surgery, radiotherapy and chemotherapy ($n = 2$), or radiotherapy alone ($n = 1$). Palliative radiotherapy or chemotherapy was given to five patients and one had 'palliative' care only. Patients with evidence of distant recurrence ($n = 11$) underwent palliative care only.

Table 11.1 *Vulvar cancer: sites of recurrence*

Reference	No.	Vulva only	Groin	Pelvis/distant
Heaps[3]	21	21	–	–
Hopkins[10]	34	24	10	–
Podratz[13]	59	30	–	–
Rhodes[16]	109	47	49	13
Simonsen[22]	41	29	12	–
Stehman[7]	37	21	12	4
Tilmans[9]	40	17	12	11
Total	**341**	**189 (55%)**	**95**	**28**

Overall median survival from the time of retreatment was only 8 months with a range of 1–144 months, indicating a subgroup of patients with recurrent disease who will do well. Once again survival was related to site of recurrence with a median survival of 13 months (range 2–49 months) for patients with an isolated vulvar recurrence, compared with 10, 4 and 5 months for those with groin, pelvic and distant recurrences, respectively.

These studies demonstrate the importance of recognizing groin node involvement at the time of relapse, because it may be appropriate to offer adjunctive groin irradiation in some patients not previously treated in this fashion. However, Hopkins reported no survivors in six node-positive patients who were treated with radiotherapy after surgery for recurrence.[10]

Irradiation alone has been used as the primary therapy at relapse.[23,24] In the study by Prempree and Amornmarn,[24] the size of the recurrent tumour was of prognostic significance, with all 10 patients who had a vulvar recurrence larger than 5 cm or large nodal metastases dying from the disease. They concluded that radiotherapy was likely to control recurrent groin disease only when nodes were smaller than 2 cm in diameter. In the report from Pao and colleagues[23] the salvage rate was only 21 per cent.

Patients with extensive local recurrence involving the anal sphincter or canal, or urethra and bladder, may be candidates for pelvic exenteration or 'ultra-radical surgery'. An extremely radical approach has been advocated in certain circumstances where pelvic side-wall infiltration without evidence of distant metastases has occurred.[25] In a series of 48 patients, there were six with recurrent vulvar cancer. In their CORT programme (combined operative and radiotherapeutic treatment), the aim was to complete a total resection of macroscopic tumour at the pelvic side wall, with preservation of the bony pelvis and neurovascular supply to the leg, grafting of abdominal or thigh tissue to the operative field to allow further high-dose radiotherapy to the area, reconstruction of pelvic organ function and postoperative brachytherapy via guide tubes implanted into the pelvic wall. Patient selection, both from the point of view of tumour extent and also, more importantly, with regard to individual appreciation of the consequences of such extensive surgery, is paramount in such situations, although in the overall group there were no treatment-related deaths with a 50 per cent 3-year survival. Mean quality of life values for a number of indices (physical, functional, social and emotional well-being) after CORT ranged from 62 per cent to 80 per cent.

CHEMOTHERAPY

The results of incorporating chemotherapy in combination with surgery and/or radiotherapy for 'high-risk' primary disease and recurrent cancer have been reported, but overall patient numbers are small. This, coupled with the number of regimens reported, makes it difficult to draw any firm conclusions about the role of cytotoxic therapy in recurrent vulvar cancer.

Interest in the use of chemotherapy began with a report of a combination of preoperative radiotherapy and chemotherapy (cisplatin and mitomycin C used as radiosensitizers) in squamous cancer of the anal canal.[26] Similar approaches to large-volume primary vulvar cancers have been reported.[27,28] In the study by Lupi and colleagues,[28] patients were treated with two cycles of chemotherapy comprising mitomycin C 15 mg/m^2 i.v. on day 1 with a 24-hour intravenous infusion of 5-fluorouracil on days 1 and 5 and concurrent radiotherapy of up to 36 Gy to the pelvic and inguinal region. A second chemotherapy cycle was given 2 weeks later with a further 18 Gy of radiotherapy. The report contained data on seven patients with recurrent disease – six with a clinically isolated vulvar lesion and one with recurrent groin disease. Surgery included radical excision of the vulvar lesion with bilateral inguinofemoral lymphadenectomy in six patients, and radical vulvectomy alone in one. A pathological complete remission was achieved in five patients.

FOLLOW-UP

Recommendations regarding frequency of follow-up suggest 3-monthly intervals for 2 years or so with 6-monthly intervals for the next 3 years.[18] Pelvic and groin examination should, clearly, be carried out at each visit. The role of routine cervical and vaginal cytology remains to be determined but, in view of the risk of multifocal intraepithelial neoplasia affecting the rest of the squamous epithelium, such investigations seem reasonable.

CONCLUSIONS

Treatment, other than palliation, of recurrent vulvar cancer is an uncommon clinical problem, because of the rarity of the primary disease and the age of patients who might have such a condition. General gynaecologists are unlikely to see more than a dozen or so cases in a lifetime of practice. Therefore, if there was ever a case for referral to a specialist centre, a patient with recurrent vulvar cancer would be one. Management options are many but their application must be made by a multidisciplinary team, possibly consisting of a gynaecological surgeon, radiation and medical oncologists, a palliative care physician, community nurse specialists and a pain relief physician. The potential longevity of patients with vulvar cancer demands a multidisciplinary approach.

REFERENCES

1   Rodriguez M, Sevin B-U, Averette HE et al. Conservative trends in the surgical management of vulvar cancer: a University of Miami patient care evaluation study. *Int J Gynecol Cancer* 1997; **7**: 151–7.

2   Hacker NF, Berek JS, Lagasse LD, Leuchter RS, Moore JG. Management of regional lymph nodes and their prognostic influence in vulvar cancer. *Obstet Gynecol* 1983; **61**: 408–12.

3   Heaps JM, Fu YS, Montz FJ, Hacker NF, Berek JS. Surgical–pathologic variables predictive of local recurrence in squamous cell carcinoma of the vulva. *Gynecol Oncol* 1990; **38**: 309–14.

4   Hacker NF, van der Velden J. Conservative management of early vulvar cancer. *Cancer* 1993; **71**: 1673–7.

5   Hacker NF. Vulvar cancer. In: Berek JS, Hacker NF (eds). *Practical gynecologic oncology,* 2nd edn. London: Williams & Wilkins, 1994: 403–39.

6   Iversen T, Aas M. Lymph drainage from the vulva. *Gynecol Oncol* 1983; **16**: 179–82.

7   Stehman FB, Bundy BN, Ball H, Clarke-Pearson DL. Sites of failure and times to failure in carcinoma of the vulva treated conservatively: a Gynecologic Oncology Group study. *Am J Obstet Gynecol* 1996; **174**: 1128–33.

8   Iversen T, Aalders JG, Christensen A, Kolstad P. Squamous cell carcinoma of the vulva: a review of 424 patients 1956–1974. *Gynecol Oncol* 1980; **9**: 271–9.

9   Tilmans AS, Sutton GP, Look KY, Stehman FB, Ehrlich CE, Hornback NB. Recurrent squamous carcinoma of the vulva. *Am J Obstet Gynecol* 1992; **167**: 1383–9.

10 Hopkins MP, Read GC, Morley GW. The surgical management of recurrent squamous cell carcinoma of the vulva. *Obstet Gynecol* 1990; **75**: 1001–5 .

11 Binder SW, Huang I, Fu YS, Hacker NF, Berek JS. Risk factors for the development of lymph node metastases in vulvar squamous cell carcinoma. *Gynecol Oncol* 1990; **37**: 9–16.

12 Origoni M, Sideri M, Garsia S, Carinelli SG, Ferrari AG. Prognostic value of pathological patterns of lymph node positivity in squamous cell carcinoma of the vulva stage III and IV FIGO. *Gynecol Oncol* 1992; **45**: 313–16.

13 Podratz K, Symmonds RE, Taylor WF. Carcinoma of the vulva: analysis of treatment failures. *Am J Obstet Gynecol* 1983; **143**: 340–7.

14 Lawton FG. Gynaecological cancer in the elderly. *The Diplomate* 1996; **3**: 286–91.

15 Lawton FG, Hacker NF. Surgery for invasive gynecologic cancer in the elderly female population. *Obstet Gynecol* 1990; **76**: 287–9.

16 Rhodes CA, Cummins L, Shafi MI. The management of squamous cell vulvar cancer: a population based retrospective study of 411 patients. *Br J Obstet Gynaecol* 1998; **105**: 200–5.

17 Lingard D, Free K, Wright RG, Battistutta D. Invasive squamous cell carcinoma of the vulva: behaviour and results in the light of changing management regimens. *Aust NZ J Obstet Gynaecol* 1992; **32**: 137–45.

18 Homesley HD. Management of vulvar cancer. *Cancer* 1995; **76**: 2159–70.

19 Ferenczy A. Intraepithelial neoplasia of the vulva. In: Coppleson M (ed). *Gynecologic oncology.* Edinburgh: Churchill Livingstone, 1992: 443–63.

20 Jones RW, Rowan DM. Vulvar intraepithelial neoplasia III: A clinical study of the outcome in 113 cases with relation to the later development of invasive vulvar cancer. *Obstet Gynecol* 1994; **84**: 741–5.

21 Kagie MJ, Kenter GG, Hermans J, Trimbos JB, Fleuren GJ. The relevance of various vulvar epithelial changes in the early detection of squamous cell carcinoma of the vulva. *Int J Gynecol Cancer* 1997; **7**: 50–7.

22 Simonsen E. Treatment of recurrent squamous cell carcinoma of the vulva. *Acta Radiol Oncol* 1984; **23**: 345–8.

23 Pao WM, Perez CA, Kuske RR, Sommers GM, Camel HM, Galaktos AE. Radiation therapy and conservation surgery for primary and recurrent carcinoma of the vulva: report of 40 patients and a review of the literature. *Int J Radiat Oncol Biol Phys* 1988; **14**: 1123–32.

24 Prempree T, Amornmarn R. Radiation treatment of

recurrent carcinoma of the vulva. *Cancer* 1984; **54**: 1943–9.

25 Hockel M, Schlenger K, Hamm H, Knapstein PG, Hohenfellner R, Rosler HP. Five year experience with combined operative and radiotherapeutic treatment of recurrent gynecologic tumors infiltrating the pelvic wall. *Cancer* 1996; **77**: 1918–33.

26 Nigro ND, Seydel G, Considine B, Vaitkevikius VK, Leichman L, Kinzie JJ. Combined preoperative radiation and chemotherapy for squamous cell carcinoma of the anal canal. *Cancer* 1983; **51**: 1826–9.

27 Berek JS, Heaps JM, Fu YS, Juillard GF, Hacker NF. Concurrent cis-platin and 5-fluorouracil chemotherapy and radiation therapy for advanced stage squamous carcinoma of the vulva. *Gynecol Oncol* 1991; **42**: 197–201.

28 Lupi G, Raspagliesi F, Zucalli R et al. Combined preoperative chemoradiotherapy followed by radical surgery in locally advanced vulvar carcinoma. A pilot study. *Cancer* 1996; **77**: 1472–8.

12

Reconstructive surgery in the management of vulvar cancer

JH SHEPHERD, JO HEROD

The mainstay of treatment for invasive carcinoma of the vulvar is wide surgical excision. This was first shown to be a feasible procedure by Antoine Basset at the turn of the century. He demonstrated that, in cadavers, a radical resection of vulval tumours was possible. He did not, however, face the challenge of closing tissue defects following his radical wide excision and *en bloc* dissections. It was Taussig who demonstrated the need for radical surgery with groin lymphadenectomy and, subsequently, Stanley Way, in the early 1950s, who championed the procedure of radical vulvectomy with bilateral groin and pelvic lymphadenectomy. Many of his wounds either could not be closed by primary intention or broke down and were left to granulate and heal by secondary intention over a 3- to 4-month period.

To his credit, Way prophesied that his radical surgery would be replaced by less morbid and more conservative approaches, thus reducing wound breakdown and other complications. Partly as a result of earlier diagnosis, but also with improving techniques, his prophetic words have proved to be true. It is now realized that the traditional 'radical vulvectomy' and bilateral groin and pelvic lymphadenectomy procedure are not necessary for most vulvar tumours.

Halstead's principles of cancer surgery still apply to vulvar cancer as much as to any other solid tumour. The primary lesion needs to be widely excised with adequate clear margins and the primary station of lymph node spread needs to be resected *en bloc*. Thus, a radical wide excision of a vulvar tumour may involve excision of a lesion measuring 1–2 cm and a partial vulvectomy or, alternatively, for much larger lesions involving both sides of the vulva, a traditional radical vulvectomy procedure. If it is possible to obtain primary closure with appropriate incisions, then this is carried out, but, if it is not, careful attention needs to be paid to obtaining skin closure by utilizing rotational flaps or grafts. It is no longer acceptable to leave wounds open to heal by secondary intention, except in the most unusual circumstances and, with the use of appropriate reconstructive surgery, it should now be possible to close almost any defect of the skin or underlying tissue.

PRINCIPLES OF RECONSTRUCTIVE SURGERY

The principles that are important in reconstructive surgery can essentially be applied to any surgery. Failure to observe them will result in potentially severe postoperative complications with extreme morbidity for the unfortunate patient (Fig. 12.1). For successful wound healing three important criteria must be met:

1 The tissues must have an adequate blood supply.
2 The wound edges must be approximated without tesion.
3 Infection must be avoided.

The principles of vulvar surgery are to obtain adequate wide clearance of the tumour, while maintaining a good blood supply to the recipient tissue and, if donor graft tissue is used, then this must also be well vascularized. Tension on the skin edges must be avoided and, at the same time, haemostasis must be adequate. Avoidance of haematoma and sub-fascial or graft collections is prevented not only by adequate haemostasis but also by suitable drainage. If haematoma formation occurs, this will increase the tension across wounds and also increase the risk of postoperative wound infection. The risk of infection will also be reduced by adequate preparation, with local toileting, debridement and antibiotic cover. Careful attention to the type of dressing used will avoid pressure necrosis.

All tissues used for reconstruction should be handled with care and in the least traumatic way. The choice of flap or graft needs to be carefully considered and tailored accurately to the size of the deficit to be filled. Suture technique should be meticulous, with skin sutures being correctly tensioned and incorporating the epidermis and dermis, while avoiding the subcutaneous layer that may carry the vascular supply. The choice of suture is, of course, subject to personal preference. Silk sutures were traditionally used to close the skin, although most reports now advocate the use of interrupted 3/0 absorbable sutures (e.g. polyglycolic acid sutures) for both the cutaneous and the subcutaneous layers.

Attention to detail in all aspects of surgical technique is vital, including preoperative preparation, intraoperative fastidious technique, and postoperative nursing care and supervision. It is a combination of all these factors that ensures successful tissue healing and recovery.

Preoperative planning

The importance of this process cannot be overstated and it is vital to the success of a reconstructive procedure. It will be necessary to assess the extent of the disease that is present to determine the nature of the excision required. To this end, a careful examination under anaesthesia is usually required, with recourse to cystoscopy, sigmoidoscopy and biopsies of tissue as indicated by the particular clinical picture. Ideally, all clinicians who will be involved in the proposed treatment should be present at this examination. Additional information may be gained from imaging studies and, in particular, by the improving magnetic resonance imaging (MRI) techniques that are now available. In this way, the perineum, vulva and underlying muscle groups can be well assessed in order to obtain a more precise image of the extent of disease. Attention must also be paid to the mobility and condition of the tissues that could be used for reconstruction. The presence of scars from previous surgery or radiation damage may mean that the method or type of flap that could normally be chosen is inappropriate. This may also apply if urinary and/or faecal stomas are present or proposed.

The patient must be adequately prepared for the proposed operation with the usual preoperative investigations, including cross-matching of appropriate volumes of blood. Antibiotic and anti-thromboembolic prophylaxis should be prescribed, with the use of sequential compression devices advisable during the surgery itself. Bowel preparation is appropriate in most cases, to reduce the chance of soiling of the wounds during the operation and in the early

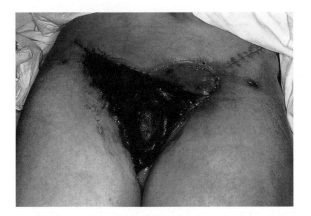

Figure 12.1 *Total necrosis of a rectus abdominis flap. This figure also appears in the colour plate section.*

postoperative phase, and some operators would wash out the rectum carefully immediately before commencing surgery. Consideration should also be given to arranging a high dependency or intensive care facility after the procedure, until care on a normal surgical ward can be resumed.

RECONSTRUCTIVE TECHNIQUES

It is possible, after the excision of most vulvar cancers, to achieve primary closure of the remaining deficit. This may require careful thought about the placement of incisions and adequate undercutting of the skin edges. Reconstructive techniques may be chosen either because closure would not be possible without undue tension, or in an attempt to improve the function and cosmetic appearance of the vulva and vagina after surgery. There are also occasions, if previous radiotherapy has compromised small vessel vascularization, when it is useful to bring in fresh, uncompromised tissue to the affected area.

Different surgeons will have their preferred methods of reconstruction, but a useful rule of thumb is that the simplest method required is likely to be the best option. Tissues utilized for reconstruction may include skin alone or cutaneous, fasciocutaneous or myocutaneous flaps. The available methods will be described, beginning with the simpler techniques that will be adequate for use in most cases requiring reconstruction, and moving on to more complicated procedures that will be needed only rarely (Table 12.1).

Split-thickness skin grafts

This simple technique has been advocated for covering defects left by the skinning vulvectomy procedures sometimes required for multifocal vulvar intraepithelial neoplasia (VIN)[1] or for Paget's disease of the vulva.[2] However, it is less suitable for use after the excision of invasive vulvar lesions. Contracture of grafts and scarring can frequently be problematic, but it is their lack of subcutaneous tissue that is their main disadvantage. The subcutaneous tissue is important both for sexual function and for the cosmetic appearance of the reconstructed vulva. Split-thickness skin grafts are usually taken from the buttock or thigh. These are excised using Humby knives (Fig. 12.2) and then placed over the recipient site, often after meshing (Fig 12.3). The grafts are than secured in place with a number of fine sutures and tulle gras dressing.

Local advancement and transposition flaps

Smaller defects on the vulva can be filled with axial, lateral or rotational skin flaps. These flaps contain cutaneous, subcutaneous and sometimes fascial tissues. They must be broad based in order to ensure an adequate blood supply, and a maximum length to base ratio of 3:1 is recommended to ensure viability. Incisions should be made perpendicular to the skin surface to avoid compromising the vascular supply of the skin edges. The incisions are carried down to the deep fascia. Flaps are then raised by cutting through the subcutaneous tissues while taking care to maintain an even thickness. Some advocate the use of sharp dissec-

Table 12.1 *Methods of reconstructing*

1. Split-thickness skin grafts
2. Local advancement and transposition flaps
    VY-plasty
    Rhomboid flap
    Mons pubis flap
    Lateral transposition flap
    Inferior gluteal flap
3. Local myocutaneous flaps
    Tensor fascia lata
    Gluteus maximus
    Gracilis
4. Distant myocutaneous flaps
    Rotational: rectus abdominis
    Free graft: latissimus dorsi

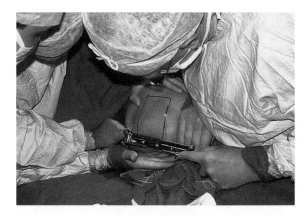

Figure 12.2 *Use of a traditional Humby knife to take a split-thickness skin graft from the thigh. This figure also appears in the colour plate section.*

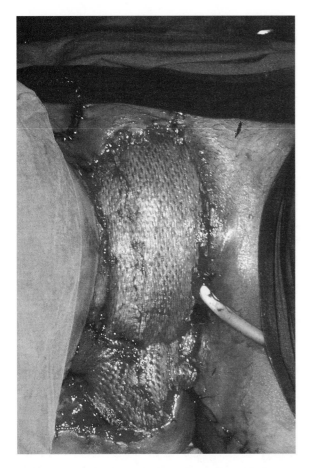

Figure 12.3 *Split-thickness skin graft on vulva. This figure also appears in the colour plate section.*

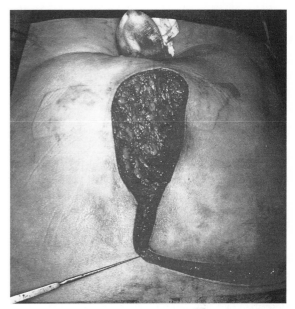

Figure 12.4 *Large cutaneous advancement flap from above the right gluteus maximus used to fill a defect in the natal cleft. This figure also appears in the colour plate section.*

tion rather than electrocautery, in the belief that this will better preserve the vascular supply to the flap. The skin edges surrounding the flap should also be undermined to optimize their mobility for closure.

The vascular supply to the skin of the perineum and inner thigh is plentiful and derived from the subfascial plexus. This plexus is fed by branches of the internal pudendal, superficial and deep femoral arteries, and also by musculocutaneous perforators.[3] An experienced operator can essentially tailor-make cutaneous or fasciocutaneous flaps to cover most small and moderate-sized defects (Fig. 12.4). A number of particular techniques have been described, including the following.

THE VY ADVANCEMENT[4,5]

This is a simple and rapid procedure whereby a 'V'-shaped incision is made, allowing mobilization and medial advancement of a triangular cutaneous flap. The repair is made in a 'Y' configuration after mobilization.

RHOMBOID OR 'LIMBERG' FLAPS[6,7]

For these, a paddle of skin is formed by making a 'V'-shaped incision immediately adjacent to a surgical defect. The paddle is in the shape of a rhomboid, i.e. a four-sided figure with sides of equal length. The paddle is then mobilized, advanced and rotated into the defect. It is suitable for covering defects up to 4 cm in diameter, although bilateral flaps can be used to cover a larger area. They are particularly well adapted to defects in the posterior vulva and perianal area, although unsuitable for use on the anterior vulva.

THE MONS PUBIS FLAP[8]

This is a flap that uses tissue from above the mons pubis. This tissue has a similar thickness of subcutaneous tissue to vulvar skin and, as it is hair bearing, has a similar appearance. It derives a blood supply from branches of the superficial external pudendal artery, which supplies the skin of the lower medial portion of the anterior abdominal wall. There is an extensive anastomosis between the vessels on each side. The flap is developed above and medial to the inguinal crease on the contralateral side of the mons pubis to the defect that is to be filled. The base of the flap is situated in the midline, directly above the defect. The site of origin and appearance of the flap make it suitable for filling anterior defects or the defect left after hemivulvectomy, although it is probably limited to filling defects no larger than 7.5 × 5 cm.

LATERAL TRANSPOSITION FLAP

These are very simple cutaneous flaps using skin from the labia majora or lateral perineum that is particularly useful for filling larger defects of the introitus or posterior or lateral vagina (Figs 12.5 and 12.6). The blood supply is derived from branches of the internal pudendal and inferior rectal arteries. As long as the length of the flap is no more than three times the width of the base, vascularity should be satisfactory. A variety of this flap in the midline was recently described by Davison and colleagues.[9]

INFERIOR GLUTEAL FLAP[10]

This flap is a fasciocutaneous flap that is derived from the skin and fascia overlying the gluteus maximus muscle. It is basically a larger version of the lateral transposition flap, described above, which can be used to fill difficult, extensive vulvar or perineal defects up to an area of approximately 110 cm.[2] The blood supply is derived from branches of the inferior gluteal vessels. It has been reported that exclusion of the inferior gluteal nerve from the flap may avoid difficulties with postoperative pain reported by Achauer and colleagues.[11]

Local myocutaneous flaps

To cover large defects of the entire vulva, larger myocutaneous flaps may be used. These flaps, by including muscle fibres, will bring a more certain blood supply and increased tissue bulk for deeper defects. They can be developed locally or from a distance. The flaps, which may appear bulky at first, will usually undergo atrophy to some extent in their muscular portion over the first few months after surgery. This usually results in an improvement of the final contour of the reconstructed area. Local myocutaneous flaps include the following.

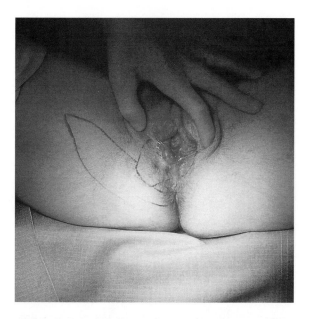

Figure 12.5 *Preoperative marking for a lateral transposition cutaneous flap from the right thigh. This figure also appears in the colour plate section.*

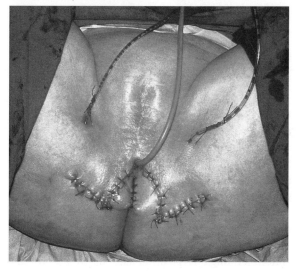

Figure 12.6 *Bilateral transposition cutaneous flaps. This figure also appears in the colour plate section.*

TENSOR FASCIA LATA FLAP[12]

This flap is of particular use to cover large defects in the groins and anterior vulva. The flap is developed on the lateral aspect of the thigh, and incorporates the skin and tensor fascia lata muscle with its vascular pedicle arising from the lateral femoral circumflex artery. This flap can be 20 cm or more in length, and

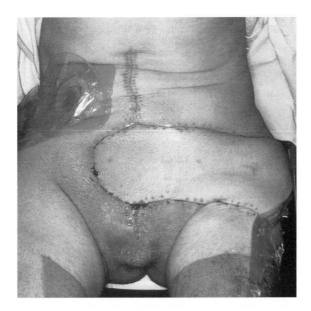

Figure 12.7 *Large tensor fascia lata fasciocutaneous flap rotated from the left thigh. This figure also appears in the colour plate section.*

can therefore be rotated medially towards the groin and vulvar region (Fig. 12.7).

GLUTEUS MAXIMUS FLAP[10,12]

This flap is developed in a similar fashion to the inferior gluteal fasciocutaneous flap described previously. However, a portion of the gluteus maximus muscle, together with its underlying blood supply, is incorporated into the flap. Large flaps up to 8–20 cm can be fashioned unilaterally or bilaterally (Fig. 12.8). These flaps can also be used to reconstruct the pelvic floor after anterior, posterior or total exenteration.

GRACILIS FLAP[13,14]

Bilateral flaps derived from the gracilis muscle and overlying tissues of the inner thigh were initially developed for use in the creation of a neovagina. However, they can also be used to fill large surgical defects on the vulva and perineum. The flap is developed immediately below a guideline drawn from the pubic tubercle to the medial femoral condyle at the knee. The flap to be taken is outlined on the skin, and an incision carried down to the level of the gracilis fascia. The gracilis muscle is then identified and is transected about 3 cm beyond the distal margin of the skin paddle using electrocautery. The vascular pedicle of the flap is at its proximal end, and is derived from the medial circumflex femoral artery and the terminal branches of the

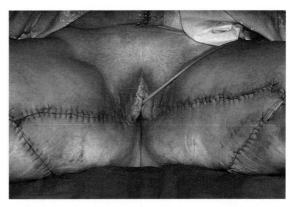

Figure 12.8 *Bilateral gluteus maximus flaps. This figure also appears in the colour plate section.*

obturator artery. Once the flap has been developed, a skin tunnel is fashioned to allow the flap to be rotated and advanced into the area where the defect is to be filled. This is a crucial part of the procedure because the vascular supply can easily be compromised as it is rotated. Often part of the blood supply is sacrificed, but clearly, this can lead to problems with necrosis as reported by Chen and collegues[14] in seven of a reported series of 11 patients. It does appear that the muscular component of the flap usually retains a satisfactory blood supply, which enhances secondary healing. One advantage of this flap, cited by its proponents, is that it is derived from tissue that is outside the usual radiotherapy fields for vulvar and perineal disease in patients previously exposed to this treatment modality.

Distant myocutaneous flaps

The use of distant flaps provides another means of filling large tissue defects with tissue that is rich in blood supply and derived from outwith potential radiotherapy fields. As a general rule, it is always preferable to use local techniques where possible, so distant flaps will be used only in exceptional circumstances. The techniques include the following.

RECTUS ABDOMINIS FLAPS[12,15,16]

This flap was first described for breast reconstruction, but both transverse and vertical rectus abdominis flaps can be mobilized and brought down to the pelvis or to the vulva for use in reconstruction. The blood supply is plentiful and derived from the superior and inferior epigastric arteries; as a result of the extensive anastomoses present, however, the entire muscle can be supplied from either vessel alone. This means that the surgery required is relatively simple, although care must be taken to avoid kinking the blood supply when relocating the flap into the pelvis. These flaps are often well suited to the creation of a new pelvic floor or neovagina after pelvic exenteration (Fig. 12.9). They are also of value for filling large defects after radical vulvectomy, particularly if any of the perivulvar tissue has received prior radiation. Another area of value is after the removal of large areas of skin over the pubis. Its major drawback is the need for an abdominal incision and the repair of the muscle donor site. If large areas of vulva are removed, it is possible to use bilateral rectus abdominis flaps although, as the muscle is wide, smaller defects can be covered by splitting the flap around the urethra and vagina rather like an 'inverted pair of trousers'.

A modification of the myocutaneous rectus abdominis flap is the transversus and rectus abdominis

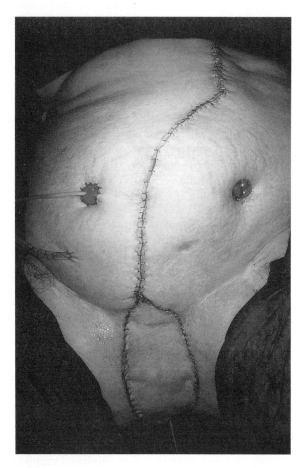

Figure 12.9 *Rectus abdominis flap used to form pelvic floor after total pelvic exenteration. This figure also appears in the colour plate section.*

musculoperitoneal (TRAMP) composite flap.[17] This flap is derived from the rectus muscle and tissues deep to it. It can be tubularized after mobilization into the pelvis to create a neovagina lined by peritoneum in vulvovaginal reconstruction.

LATISSIMUS DORSI FLAP[18]

This flap, which again is utilized in thoracic reconstruction, can, on occasion, be brought down to the lower abdominal wall or pelvis if other flaps are unsuitable. A free graft transposition is required with microscopic reanastomosis of the vascular supply to the femoral vessel. A large defect can thus be filled with fresh tissue from outside the previous treatment field.

PELVIC EXENTERATION

Reconstructive techniques play an important part in exenterative surgery. Indeed, this is often the most difficult and challenging part of the procedure. Careful thought and planning should therefore be given to these matters preoperatively. Reconstructive surgery may involve the formation of a new vagina after colpectomy or the placement of fresh tissue into the pelvis to fill a defect after removal of the pelvic floor. The introduction of fresh, healthy, non-irradiated tissue into the pelvis will aid healing in these circumstances and improve the quality of life postoperatively. Typically, myocutaneous flaps will be best suited to these purposes. Formation of a neovagina not only provides the opportunity for sexual rehabilitation, but also enhances healing in the pelvic cavity, and may reduce morbidity from chronic drainage and fistula formation.[19] Exenteration for vulvar cancer is an accepted surgical procedure for certain advanced or recurrent cases.[20]

POSTOPERATIVE CARE

As with preoperative planning and the surgery itself, meticulous attention to detail is important in the postoperative phase. The care taken at this stage will optimize the chances of a satisfactory outcome to the surgery and hopefully minimize the chances of complications. The antibiotic and anti-thromboembolic prophylaxis commenced at the time of surgery will be continued after the procedure has been completed.

Antibiotics are appropriate for 48–72 hours postoperatively, and subcutaneous heparin with thromboembolic prevention support stockings should be continued until full mobility is resumed. Patients should be nursed on a suitable bed and an air-fluidized (Clinitron) bed is ideal for these cases. This will minimize the risk of pressure necrosis occurring. A period of strict bedrest will be necessary immediately postoperatively with most authors advocating 3–5 days as appropriate. Particular attention should be directed at avoiding shearing forces that could disrupt wounds. Wounds should frequently be assessed to detect ischaemia and/or necrosis and cleansed two to three times each day with physiological (0.9 per cent) saline before air drying. Any soiling of the wound should be dealt with immediately by this same method. To help avoid this problem the prescription of agents such as Lomotil (co-phenotrope) is sometimes used to delay the onset of bowel motions. A urinary catheter is appropriate in most cases for a number of days after surgery and can be removed once the patient is adequately mobile and can get to the toilet and pass urine.

POSTOPERATIVE COMPLICATIONS

The majority of patients who require major vulvar reconstruction are, of course, elderly and will often be in less than perfect health. These women will be prone to all the usual complications of surgery, and particularly the threat of venous thromboembolism. The specific problems that relate to the vulvar reconstruction itself are those of infection and ischaemia leading to wound separation and breakdown. This is a particular problem in those who have previously been treated by radiotherapy to the surgical site, because this may have compromised the local small vessel vasculature.

Small areas of ischaemia and subsequent necrosis at the tip of the flaps are very common and will almost always heal by secondary intention, as long as there is scrupulous wound care. Larger areas of necrosis may necessitate debridement to enable healing to occur, again by secondary intention. In situations such as this, however, the potential threat of necrotizing fasciitis should be recognized because, if this should occur, delay in recognition and appropriate therapy could be fatal.

In the long term, contractures of the scars are sometimes problematic and may require further surgery to correct the problem. This seldom requires surgery more complex than simple advancement or 'Z'-plasty procedures. More frequent are the psychological and sexual difficulties that have been covered elsewhere in this text; they are summarized below with particular regard to reconstruction.

PSYCHOLOGICAL AND PSYCHOSEXUAL ASPECTS OF VULVAR RECONSTRUCTIVE SURGERY

There has been an increasing awareness of the potential psychological and psychosexual problems that may be associated with gynaecological surgery. This is of particular importance when carrying out reconstructive surgery for cancer or pre-cancer of the vulva. There will, of course, be many anxieties relating to the diagnosis of cancer, and the potential success or failure of the treatment. In addition, there are problems that relate to a woman's body image and the physical or psychological sexual difficulties that may follow surgery. As with most things in life, prevention is better than cure and it is vital that counselling, designed to prevent or minimize such difficulties, is an integral part of the whole management process.

Patients will be helped by a careful explanation of all matters relating to investigation, treatment and potential postoperative problems. These discussions should begin at the very first consultation. Explanations will be required throughout the management pathway as various problems arise or as the woman desires more information. This counselling process takes place on more than one occasion, with the objective of allowing the patient to arrive at a position of full understanding of the impact of the proposed surgery on her future life. This is of particular importance where stoma formation is indicated or even a possibility, and obviously where surgery may affect sexual function. Ideally, one member of the team should have specific skills and training and above all time to devote to this aspect of the patient's care.

Where vaginal reconstruction is proposed, the process of sexual rehabilitation should be carefully outlined before surgery. After surgery, it will be necessary to start the process using vaginal dilators and to encourage an early resumption of coitus as soon as the woman and her partner feel emotionally prepared. This will help to avoid problems with vaginal stenosis. A specialist nurse is well suited to supervise this important aspect of the rehabilitation process.

WHO SHOULD PERFORM VULVAR RECONSTRUCTIVE SURGERY?

Vulvar cancer is uncommon, with approximately 800 new cases registered annually in the UK. The highest standards of care will be produced in these few cases only if they are managed in a small number of specialist centres. This will allow a team of expert surgeons (of differing disciplines), medical and clinical oncologists, radiologists, pathologists and specialist nurses to attend to the many and complex demands that the management of such patients often pose. The fact that few cases will require reconstruction is an even stronger argument for developing specialist centres for the care of women with vulvar cancer.

Simple advancement techniques and the use of transposition flaps should be within the surgical expertise of a gynaecological oncologist. However, even in specialist centres, more difficult cases should be managed by a combination of gynaecological and plastic surgeons.

REFERENCES

1 Rutledge F, Sinclair M. Treatment of intra-epithelial neoplasia of the vulva by skin excision and graft. *Am J Obstet Gynecol* 1968; **102**: 806–18.

2 DiSaia PJ, Dorion GE, Cappucini F, Carpenter PM. A report of two cases of recurrent Paget's disease of the vulva in a split thickness graft and its possible pathogenesis-labeled retrodissemination. *Gynecol Oncol* 1995; **57**: 109–12.

3 Cormack GC, Lamberty BGH. The blood supply of the thigh skin. *Plast Reconstr Surg* 1985; **75**: 342–6.

4 Reid R. Local and distant skin flaps in the reconstruction of vulvar deformaties. *Am J Obstet Gynecol* 1997; **177**: 1372–83.

5 Tateo A, Tateo S, Bernasconi C, Zara C. Use of V-Y flap for vulvar reconstruction. *Gynecol Oncol* 1995; **62**: 203–6.

6 Helm CW, Hatch KD, Partridge EE, Shingleton HM. The rhomboid transposition flap for repair of the perineal defect after radical vulvar surgery. *Gynecol Oncol* 1993; **50**: 164–7.

7 Burke TW, Morris M, Levenback C, Gershensen DM, Wharton JT. Closure of complex vulvar defects using local rhomboid flaps. *Obstet Gynecol* 1994; **84**: 1043–7.

8 Potkul RK, Barnes WA, Barter JF, Delgado G, Spear SL. Vulvar reconstruction using a mons pubis pedicle flap. *Gynecol Oncol* 1994; **55**: 21–4.

9 Davison PM, Sarhanis P, Foden-Schroff J, Kilby M, Redman CW. A new approach to reconstruction following vulval excision. *Br J Obstet Gynaecol* 1996; **103**: 475–7.

10 Loree TL, Hemppling RE, Eltabbakh GH, Recio FO, Piver MS. The inferior gluteal flap in the difficult vulvar and perineal reconstruction. *Gynecol Oncol* 1997; **66**: 429–34.

11 Achauer BM, Braly P, Berman ML, DiSaia PJ. Immediate vaginal reconstruction following resection for malignancy using the gluteal thigh flap. *Gynecol Oncol* 1984; **68**: 521–32.

12 Knapstein PG, Friedberg V. Reconstructive operations of the vulva and vagina. In: Knapstein PG, Friedberg V, Sevin B-U (eds). *Reconstructive surgery in gynecology*. New York: Thième Medical Publishers, Inc, 1990: 11–70.

13 Burke TW, Morris M, Roh MS, Levenback C, Gershensen DM. Perineal reconstruction using single gracilis myocutaneous flaps. *Gynecol Oncol* 1995; **57**: 221–5.

14 Chen SHT, Hentz VR, Wei F-C, Chen Y-R. Short gracilis myocutaneous flaps for vulvoperineal and inguinal reconstruction. *Plast Recontr Surg* 1995; 95: 372–7.

15 Shepherd JH, Van Dam P, Jobling T, Breach N. The use of rectus abdominis musculo-cutaneous flaps following radical excision of vulva cancer. *Br J Obstet Gynaecol* 1990; **97**: 1020–5.

16 Patsner B, Hetzler P. Post-radical vulvectomy reconstruction using the inferiorly based transverse rectus abdominis (TRAM) flap: A preliminary experience. *Gynecol Oncol* 1994; **55**: 78–81.

17 Hockel M. The transverse and rectus abdominis musculoperitoneal (TRAMP) composite flap for vulvovaginal reconstruction. *Plast Reconstr Surg* 1996; 97: 455–9.

18 Neven P, Shepherd JH, Tham KF, Fisher C, Breach N. Reconstruction of the abdominal wall with a latissimus dorsi musculocutaneous flap. A case of massive abdominal wall metastasis from a cervical cancer requiring palliative resection. *Gynecol Oncol* 1993; **49**: 403–6.

19 Hopkins MP, Morley GW. Pelvic exenteration for the treatment of vulvar cancer. *Cancer* 1992; **70**: 2835–8.

20 Cavanagh D, Shepherd JH. The place of pelvic exenteration in the management of advanced carcinoma of the vulva. *Gynecol Oncol* 1982; **13**: 318–22.

13

Rare tumours of the vulva

CW HELM

Vulvar cancers as a whole are not common but, as invasive squamous cell carcinoma and vulvar intraepithelial neoplasia (VIN) represent more than 80 per cent of vulvar tumours, all others may be classed as rare (Table 13.1). The data of the Surveillance, Epidemiology and End Results (SEER) programme for nine population-based cancer registries, covering about 10 per cent of the US population, found that, excluding squamous intraepithelial neoplasia, the relative distribution of invasive and preinvasive cancers was squamous cell carcinoma 78.2 per cent, basal cell carcinoma 6.8 per cent, melanoma 6.7 per cent, Paget's disease 4.1 per cent, adenocarcinoma 2.03 per cent, sarcoma 1.1 per cent, and other 0.93 per cent.[1]

There is a general lack of definitive information about these rare tumours and data come from reports of small numbers of patients. Randomized controlled trials of treatments are not practical and guidelines are, in many cases, based on theory and extrapolation of data gleaned from the study of similar tumours occurring outside the vulva and from squamous cell carcinoma of the vulva.

The investigation of patients with such rare tumours is similar to that for invasive squamous cell carcinoma. The aim, through history, clinical examination and special investigations, is to determine the extent of the primary tumour of the vulva and possible metastases, and to look for the presence of associated tumours on the vulva and elsewhere.

The pathology of these rare lesions has been discussed in detail in Chapters 2 and 3. This chapter attempts to integrate the pathology with the clinical manifestations and management of rare tumours. Some duplication is unavoidable.

PAGET'S DISEASE OF THE VULVA

Paget's disease of the vulva (PDV) is a type of intraepithelial neoplasia[2] that arises from multipotential stem cells in the epidermis and epidermally derived adnexal structures.[3] The first report of the condition was on the mammary areola by Sir James Paget in 1874,[4] but the first case involving the vulva was not described until 1901.[5] PDV (Fig. 13.1) represents approximately 4.1 per cent of all malignant tumours of the vulva[1] excluding squamous intraepithelial neoplasia (VIN). It is approximately 24 times less common than vulvar squamous carcinoma in situ.[1]

Table 13.1 *Rare preinvasive and invasive tumours of the vulva*

Preinvasive
    Paget's disease
    Dysplastic naevus
    Congenital naevus
Invasive
Primary
    Melanoma
    Basal cell carcinoma
    Verrucous carcinoma
    Adenocarcinoma
    Bartholin's gland carcinoma
    Sarcoma
    Merkel cell carcinoma
Secondary
    Metastatic

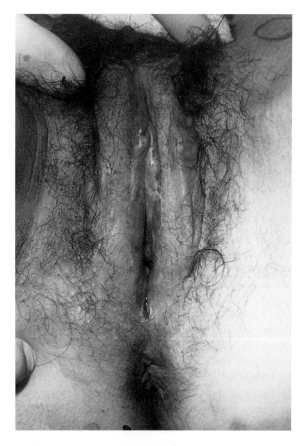

Figure 13.1 *Extensive Paget's disease of vulva with underlying adenocarcinoma of the left vulva.*

Age, site, presentation and diagnosis

PDV affects mainly postmenopausal women of European origin[6,7] with a mean age at diagnosis of 64 years.[8] The youngest reported case was in a 24-year-old African–American woman.[9] It begins on the apocrine gland-bearing regions of the vulva, genital folds and perianal region, and may be multifocal.[10]

The condition presents with pruritus in over 50 per cent,[6,7] together with soreness, burning, bleeding and pain.[8,11,12] It may either appear as red velvety areas with white islands of hyperkeratosis or be pinkish and scaly. The diagnosis is made by biopsy and there is a distinctive histological appearance with pathognomonic 'Paget' cells.[3]

Association with underlying and extravulvar malignancy

PDV is thought to be commonly associated with an underlying subjacent glandular apocrine adenocarcinoma[13] (Table 13.2) analogous to the situation with Paget's disease of the breast. In a review of the English literature between 1962 and 1982, Chanda[8] (Table 13.2) found that 24 per cent of 194 patients with extramammary Paget's disease, including 109 with PDV, were associated with a concurrent underlying cutaneous adnexal carcinoma. Helwig and Graham,[14] in a review of material at the Armed Forces Institute of Pathology in Washington, DC, reported that 13 of 40 (33 per cent) patients with anogenital Paget's disease had associated underlying cutaneous adnexal carcinoma. They emphasized the need to differentiate between direct involvement of adnexal structures by Paget cells within an intact basement membrane and true invasive adenocarcinoma.

Progression of PDV itself to invasive adenocarcinoma can occur but is thought to be rare.[10] Cappuccini and colleagues[16] described a case of non-invasive PDV that metastasized to the bone marrow in the absence of an underlying adenocarcinoma. Parmley and colleagues[17] reported three cases of non-invasive PDV with metastases to the vertebrae, ribs and bone of the pelvis. There have also been reports of women with minimally invasive PDV with involvement of the lymph vascular space[18] and some with minimally invasive PDV with 1 mm of invasion who developed extensive inguinofemoral lymph node metastases.[19]

In Chanda's review,[8] 9 per cent of 109 cases of PDV (Table 13.2) were associated with a concurrent malig-

Table 13.2 *Proportion of cases of Paget's disease of the vulva associated with another malignancy*

Timing and site of malignancy	Percentage cases from		
	Chanda[8] (n = 109)	Helwig[14] (n = 40[a])	Degefu[15] (n = 200)
Concurrent			
Underlying cutaneous	24[b]	33	
Internal	9[c]		
Non-concurrent			
Internal	19		
Concurrent and non-concurrent			
Urogenital	16		15
Breast	10		
Total internal malignancy (concurrent/non-concurrent)	28	18	

[a] Anogenital Paget's disease.
[b] 24 per cent of 194 cases of Paget's disease, the majority involving vulva, penis, scrotum, groin or perianal region.
[c] Including one Bartholin's gland carcinoma.

nancy in the cervix (squamous cell carcinoma and adenocarcinoma), breast, Bartholin's gland and gallbladder. In addition, 21 (19 per cent) other non-concurrent malignancies occurred making a total of 28 per cent who had a concurrent or non-current internal malignancy. Degefu and colleagues[15] reviewed the literature and found that 30 of 200 cases (15 per cent) of PDV reported had other concomitant or coincidental urogenital malignancies, most commonly in the vulva, 33 per cent (three melanomas, three squamous cell carcinomas, two Bartholin's gland carcinomas and two hidradenocarcinomas); cervix, 27 per cent (six invasive squamous cell carcinomas, two endocervical carcinomas); bladder, 13 per cent; ovary, 10 per cent; and single cases of urethral, vaginal, endometrial, ureteral and renal carcinomas. Perianal Paget's disease has been associated with an underlying rectal carcinoma.[14,20] Chanda[8] reported that 27 of 31 (87 per cent) of concurrent and non-current internal malignancies, reported in association with Paget's disease of the vulva, were in the female genitourinary system or breast with 55 per cent in the genitourinary system alone.

Management

The management of PDV is defined by the need to exclude invasive PDV, an underlying adnexal adenocarcinoma and a concurrent carcinoma in the vulva and elsewhere, particularly the breast, urinary tract, genital tract and rectum. Special investigations to be considered include mammography, cervical smear, colposcopy, urine cytology, cystoscopy, intravenous urogram, proctosigmoidoscopy and computed tomography (CT) or a magnetic resonance imaging (MRI) scan of the abdomen and pelvis.

The need to exclude invasive PDV and an underlying adnexal adenocarcinoma means that the tumour must be excised. If such a tumour is known to be present, then treatment should be as for an invasive adenocarcinoma of the vulva. If it is not known whether or not there is an underlying carcinoma, the vulvar skin and underlying appendages should be removed.[21] Previously, radical vulvectomy was preferred[12,17] but others have performed more conservative surgery, including skinning vulvectomy with split-thickness skin graft, hemivulvectomy or simple vulvectomy.[22] Bergen and colleagues[22] have shown that hair follicles and sweat glands do not extend more than 4 mm from the surface of the epidermis, and conclude that excision of the skin of the vulva with some of the underlying fat is adequate to include all subcutaneous glands. Of 14 patients, only one patient recurred who had had negative margins at the time of original surgery.[22] Excision may have to be extensive if the disease extends to the buttocks, perineum or vagina and, as PDV has been documented histologically in apparently normal skin on the contralateral vulva, some gynaecologists favour total vulvectomy[20] rather than local excision of visible tumour.

Wide margins around the visible abnormality seem sensible because the histological abnormality extends much wider than the visible abnormality.[23] Although Feuer and colleagues[18] suggested a minimum 0.5 cm margin, others suggest 2–3 cm. Frozen sections to delineate the margin of tumour at surgery may be misleading, particularly as a result of skip lesions.[23] If there is a desire to preserve the clitoris, this area can be preserved and treated with laser ablation.[22] Inguinal node dissection is unnecessary unless an invasive adenocarcinoma is found.

Outcome

When an underlying carcinoma is present, the prognosis is poor[7,8,12,13,17,24] and in recent reports survival of 0 per cent at 2 years and 27.7 per cent at 6.2 years has been found.[25,26]

Patients with non-invasive PDV do not die of their disease, but do develop recurrent disease and may develop invasive carcinoma. Interestingly, Paget's disease may recur in an area previously totally excised and transplanted with autologous skin.[6,27–30] Friedrich[31] reported that the recurrence rates for all patients with PDV treated surgically, regardless of extent of histological involvement, was 12.4 per cent and, from a review of the world literature, Breen and colleagues[7] reported a recurrence rate after all forms of surgery of 11.6 per cent. Individual series have reported recurrence rates as high as 54 per cent.[26] Breen and colleagues[7] reviewed the results of therapy in 98 patients, and noted no recurrences in five patients treated with local excision, nine of 49 (18 per cent) treated with simple vulvectomy and 3 of 44 (6.8 per cent) treated with modified or radical vulvectomy. Recurrence rates are thought to be similar for microinvasive PDV.[25] Usually, recurrences are amenable to local therapy[12] and treatment options include further local excision, laser ablation and topical 5-fluorouracil (5-FU) cream.[32]

The development of recurrent PDV and invasive carcinoma may take between 8 and 10 years;[10,13,25] so long-term follow-up is mandatory.

MALIGNANT MELANOMA

Melanoma is a malignant tumour of melanocytes of neural crest origin, which are normally found in the basal portion of the epidermis. Malignant melanoma of the vulva (MMV) was first reported in 1861.[33] It represents 1.3 per cent of all melanomas in women[34] and 3.6–6.7 per cent of all vulvar malignancies.[1,35] Studies from individual centres suggesting rates of almost 10 per cent may reflect referral bias.[36,37] Inci-

dence rates of 0.108/100 000 per annum are reported from the USA[34] and 0.08/100 000 per annum for the West Midlands in the UK.[35]

Age, site, presentation and diagnosis

In studies with more than 25 patients over the last 30 years the mean age was 60 years with a range from 10 years to 96 years.[34–36,38–43] Approximately one-third of patients are premenopausal[36] and many series report patients aged 20 years or younger.[38,41–45]

Of the MMVs 70 per cent arise in, or involve, the mucosal surfaces of the vulva with 25 per cent involving just one labium majus and 10 per cent the clitoris (Figs 13.2 and 13.3).[35–37,39,40] Although MMVs may be

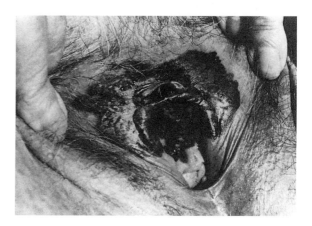

Figure 13.2 *Extensive superficial spreading vulvar melanoma. (Reproduced with permission from Silvers and Halperin.[46])*

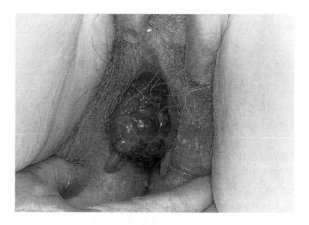

Figure 13.3 *Fungating, black, nodular melanoma of the vulva. (Reproduced with permission from Lynch and Edwards.[47])*

an incidental finding, many present with a mass or lump, pruritus, discharge or bleeding, or even occasionally as a swelling from metastasis in the groin.[35,40] Some patients may note changes in pre-existing moles.[40]

Predisposing conditions

MMVs are two to four times more common in European than in African–American women.[34,48] The incidence rises with age, but does not appear to have increased over time within the USA, and there is no increased incidence in the hotter, southern states.[34]

There is little information about familial MMVs, although some papers report a family history of melanoma in those with MMV.[36,38] Cutaneous melanoma occurs at a younger age in patients with a family history of melanoma compared with those with no family history: 44.8 years versus 49.7 years.[49] These patients are also more likely to have multiple lesions and better survival. Evidence linking MM to pregnancy is thought to be questionable.[50]

Pre-cancerous conditions

Pigmented lesions on the vulva are common, often remain unnoticed by the patient and are usually benign.[51,52] Such benign lesions include seborrhoeic keratosis, haemangioma, lentigo, dermatofibroma, extramammary breast tissue, melanosis and pigmentation associated with hormones and following inflammation.[47] More malign lesions include VIN, acanthosis nigrans, melanoma and Kaposi's sarcoma.[47] Rock and colleagues[52] screened 303 consecutive new patients during routine gynaecological examination and found that 10.3 per cent had pigmented lesions of the vulva and 2.3 per cent (7 of 303) had naevocytic naevi, one of which was a premalignant dysplastic naevus.

There are three types of acquired benign naevi histologically. Intradermal and compound types are generally soft, dome shaped, papular, sharply marginated, evenly pigmented, tan to dark brown in colour and less than 10 mm in diameter, whereas junctional naevi are sharply marginated pigmented lesions 2–10 mm in diameter, which are flat and range in colour from tan to dark brown to black.[47,52] The risk of malignant transformation is increased in the dysplastic naevus. Clinically, dysplastic naevi tend to be flat or slightly raised and demonstrate one or more atypical features including irregular borders, indistinct margin, large size (>5 mm) and variegated pigmentary patterns, including speckling and reddish hues.[47,53] These lesions have been described on the vulva.[51,54] Dysplastic naevi are more common in patients with multiple torso and limb naevi[51] and in those with familial dysplastic naevus syndrome.[53]

Congenital naevi are present at birth; the common cutaneous naevus usually appears in young adult life whereas cutaneous dysplastic naevi appear in adolescence and may continue to appear even after the age of 35 years.[50] Congenital naevi are brown lesions that show some degree of surface irregularity and tend to be larger than acquired naevi.[47] Larger congenital lesions are characterized by a more irregular surface, border and colour, but they do not enlarge except in proportion to growth of the skin. At puberty they become thicker and darker.[47] The lifetime risk of developing malignant melanoma in a congenital naevus is estimated at 5–20 per cent when the lesion is larger than 2 cm.[50]

Management of pigmented lesions

It is not necessary to remove all pigmented lesions on the vulva, particularly benign naevi, but biopsy should always be performed if there is clinical doubt.[47] All congenital naevi and those thought to be junctional or dysplastic should be removed.[50] This means pigmented lesions larger than 5 mm with irregular borders, indistinct margin and variegated pigmentary patterns including speckling and reddish hues. In addition, pigmented lesions, whose size or pigmentation is increasing, are causing irritation or pain or are ulcerated or bleeding should also be excised.

Patients with dysplastic naevi who have a family history of dysplastic naevi or melanoma and/or have other cutaneous lesions with similar appearance should be followed closely by a skin cancer specialist.

Prognostic features and survival

The following prognostic features have been reported: depth of invasion;[35,37,40,42,43,45,55–59] ulceration;[35,42,57,59] cell type (epithelioid worse than spindle);[35] tumour growth pattern (nodular worse than superficial spreading);[40,57] mitotic rate;[35,42,57] inflammatory response;[35,57] involvement of the lymph vascular space;[59] lesion size smaller than 2 cm;[39] DNA ploidy;[59] increasing age;[35,43,45,58] node status;[36,42,43,45,55,56,58–60] clinical staging, based on the 1971 staging of the

International Federation of Gynaecology and Obstetrics (FIGO) (I/II versus III/IV);[35] and the 1992 staging of the American Joint Committee on Cancer (AJCC).[58]

Studies that have examined prognostic factors in MMV with regression or multivariate analysis indicate that varying factors are most important for survival/recurrence-free survival: FIGO (1971) stage (I/II versus III/IV) and cell type;[35] age, tumour thickness and groin node metastasis;[43] ulceration, depth of invasion and node status;[42] groin node metastasis, invasion of endothelium-lined spaces, clitoral involvement and multifocal tumour;[59] and AJCC staging.[58]

Depth of invasion

Clark[61] defined five levels of invasion into the epidermis and dermis of cutaneous malignant melanoma, which correlated with survival (Fig. 13.4), but there were difficulties applying these levels to the vulva because the transition between papillary dermis and reticular dermis was rather subjective.[46] Breslow[62] reported that prognosis was related to tumour size, tumour thickness and Clark's levels. Chung and colleagues[37] incorporated tumour thickness into a modification of Clark's definition for levels II, III and IV (Fig. 13.4). Which method of classifying depth of invasion to use is a matter of convenience, but a report from Chung's original hospital found that Chung's levels are a more accurate predictor of survival and risk of nodal disease than Breslow's tumour thickness[43] (Tables 13.3, 13.4 and 13.5).

Staging

The AJCC system[68] incorporates tumour thickness/Clark's levels. The FIGO and TNM systems use lesion size as a discriminant of stage, and this has not been shown to be a significant factor in outcome for MMVs. In a prospective study of MMV examining many clinicopathological factors, AJCC staging for cutaneous melanoma had the most significant correlation with recurrence-free interval whereas FIGO clinical staging

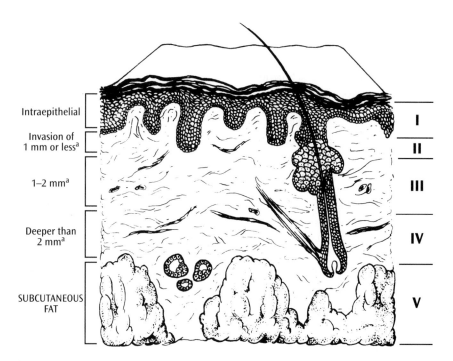

Intraepithelial — I

Invasion of 1 mm or less[a] — II

1–2 mm[a] — III

Deeper than 2 mm[a] — IV

SUBCUTANEOUS FAT — V

[a] As measured from granular layer of surface epithelium

Figure 13.4 *Levels of involvement in melanoma of the vulva. Level I (melanoma confined to the surface epithelium and pilar sheath) and level V (tumour extension into the underlying adipose tissue) are identical to Clark's levels I and V. Levels II, III and IV are determined by measurements from the granular layer of the vulvar skin or outermost epithelial layer of the squamous mucosa. (Reproduced with permission from Chung et al.[37])*

Table 13.3 *Melanoma of the vulva – survival by tumour thickness*

Reference	Year	No.	Tumour thickness								Follow-up
			<0.76 mm		0.76–1.5 mm		1.51–3 mm		>3.0 mm		
			No.	(%)	No.	(%)	No.	(%)	No.	(%)	
Podratz[40a]	1983	48	3	(100)	7	(92)	15	(90)	23	(23)	16 months to 29 years (Kaplan–Meier)
Beller[44]	1986	13	1	(100)	1	(100)	4	(75)	7	(43)	34–120 months
			<0.75 mm		0.75–1.5 mm						
Trimble[43]	1992	65	12	(48)	10	(79)	9	(56)	34	(44)	Median 193 months (Kaplan–Meier)
							1.6–3.0 mm		>3.10 mm		
Woolcott[41]	1988	25			3	(100)	7	(57)	15	(40)	Minimum 60 months
									> 3–≤5 mm		
Scheistrøen[59b]	1995	36	5	(80)	9	(89)	11	(54)	11	(54)	Median 99 months (67–374 months) (Kaplan–Meier)

[a] Figures estimated from survival curve.
[b] >5 mm thickness, $n = 34$, survival rate 27%.
Bradgate[35] reported age-adjusted 5-year survival rates in the following tumour thickness groups: 0–4 mm, $n = 13$, 59%; 4.1–8.0 mm, $n = 19$, 38%; 8 mm, $n = 14$, 10%.

Table 13.4 *Melanoma of the vulva: 5- and 10-year survival rates by Clark's and Chung's levels*

Reference	Year	No.	Group[a]										Follow-up
			I		II		III		IV		V		
			No.	(%)	No.	(%)	No.	(%)	No.	(%)	No.	(%)	
Clark's levels (5-year)													
Podratz[40]	1983	48			6	(100)	7	(83)	11	(81)	24	(28)	16 months to 29 years (Kaplan–Meier)
Jaramillo[56]	1985	9			1	(100)	2	(50)	5	(40)	1	(0)	Minimum 60 months
Benda[63]	1986	13	1	(100)	2	(50)	6	(0)	3	(33)	1	(0)	52–125 months
Bradgate[35]	1990	43			2	(100)	2	(0)	32	(41)	7	(17)	48 months to 25 years
Chung's levels (5-year)													
Benda[63]	1986	13	1	(100)	2	(50)	3	(0)	6	(17)	1	(0)	52–125 months
Trimble[43]	1992	47	1	(100)	12	(81)	8	(87)	20	(4)	6	(33)	Median 193 months (Kaplan–Meier)
Clark's levels (10-year)													
Podratz[40]	1983	48			6	(100)	7	(83)	11	(65)	24	(23)	16 months to 29 years
Chung's levels (10-year)													
Trimble[43]	1992	47	1	(100)	12	(81)	8	(87)	20	(11)	6	(33)	Median 193 months Kaplan–Meier

[a] The number (and percentage) surviving.

Table 13.5 *Malignant melanoma: overall survival*

Reference	Year	No.	Treatment	%	Follow-up (months)
Yackel[39]	1970	21	S	33	Min. 60
Morrow[36]	1972	14	S mainly	50	Min. 60
Chung[37]	1975	33	S mainly	30	Min. 60
Edington[66]	1980	15	S	8	33
Ariel[64]	1981	40	S	32	Min. 60
Podratz[40]	1983	48	S mainly	54	16 months to 29 years (Kaplan–Meier)
Benda[63]	1986	13	S mainly	27	52–125
Bouma[60]	1982	9	S	44	Min. 60
Johnson[57]	1986	18	a	22	32 (2–157)
Davidson[67]	1987	22	Ss	27	
Woolcott[41]	1988	32	Ss	44	Min. 60
Bradgate[35]	1990	50	Ss	35	4–25 years (age-adjusted)
Tasseron[42]	1992	30	Ss	56	b(Kaplan–Meier)
Look[65]	1993	16	S mainly	30	Median 24 (3–143) (Kaplan–Meier)
Scheistrøen[59]	1995	75	Ss[b]	46	Median 99 (67–374) (Kaplan–Meier)

S, radical surgery including radical vulvectomy; S mainly = mainly radical surgery; Ss, roughly equal numbers with radical and non-radical surgery.
a Information not given.
b Patients treated with radiation.

was not a factor.[58] The Gynecologic Oncology Group (GOG) has recommended that the AJCC system should be used for MMVs.

Treatment

Treatment of MMVs is a balance between trying to achieve locoregional control while minimizing treatment morbidity.[35] Paralleling the move to radical surgery for squamous cell carcinoma of the vulva,[69] the standard treatment for MMVs became radical vulvectomy with bilateral groin and pelvic node dissection.[36,37,39,40,55,56,66,70,71] In 1987, Davidson and colleagues[67] reported on 32 patients with MMVs and MM of the vagina, finding no difference in outcome whether the patients underwent radical surgery (radical vulvectomy alone, radical vulvectomy combined with groin and iliac node dissection or anterior exenteration) or simple vulvectomy, or local excision alone or with adjuvant radiotherapy. The authors suggested local excision of the primary lesion alone, with groin dissection only for clinically evident disease in the groins. Radical surgery should be considered for those with bulky primary lesions or extensive local recurrence. Subsequently, most reports suggested no difference in survival for wide local excision and hemivulvectomy versus radical surgery,[35,41–43,45,59] although the total number of patients treated was

small and none of the studies was prospective or randomized (see Table 13.5).

Surgical excision margins

Historically, cutaneous melanomas were excised with wide margins of 5–15 cm,[45] but less wide excision with a margin of 1–2 cm appears to be adequate for cutaneous melanomas less than 2 mm thick and with a diameter of less than 2 cm.[62,72,73]

There are few specific data on excision margins in MMVs. Podratz and colleagues[40] noted a worse outcome for medial tumours versus lateral tumours, and speculated that this may be associated with less good margins achievable for medially based lesions. Rose and colleagues[45] found that three of six patients undergoing conservative surgery with margins that were less than 2 cm or unspecified recurred, compared with only one of six patients with a margin of more than 2 cm[45]. Trimble and colleagues[43] advocated radical local excision to obtain margins of 1–2 cm for thin melanomas, Chung level II (1 mm or less invasion) and 3 cm for thicker melanomas, Chung levels III and IV. Chung level I can be treated with simple excision and close follow-up. Even in thin lesions of less than 0.76 mm, the margin must be adequate because there are reports of recurrence in such patients.[45,74] Tasseron and colleagues[42] proposed that a margin of 2–3 cm with local excision is sufficient for all.

Management of regional lymph nodes

Histologically negative groin lymph nodes are associated with a survival rate of 38–73 per cent and positive nodes with 0–40 per cent.[35,39,40,43,66] Capillary–lymphatic space (CLS) involvement and central primary lesions are the most significant independent predictors of positive groin nodes as identified by multiple regression.[58] In an analysis of 71 patients with MMVs entered into a GOG protocol, GOG performance status, FIGO (1969) staging, tumour size and tumour location (central including bilateral, clitoral, urethral, vaginal, perineal or anal versus non-central), CLS involvement and Breslow's depth of invasion were significantly associated with lymph node metastasis.[58] Of patients with positive CLS involvement or central primary lesions, 31.8 per cent have positive groin nodes.[58]

For cutaneous melanoma involving the extremities, elective regional lymph node dissection for clinically uninvolved nodes has not been shown to give survival benefit over delayed lymph node dissection when the nodes become clinically enlarged.[75,76] Elective node dissection in all patients with MMV was questioned by Chung and colleagues,[37] who suggested that it was unnecessary in Chung level II (thickness ≤1 mm). Instances of lymph node involvement with tumour thickness less than 0.76 mm or Clark's level II are rare but do occur.[43] Trimble and colleagues[43] suggested that lesions thicker than 0.76 mm (Clark's level III) benefited from prophylactic elective groin node dissection, because long-term survival may be achieved with positive nodes and Podratz and colleagues[40] reported a 31 per cent 10-year survival rate in the presence of microscopically involved groin nodes, when prophylactic groin node dissection was carried out with radical vulvectomy. They also reported that only one of 44 patients with ipsilateral or bilateral groin node dissection developed recurrence in the groins. Thus, the evidence suggests that a groin node dissection should be considered in MMV for lesions with a depth of invasion of more than 0.76 mm (Clark's level III), either ipsilateral for lateralized lesions or bilateral for central lesions.

The removal of clinically involved nodes may also be beneficial in MMVs.[40–43]

Survival

The overall survival rate is between 8 per cent and 56 per cent in published series (see Table 13.5). Survival in relation to tumour thickness, Clark's levels and Chung's levels is given in Tables 13.3 and 13.4.

Recurrences

After primary therapy, recurrences are common with rates varying from 51 per cent[40] to as high as 93 per cent.[66] Podratz and colleagues[40] reported that 62 per cent who developed recurrence initially did so locally, most commonly in the vulva and vagina; 37 per cent initially developed distant metastases, most commonly to the lungs and bone. Of patients with recurrences, 29 per cent had involvement of multiple sites.[40] This concurs with the findings of others.[36,41] Phillips and colleagues,[58] reporting on GOG data, found that 49.3 per cent of 71 patients developed recurrent disease, 28 per cent in the vulva or vagina, 26 per cent in the groins and 40 per cent distant.[58] The median time to recurrence was 12 months and, even if patients had local recurrences initially, they die with distant disease. Late recurrences occurring at between 10 and 19 years are well documented.[35,37,41,42] It may be difficult to exclude a second primary in this situation. Adjuvant interferon -α2b can be used for patients with recurrence.[77]

The outcome after recurrence is poor. The median survival after recurrence was 5.9 months (range 2–21 months).[65] Podratz and colleagues[40] reported a 5 per cent probability of surviving 5 years after recurrence.

Adjunctive treatment

Malignant melanoma is resistant to standard radiotherapy and chemotherapy. Interferon -α2b (has been shown to increase disease-free and overall survival for patients with node-positive disease[77] and is recommended for use in patients with this disease. Median disease-free survival increased from 1 to 1.7 years, and overall survival from 2.8 to 3.8 years. Interferon -α2b can also be used for patients with other forms of locoregional disease, including disease in transit, satellites or local recurrence. Those with disease that is more than 4 mm thick and with negative nodes should be entered into clinical trials for evaluation of this treatment.[78]

Melanoma that has spread to distant sites is infrequently curable with standard therapy, although long-term survival is sometimes achieved by surgical resection of metastases to the lungs, gastrointestinal tract and brain.[79] Radiotherapy may be used for palliation of brain, bone and visceral metastases. Patients with advanced disease should be entered into clinical trials.

BASAL CELL CARCINOMA

Basal cell carcinoma of the vulva (BCCV) was first reported in 1926.[80] It represents 0.8–14.7 per cent of all vulvar malignancy in older reports[81] and 4.9 per cent and 6.8 per cent, respectively, in more recent studies.[1,81]

Age, site, presentation and diagnosis

The mean age at diagnosis is 69 years (range 34–95 years).[81–86] BCCV occurs mainly on the anterior vulva and mons pubis. The least common site is the non-hair-bearing skin on central vulvar structures.[84]

Of the lesions, 82 per cent are less than 2 cm in their greatest dimension[84] and 89 per cent are confined to the vulva at the time of diagnosis[81] (Fig. 13.5). Symptoms are non-specific irritation, soreness and pruritus. BCCV can have several different clinical appearances, including a nodule (Fig. 13.5), polyp,

ulcer, or an area of pigmentation or depigmentation[81,87] and even a large, pedunculated exophytic mass.[87] The variability of physical findings makes the clinical diagnosis difficult and it is unusual to be diagnosed before biopsy.[81,87]

Aetiology and association with other malignancies

The aetiology of BCCV is obscure. Ultraviolet irradiation and sunlight, which have been linked to BCC of the face and extremities, is not likely to play a role in the vulva. Exposure to arsenical compounds, irradiation, chronic irritation, trauma and chronic infection have been implicated.[83–85,88] Lichen sclerosus is not considered to be a predisposing factor.[83,85,88]

An association with other malignancies has been reported. Benedet and colleagues[84] found that 39 per cent of patients had either another BCC or some other tumour, including cancer of the ovary, cervix, lung, colon and breast, and lymphoma and squamous cell carcinoma of the vulva.[84] It may occur adjacent to a squamous cell carcinoma of the vulva[85] and adequate biopsy is thus necessary to be sure that this more aggressive carcinoma is not present. The author has experience of a case in which preoperative biopsy reported a BCC and the definitive pathology report

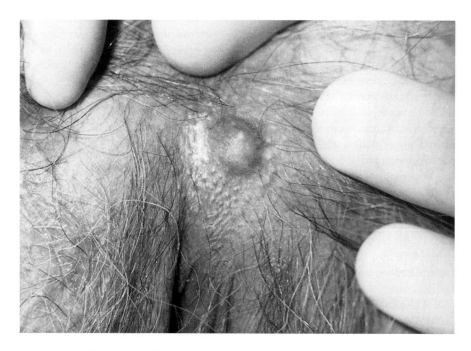

Figure 13.5 *Recurrent basal cell carcinoma of the vulva.*

indicated a squamous cell carcinoma, and another patient with the opposite scenario. This could lead to both under- and over-treatment.

Treatment

There is broad consensus that initial treatment of the primary lesion should be wide local excision.[81–86,88] The exact margin necessary has not been established but may be just a clear histological margin. Provided that the tumour is in a convenient situation, it is always best to aim for a minimum 1 cm margin as with squamous cell carcinoma.[89] If the tumour is locally extensive, then more extensive surgery may be necessary to achieve clear margins.

Management of groin nodes

Routine dissection of the groin lymph nodes is not indicated because BCCV is a locally invasive neoplasm and metastases in the groins merit case reports.[86,88,90–93] Factors that increase the chance of nodal metastasis are tumour size over 4 cm and deep invasion into subcutaneous tissues.[81,84,86,90–95] Thus, groin node dissection is indicated only when there is a large, deeply invasive tumour or the nodes are clinically suspicious or involved.

Management of positive margins after excision

Positive margins at the time of primary surgery would be expected to increase the chance of recurrence. Feakins and Lowe[81] reported that four of 45 (9 per cent) patients with BCCV recurred and three of the four had been incompletely excised whereas the fourth had metastatic disease at the time of initial surgery. However, there were no recurrences in four of the seven patients with incomplete excision of the primary. Benedet and colleagues[84] followed seven patients with positive margins for 2–24 years without any recurrence, and they suggested that these patients could be safely followed without further excision.[84] However, if the report shows a positive margin, it would be sensible to carry out a further excision unless this would cause unacceptable dysfunction to the patient.

Recurrence

Recurrence rates vary between 0 and 21 per cent.[82,83,85,88] Two recent series report rates of 9 and 12 per cent.[81,84] Most recurrences are local and can be surgically excised. It must be remembered that a new primary BCCV can develop at a different site on the vulva.[88]

Follow-up

All patients should be followed up indefinitely after BCCV has been treated, the interval depending on the features of the lesion excised. For completely excised small lesions, a 6-monthly check-up is adequate.

Outcome

The overall outcome for patients with BCCV is excellent and the vast majority of patients die from other causes. Of 28 patients with adequate follow-up (21 for > 5 years), only one died as a result of BCCV.[84] Feakins and Lowe[81] reported on 45 patients with a mean follow-up of 59 months (range 1–112 months) and only one died from metastatic BCCV.

Role of radiation

Breen and colleagues,[83] reporting on what little there is in the literature, suggested reserving radiation for lesions so advanced that surgery was not feasible. When used after incomplete excision of a primary lesion, radiation did not affect recurrence and was associated with persistent vulvar ulceration in two patients.[81] However, on the skin there are reports of cure rates of 94–98 per cent with radiation in selected cases,[96] and Winkelmann and Llorens[93] reported complete clinicopathological remission of a 6 × 15 cm fungating BCCV with preoperative radiotherapy, and suggested that this should be considered when lesions are sufficiently large that radical surgery would otherwise be necessary to remove the tumour. There may also be a case for considering radiotherapy when surgical excision would significantly compromise subsequent function.

Management of metastatic disease

Despite the fact that patients with metastases from extravulvar BCC usually do badly, with a median survival of 10–19 months,[97,98] there are long-term survivors. The most common sites of metastasis are the lungs, bone, lymph nodes and liver. The time to diagnosis of metastasis may be up to 30 years with an average of 9.6 years.[98]

When metastasis to groin nodes occurs, surgical excision appears to give the best survival. Activity has been reported for some chemotherapy agents including 5-fluorouracil[98] and cisplatin ± doxorubicin,[99] but most patients die from their disease.

VERRUCOUS CARCINOMA

Verrucous carcinoma is a variant of squamous cell carcinoma first described by Ackerman in the oral cavity.[100] Goethals and colleagues[101] were said by Kraus and Perez-Mesa[102] to be the first to report the occurrence of verrucous carcinoma on the vulva (VCV).

Age, site, presentation and diagnosis

VCV mainly affects older women. In a review of 24 cases, the mean age was 54 years (range 29–86 years). Only three women (12.5 per cent) were younger than 40 years, whereas 71 per cent were postmenopausal.[103] VCV presents with pruritus, discomfort, discharge and bleeding associated with either ulceration and infection or a mass.[103] Clinically, the lesion appears as a warty, fungating, cauliflower-like, ulcerated mass (Fig. 13.6) similar to a large condyloma.[104,105] As the tumour increases in size, it may encroach on adjacent structures, and associated infection results in induration of the tissues and inflammatory enlargement of groin nodes.[104,106,107]

VCV most commonly arises unifocally on the labia majora, but it may be so extensive that the site of origin cannot be determined.[105] The colour may be shades of grey, white, yellow and pink.[103,104,106] The lesions are thought to be related to human papillomavirus (HPV).[108,109]

Diagnosis is made histologically, but it may be difficult for the pathologist to recognize the carcinoma unless the base of the lesion is included in the biopsy.[104] The diagnosis should be prompted particularly if there are massive condylomata acuminata resis-

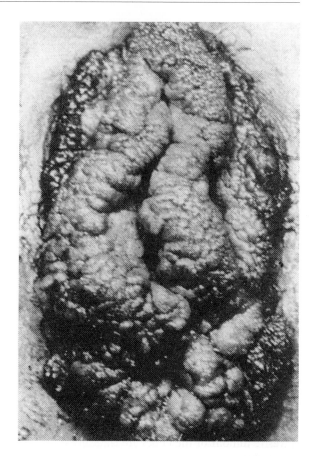

Figure 13.6 *Verrucous carcinoma of the vulva. (Reproduced with permission from Partridge, E.E., Murad, T., Shingleton, H.M et al. (1980) Verrucous lesions of the female genitalia. American Journal of Obstetrics and Gynecology, 137, 419–424.)*

tant to treatment in a patient aged over 40 years.[103] The differential diagnosis includes condyloma acuminatum and squamous cell carcinoma.

Treatment

Wide local excision is considered to be the treatment of choice.[102–104,110–112] The extent of surgery depends on the size of the lesion and care should be taken to excise all the tumour because inadequate excision will encourage recurrent disease. Inflammation around the tumour may make histological examination of the margins difficult.

Regional lymph nodes

Inguinofemoral node dissection is not indicated routinely because metastasis has not been reported in VCV.[105] In the largest series, Japaze and colleagues[103] reported that none of 17 patients undergoing groin node dissection had positive nodes. However, regional node metastases have been reported in up to 9 per cent of non-genital tumours.[101,113] It is suggested that nodes should be removed only in the case of a large primary tumour or recurrent tumour or when the nodes are clinically suspicious.[104]

Radiation

Concern about the use of radiation for verrucous carcinoma as a whole was raised by Kraus and Perez-Mesa,[102] who reported 17 cases of verrucous carcinoma of the oral cavity, larynx and genitalia treated with initial radiation. Two patients were unresponsive to radiotherapy, eleven recurred and four converted to an anaplastic lesion. Others agree that radiation does not have a significant therapeutic benefit.[103]

Outcome

As with other rare tumours, the literature on VCV is incomplete but analysis of the cases in Table 13.6

Table 13.6 *Treatment and outcome for verrucous carcinoma of vulva*

Reference	Year	No.	Treatment	Margin	Status (months)	Recurrence site
Kraus[102]	1966	1	s	a	ANC (120)	
Foye[112]	1970	1	Rs	+	ANC (31)	
Gallousis[113]	1972	1	s, R	−	DOD (16)	Perineum, I-R, gluteal fossa
		1	RVND	−	ANC a	
		1	RVND	a	ANC a	
Lucas[111]	1974	1	RVND, AE	−	DOD (8)	Groin
		1	s	a	ANC (24)	Labium
		1	R		AWD (6)	Vulva, perineum
Isaacs[104]	1976	2	s	a	ANC (48, 48)	
		1	RV, R	a	DOD (17)	a
		1	palliative S	a	DOD (12)	a
Powell[106]	1978	1	RVND	−	ANC (16)	
Zaaijman[116]	1978	1	RVND	a	ANC (12)	
Selim[115]	1979	1	RVND	−	ANC a	
Stehman[110]	1980	1	RVND	−	ANC (5)	
		1	Palliative cryotherapy	NA	DOD (15)	Suburethra
		1	Palliative R	NA	DOD (1)	Chest
Japaze[103]	1982	10	RVND	a	ANC ($\times$ 10 a)	
		1	RVND	a	ANC (120)	$\times$2 vulva, perineum, bladder or groin
		1	RVND	a	DOD (40)	$\times$3 vulva, perineum, bladder or groin
		3	s	a	ANC a	
		2	s	a	ANC (60, 84)	Vulva, perineum, bladder or groin
		1	RVND, R	a	AWD a	Vulva, perineum, bladder or groin
		4	RVND, R	a	DOD (15, 26, 48, 130)	Vulva, perineum, bladder or groin
		1	sR	a	DOD (36)	Vulva, perineum, bladder or groin
		1	R	NA	DOD a	
Brisigotti[114]	1989	2	RVND, RVND	a	ANC (48, 48)	
		1	RVND	a	AWD (204)	Urethra, vagina, perineum
		1	s	a	ANC (120)	
		1	s, R	a	AWD (84)	Urethra, vagina, perineum

s, non-radical surgery; ANC, alive without cancer; Rs, radiation; DOD, dead of disease; I-R, ischiorectal; RVND, radical vulvectomy and bilateral groin node dissection; AE, anterior exenteration; AWD, alive with disease; NA, not applicable.
[a] No mention.

suggests that, although VCV is a locally growing tumour, there are considerable recurrence and mortality rates. Of the 47 cases, 44 were apparently treated for cure and, of these, 23 per cent (10 of 44) died of VCV at 15–130 months, 68 per cent (30 of 44) were alive and free of disease at 12–120 months (in 16 cases, duration of follow-up is not mentioned) and 9 per cent (4 of 44) were alive with VCV at 6–204 months. Twenty-eight patients underwent radical surgery and in 20 of these there is no mention of the adequacy of the surgical margins. In four of five cases with negative margins, the patients were alive without VCV at follow-up and one patient died from VCV at 8 months. Nine patients underwent less than radical surgery without any radiation. Margin status is undocumented but all patients (100 per cent) were alive and free of VCV at 24–120 months (duration not mentioned in three cases). However, three (33 per cent) patients experienced recurrence. Japaze and colleagues,[103] in the only significant series of VCV, reported a 94 per cent corrected 5-year survival rate (16 of 17) in patients with VCV amenable to treatment with surgery alone. Of seven patients treated with combined surgery and radiation, including three stage IV lesions, only three (43 per cent) survived 5 years.

Recurrences

Recurrences occurred in 17 (39 per cent) patients treated for cure (Table 13.6) and these were all local. Nine of the 17 (53 per cent) who recurred died of VCV and, at last follow-up, four (23.5 per cent) were alive and free of disease between 24 and 120 months, whereas four (23.5 per cent) were alive with recurrence. In the series of Japaze and colleagues,[103] nine of 24 (37 per cent) recurred at intervals of 5–120 months in the vulva, perineum, bladder or inguinal regions. One patient had three recurrences and three had two recurrences. All the patients underwent surgery and six of the nine (66 per cent) died from VCV.[103]

Chemotherapy

The use of 5–fluorouracil and cisplatin or mitomycin C, combined with radiation, has become popular for the initial treatment of locally advanced squamous cell carcinoma of the vulva,[117] but there have been no reports of its use with VCV where it might have a theoretical role in large or recurrent tumours.

ADENOCARCINOMA AND BARTHOLIN'S GLAND CARCINOMA

Primary adenocarcinoma of the vulva represents approximately 2 per cent of all invasive vulvar malignancies.[1] As a result of its rarity, it is important to ensure that it does not represent a metastasis.[118] Most cases arise in the Bartholin's gland or sweat glands in association with Paget's disease, but separate primaries may arise.[118–121]

As information on these tumours is very sparse, treatment should be based on the same principles as for squamous cell carcinoma of the vulva. Wide surgical excision, sufficient to obtain clear margins of at least 2 cm, should be used with groin node dissection, unilateral for lateralized lesions and bilateral for central lesions.[25] Historically, outcome has been poor. Taylor and colleagues[122] reported on four patients with adenocarcinoma arising in Skene's glands who had a mean survival of 11 months. Survival of 0 per cent at 2 years and 27.7 per cent at 6.2 years has been reported for adenocarcinoma underlying Paget's disease of the vulva[25,26] and there are no effective chemotherapeutic regimens.[25,26] Radiation is mostly disappointing[25,26] although it may have a role.[17]

BARTHOLIN'S GLAND CARCINOMA (BGC)

Carcinoma involving the Bartholin's gland (BGC) represents between 3.9 per cent and 7.25 per cent of all vulvar carcinomas.[123–126] The mean age is 57 years (range 14–85 years);[125] 38 per cent are less than 50 years old.[125] The patients present either with a vulvar mass, perineal pain, swelling and drainage or with a groin lump. Delays in diagnosis have been reported in younger women, in whom a diagnosis of Bartholin's cyst or abscess has been incorrectly made in almost a quarter of patients.[125]

Diagnosis may be made by incisional or excisional biopsy or by fine needle aspiration.[127] Strict diagnostic criteria were established by Honan in 1897,[120] but more limited criteria are now accepted with the tumour having to demonstrate histological transition with elements of Bartholin's gland epithelium, and it is necessary to exclude a primary elsewhere.[124] There are many problems with historical reports on this tumour, particularly the absence of any mention of whether the criteria for diagnosis have been fulfilled.[126] The proportion of different histological types is given in Table 13.7.

Table 13.7 *Histological types of Bartholin's gland carcinoma*

Type	No.	Percentage
Squamous cell	61	48.4
Adenocarcinoma	35	27.7
Adenoid cystic	16	12.7
Adenosquamous	5	3.9
Transitional cell	3	2.3
Anaplastic	4	3.1
Unknown	2	
Total	126	

Data from Leuchter et al.[125] and Copeland et al.[126]

Treatment

Part of the significance of BGC is in the anatomical site of the Bartholin's glands, lying deeply on the inferior fascia of the urogenital diaphragm underneath the lower end of the bulbocavernosus muscles and the posterior portion of the bulb of the vestibule. Traditionally, treatment has been by radical vulvectomy with a downplay of the role of radiation.[123,125,126] Copeland and colleagues,[126] in reviewing the experience of the MD Anderson Hospital, reported that more limited surgery in combination with radiation may be worth pursuing. Seven of 12 patients who underwent hemivulvectomy or wide excision received adjunctive radiation and had no recurrences, whereas two who were not given radiation developed recurrence, although none died. The extent of surgery is defined by the site and extent of the tumour, and it may be necessary to dissect deep into the ischiorectal fossa to remove adjacent tissue, anal sphincter, rectum, vagina, and even the inferior pubic ramus and a portion of the urogenital diaphragm.[126]

Management of groin nodes

The incidence of positive groin nodes is 33–47 per cent[125,126] and may occur with tumours that are 2 cm in size.[125] The incidence of contralateral positive nodes is 4.5–14 per cent.[125,126] Copeland and colleagues[126] found that an ipsilateral groin node dissection would have picked up nodal spread in 12 of 14 (86 per cent) patients whose nodes were positive, and thus recommend performing only an ipsilateral node dissection unless the contralateral nodes are suspicious. In 25 cases in which a pelvic node dissection was done together with a groin node dissection, there was no instance of positive pelvic nodes in the absence of positive groin nodes.[125] Pelvic node dissection is therefore not routinely of value.

Outcome

Copeland and colleagues[126] reported an overall 5-year survival rate of 84 per cent for 36 patients with confirmed or possible BGC. All 10 patients treated with hemivulvectomy or wide local excision were alive at 24–48 months. Leuchter and colleagues[125] reported a 5-year disease-free survival rate of 71 per cent (10 of 14), with 12 patients undergoing at least radical vulvectomy and bilateral groin node dissection.

The survival rate is 52–87 per cent for negative groin nodes and 36–79 per cent for positive groin nodes. A single positive node is associated with a 71–83 per cent survival rate and two or more nodes with a 18–50 per cent rate.[125,126]

Radiation

Copeland and colleagues[126] found that only one of 14 (7 per cent) of the irradiated patients developed a local recurrence compared with six of 22 (27 per cent) non-irradiated patients. The difference was not statistically significant, but patients receiving radiation tended to have worse prognostic features. Leuchter and colleagues[125] reported one patient in poor medical condition who underwent radiation for extensive disease. There was no residual tumour on wide local excision after radiation, and the patient was free of disease at 5 years. Copeland and colleagues[126] recommend postoperative radiation to the vulva, inguinal nodes and pelvic nodes after an ipsilateral inguinal lymphadenectomy.

Recurrence

Patients who recur after having had positive groin nodes at the time of initial treatment do badly. Whereas all three patients who recurred after having positive nodes died, five of six patients, who recurred after having negative nodes at the time of initial treatment, recurred locally only and four of these were cured.[126] Leuchter and colleagues[125] reported a patient with two local recurrences who was alive and free of disease after two wide local excisions. Another patient with negative nodes developed distant metastases and lived for 28 months with chemotherapy.

ADENOID CYSTIC CARCINOMA OF BARTHOLIN'S GLAND (ACCB)

Adenoid cystic carcinoma (ACC) more commonly involves the salivary glands, oral cavity, nasopharynx, breast and skin. ACC of Bartholin's bland (ACCB) behaves differently to other adenocarcinomas of the vulva, being more indolent and prone to local recurrence rather than distant and regional metastasis; it also has a predilection for perineural invasion.[128] ACCB represented 0.9 per cent of invasive vulvar carcinomas at the MD Anderson Hospital between 1963 and 1985.[129]

Age, site, presentation and diagnosis

Copeland and colleagues[129] reviewed 37 cases in the literature, 20 of which had previously been reviewed by Bernstein and colleagues.[130] The median age was 42 years (range 25–76 years). The most common presentation was a palpable and usually painful mass. Seven of 14 (50 per cent) patients aged under 42 years had ACCB diagnosed in association with pregnancy. The significance of this is unclear.[129]

Treatment

The treatment of choice is wide local excision and ipsilateral groin node dissection.[129] Positive margins are associated with a poor outcome[130] and surgery may have to be radical to achieve clear margins.

Groin nodes

The incidence of involved groin nodes is 13–22 per cent.[125,129] No contralateral nodal involvement has been reported,[129] so ipsilateral groin node dissection should be sufficient.

Radiation

Radiation should be considered if the margins are positive, because it can help with local control.[129–131]

Outcome and recurrence

More than 50 per cent develop recurrence by 40 months, but in others it may develop after many years.

DePasquale and colleagues[128] reviewed 45 patients in the world literature, and found that 61 per cent of those undergoing wide local excision had recurrence versus 50 per cent undergoing radical vulvectomy.

Patients may live for extended periods after recurrence with slowly progressive disease. Despite a progression-free interval at 5, 10 and 15 years of 47, 38 and 13 per cent, respectively, the equivalent survival is 71, 59 and 51 per cent.[129] Patients developing a recurrence within 2 years do not live beyond 3 years; however, all patients developing recurrence at or after 3 years were alive at 5 years.[129]

Treatment of recurrence

Local recurrences should be excised. Adjuvant radiation contributed to local control in patients with recurrence.[129,131] There is sparse experience of chemotherapy in ACCB. Doxorubicin is reported to be the most active agent.[128]

SARCOMA OF THE VULVA

Sarcomas of the vulva (SOVs) represent less than 1 per cent of all soft-tissue sarcomas occurring in women[132] and 1.1–3 per cent of all vulvar malignancies.[1,133] There are many different types of sarcoma affecting the vulva (Table 13.8). Information is limited because of their rarity, and historical reports are difficult to compare because of changing terminology over the years.[133] Although some sarcomas have a reputation for early distant metastasis, many sarcomas of the

Table 13.8 *Types of soft-tissue sarcoma in the vulva*

Leiomyosarcoma[133]
Malignant fibrous histiocytoma[134]
Neurofibrosarcomas[133]
Rhabdomyosarcoma[133,135]
Fibrosarcoma[133,134]
Epithelioid sarcoma[133]
Liposarcoma[136]
Dermatofibrosarcoma protruberans[137]
Alveolar soft part sarcoma[138]
Malignant granular cell tumour[139]
Malignant Schwannoma[133]
Kaposi's sarcoma of the vulva[140]
Aggressive angiomyxoma[141]
Angiosarcoma[132]

vulva are slow-growing tumours associated with a protracted course and only late distant metastasis. Treatment guidelines must often be based on extrapolation from experience gained in treating similar histological types occurring at other sites.

Age, site and presentation

Although the mean age of SOVs is 38 years[133] rhabdomyosarcomas occur predominantly in children and adolescents[142] (Table 13.9).

Sarcomas most commonly arise in the labia majora[133] and patients present with a lump, discomfort or bleeding or occasionally with symptoms of metastatic disease. Tumours may be superficial, of small size, with a nodular or multinodular pattern; they may be mistaken for an infectious process which causes a delay in diagnosis, especially in younger adults.

Prognostic indicators

There is a lack of data on prognostic indicators for either soft-tissue sarcomas of the vulva overall or for individual subtypes.

Studies on pelvic sarcomas have found that the size of the primary tumour and the grade are important.[143,144] In vulvovaginal sarcoma, the tumour grade is important but not the size of the primary or histological subtype.[132] Recurrence of leiomyosarcoma of the vulva may be related to the mitotic activity, size of tumour and margin status.[145]

Treatment

Curtin and colleagues[132] summarized the principles of treatment for SOV. Initial treatment is excision to obtain a clear margin: if the tumour is low grade and completely resected the patient should just be followed; if the tumour is high grade or recurrent low grade, radiation should be given to the tumour field.

Metastatic disease should be treated by chemotherapy on a research protocol. Various types of chemotherapy have been used for metastatic sarcoma, but doxorubicin alone has been shown to be as effective as combination with ifosfamide or cyclophosphamide, vincristine and dacarbazine (CYVADIC).[146] Response rates are only 24 per cent with median duration of 46 weeks and less than a 5 per cent survival rate at 5 years.[146] A role for adjuvant chemotherapy for completely resected soft-tissue sarcoma has still not been defined. Some believe that a case has not been proved,[147] whereas a large meta-analysis suggested some possible benefit.[148]

Leiomyosarcoma

Leiomyosarcoma is the most commonly occurring SOV. It is a slowly growing indolent neoplasm with later local and distant recurrences. Of five cases treated with radical surgery, three died with distant metastases after a protracted course at 72, 180 and 192 months, and another was alive with pulmonary metastases at 22 months. Three patients had originally had one or more local excisions.[133]

Table 13.9 *Relative frequency and age of patients with sarcoma of the vulva*

Type of sarcoma	No.	Percentage	Age (years)	
			Mean	Range
Leiomyosarcoma	9	43	52[a]	40–64
Rhabdomyosarcoma	5	24	24	16–28
Neurofibrosarcoma	3	14	36	25–39
Fibrosarcoma	2	9	35	30–39
Epithelial sarcoma	1			
Dermatofibrosarcoma	1			
Total	21			

[a] Mean age no greater than 52 years based on figures given in paper.
From Curtin et al.[132] and DiSaia et al.[133]

Rhabdomyosarcoma

Rhabdomyosarcoma is the most common of all soft-tissue sarcomas; subtypes include alveolar, embryonal and pleomorphic.[135] Typically, they occur in infants and young women and are rapidly growing tumours that metastasize early.[133] When a clinician encounters atypical granular spongy tissue in what was expected to be a cyst or abscess in the vulva or perineum, rhabdomyosarcoma should be suspected.[135]

The outlook for rhabdomyosarcoma has become more promising since the introduction of chemotherapy.[149] Hays and colleagues[150] reported the experience of the Intergroup Rhabdomyosarcoma Study Group with primary rhabdomyosarcomas of the vagina, uterus and vulva in children and adolescents. Eight of nine (89 per cent) patients were disease free at 4–10 years (mean 6.4 years) and one was alive with disease at 2.5 years, after surgery, radiotherapy and chemotherapy with vincristine, actinomycin D ± cyclophosphamide ± doxorubicin.[150]

Alveolar rhabdomyosarcoma

The tendency to metastasis early encourages the use of adjuvant therapy following resection with post-operative local radiotherapy and then chemotherapy with vincristine, actinomycin D and cyclophosphamide.[135] Good outcomes are reported with resection followed by chemotherapy,[142,150] but patients with metastatic disease do badly.[135]

Embryonal rhabdomyosarcoma

Embryonal rhabdomyosarcoma, typically seen in the vagina, is very rare on the vulva.[151,152] Sarcoma botryoides is a variant of embryonal rhabdomyosarcoma arising beneath a mucous membrane and producing a typical polypoid appearance.[152] The Intergroup Rhabdomyosarcoma Study reported that four of five children and infants with embryonal rhabdomyosarcoma were disease free between 4 and 10 years, after treatment with combinations of surgery, radiotherapy and chemotherapy, including vincristine, actinomycin D ± cyclophosphamide ± doxorubicin.[150]

MISCELLANEOUS SARCOMAS

Malignant fibrous histiocytoma

Classically, this presents as a large mass in a middle-aged woman. Treatment is wide local excision. Widespread metastasis can occur.[134,153]

Dermatofibrosarcoma protuberans

This is a low-grade variant of malignant fibrous histiocytoma, which recurs locally but rarely metastasizes.[134,137,154,155] It appears as a multinodular, firm, well-circumscribed mass lying just beneath the epidermis.[137] Treatment is wide local excision. Although there is a clinical appearance of encapsulation, fine microscopic projections of the tumour may extend well beyond the apparent margins.[137]

Neurofibrosarcoma

This is a slow-growing tumour that should be treated with wide local excision. DiSaia and colleagues[133] reported on three patients with neurofibrosarcoma who were treated with local excision, and were alive and well at 18, 39 and 110 months.

Epithelioid sarcoma of vulva

This tumour is named because the cells bear a resemblance to squamous epithelioid cells. It was first reported in the vulva by Piver and colleagues[156] and then by others.[157,158] Most occur in young or middle-aged adults with the mean age in two series being 23 and 33 years.[158] The majority behave as a slow-growing painless mass which should be widely excised. In tumours at other sites, there is a high rate of recurrence.

Aggressive angiomyxoma

These are slow-growing, infiltrative tumours, which are often of a large size and have a gelatinous appearance. They occur predominantly on the vulva, vagina, pelvic floor and perineum in young women.[159] Treatment is wide local excision to obtain clear margins. They are prone to extensive local recurrence and do not metastasize. Recurrence rates are high.[141,159]

Other sarcomas

These include fibrosarcoma,[133,134] liposarcoma,[136] alveolar soft-tissue sarcoma,[138] malignant granular cell tumour,[139] malignant Schwannoma[133] and angiosarcoma;[132] they should all be treated according to the guidelines given by Curtin and colleagues.[132]

Kaposi's sarcoma

This is a malignant tumour of endothelial origin, which is more common in men than in women and rarely affects the vulva.[140,160] The forms include classic, endemic African, iatrogenic associated with immunosuppression and AIDs associated.[161] Cutaneous lesions evolve through stages of macules, papules, plaques and nodules, which are classically bluish–red in colour. Oedema and ulceration are common and the lesions are often multiple.[162] The clinical course varies from indolent and slow in the classic, more aggressive in the endemic to rapidly progressive in the AIDS-associated forms.[161] Spontaneous regression may occur.[163,164] Local lesions may be treated with radiotherapy, laser ablation, cryotherapy or intralesional chemotherapy.[163] Widespread disease is treated with various chemotherapy agents, including vincristine, vinblastine, bleomycin, doxorubicin and etoposide, sometimes combined with interferon-α and antiviral agents in AIDS-associated disease.

Good responses to chemotherapy have been reported for skin lesions,[165] but the outcome is poor for patients with HIV infection, particularly if they develop opportunistic infection.[163]

Treatment of lung metastases

Resection of sarcoma that has metastasized only to the lung should be considered if complete clearance of the metastases looks possible. The surgery is made easier by the fact that 80 per cent of metastases are situated peripherally in the lungs. Van Geel and colleagues reported on the experience of the European Organization for Research and Treatment of Cancer – Soft Tissue and Bone Sarcoma Group.[166] Overall 5-year survival and disease-free survival rates post-metastasectomy were 38 and 35 per cent and at 10 years they were 26 and 28 per cent. Median follow-up after surgery was 2.5 years. Good prognostic factors were found to be disease free from initial treatment for over 2.5 years, grade less than III, radical resection or treatment of initial sarcoma and age less than 40. The site of the primary tumour, histological type, the number of metastases and whether the metastases were unilateral or bilateral were not significant factors.

MERKEL'S CELL CARCINOMA

Merkel's cell carcinoma is a neuroendocrine carcinoma that is thought to originate from touch-sensitive receptor cells, Merkel's cells, in the basal layer of the epidermis.[167] It most commonly occurs on the face, scalp extremities and trunk in older patients, but it rarely involves the vulva.[127,167–174]

This tumour behaves aggressively with early local and distant spread and a poor outcome. Ten cases have been reported and reviewed.[167,174] The mean age was 57 years (range 28–74 years) and the size 1.5–9 cm. Initial surgery varied between wide local excision and radical vulvectomy and lymphadenectomy. One patient was lost to follow-up, one was alive and well at 13 months, one was alive with distant metastases at 5 months and seven (70 per cent) developed distant metastases and died within 2.5 years. Radiotherapy is not effective for primary therapy of lesions at other sites[175] but may play a role for lymph node involvement and local recurrences on the vulva.[173]

It is difficult to recommend radical surgery when the outcome is so poor[167] and, as with other vulvar tumours, surgery should be tailored to the size of the tumour, with at least wide local excision and lymphadenectomy. The use of adjuvant chemotherapy should be considered, using agents similar to those for small cell carcinoma of the lung based on cisplatin and etoposide.[171–173] However, although good responses are reported for cisplatin and etoposide at other sites,[176] response to chemotherapy for vulvar tumours has been poor.[171–173,177]

METASTASES TO THE VULVA

Metastatic tumours to the vulva are rare, as evidenced by the absence of a single case in a report of postmortem examinations of 1000 patients who had carcinoma of epithelial origin.[178] Dehner reported that metastatic disease represented 8 per cent of 262 cases of vulvar malignancy[179] with 73 per cent of the metastases coming from the reproductive tract and 18 per cent from the renal tract; 46 per cent were from squamous cell carcinoma of the cervix, 18 per cent from endometrial carcinoma, 9 per cent from urethral and renal carcinomas, and the remainder from carcinomas of the vagina, ovary and breast and one lymphoma. Metastases to the vulva originate from the bladder,[180] stomach,[181] melanoma,[182] breast,[179,183] lymphoma,[179,184] vagina, ovary, choriocarcinoma, rectum, lung and neuroblastoma,[179] and potentially from other sites. They most commonly involve the labia majora followed by the clitoris, labia minora and perineum. They may be single or multiple, and present with the common symptoms of vulvar malignancy, painless lump, discomfort, ulceration or bleeding.

Metastases to the vulva are associated with a poor outcome[179] and management must be in the light of the primary site and other disease.

REFERENCES

1 Sturgeon SR, Brinton LA, Devesa SS et al. In situ and invasive vulvar carcinoma incidence trends (1973–1987). *Am J Obstet Gynecol* 1992; **166**: 1482–5.

2 Wilkinson EJ. Report of the ISSVD Terminology Committee. *J Reprod Med* 1986; **31**: 973–4.

3 Wilkinson EJ, Friedrich EG. Diseases of the vulva. In: Kurman RJ (ed). *Blaustein's Pathology of the Female Genital Tract*. New York: Springer-Verlag, 1987: 36–96.

4 Paget J. On disease of the mammary areola preceding cancer of the mammary gland. *St Bartholomew's Hospital Reports* 1874: **10**: 87–9.

5 Dubreuilh W. Paget's disease of the vulva. *Br J Dermatol* 1901; **13**: 407–13.

6 Beecham CT. Paget's disease of the vulva. *Obstet Gynecol* 1976; **47S**: 55–8.

7 Breen JL, Smith CI, Gregori CA. Extramammary Paget's disease. *Clin Obstet Gynecol* 1978; **21**: 1107–15.

8 Chanda JJ. Extramammary Paget's disease: prognosis and relationship to internal malignancy. *J Am Acad Dermatol* 1985; **13**: 1009–14.

9 Stapleton JJ. Extramammary Paget's disease of the vulva in a young black woman. *J Reprod Med* 1984; **29**: 444–6.

10 Hart WR, Millman JB. Progression of intraepithelial Paget's disease of the vulva to invasive carcinoma. *Cancer* 1977; **40**: 2333–7.

11 Boehm F, Morris JM. Paget's disease and apocrine gland carcinoma of the vulva. *Obstet Gynecol* 1971; **38**: 185–92.

12 Creasman WT, Gallagher HS, Rutledge F. Paget's disease of the vulva. *Gynecol Oncol* 1975; **3**: 133–48.

13 Lee SC, Roth LM, Ehrlich C et al. Extramammary Paget's disease of the vulva. *Cancer* 1977; **39**: 2540–9.

14 Helwig EB, Graham JH. Anogenital (extramammary) Paget's disease. *Cancer* 1963; **16**: 387–403.

15 Degefu S, O'Quinn AG, Dhurandhar HN. Paget's disease of the vulva and urogenital malignancies: A case report and review of the literature. *Gynecol Oncol* 1986; **25**: 347–54.

16 Cappuccini F, Tewari K, Rogers LW et al. Extramammary Paget's disease of the vulva: metastases to the bone marrow in the absence of an underlying adenocarcinoma. *Gynecol Oncol* 1997; **66**: 146–50.

17 Parmley TH, Woodruff JD, Julian CG. Invasive vulvar Paget's disease. *Obstet Gynecol* 1975; **46**: 341–6.

18 Feuer GA, Shevchuk M, Canalog A. Vulvar Paget's disease: The need to exclude an invasive lesion. *Gynecol Oncol* 1990; **38**: 81–9.

19 Fine BA, Fowler LJ, Valente PT et al. Minimally invasive Paget's disease of the vulva with extensive lymph node metastases. *Gynecol Oncol* 1995; **57**: 262–5.

20 Friedrich EG, Wilkinson EJ, Steingraeber PH et al. Paget's disease of the vulva and carcinoma of the breast. *Obstet Gynecol* 1975; **46**: 130–4.

21 Woodruff JD. Paget's disease of the vulva. *Obstet Gynecol* 1955; **5**: 175–85.

22 Bergen S, DiSaia PJ, Liao SY et al. Conservative management of extramammary Paget's disease of the vulva. *Gynecol Oncol* 1989; **33**: 151–6.

23 Gunn RA, Gallagher HS. Vulvar Paget's disease: a topographic study. *Cancer* 1980; **46**: 590–4.

24 Taylor PR, Stenwig JT, Klausen H. Paget's disease of the vulva. *Gynecol Oncol* 1975; **3**: 46–60.

25 Kodama S, Kaneko T, Saito M et al. A clinicopathologic study of 30 patients with Paget's disease of the vulva. *Gynecol Oncol* 1995; **56**: 63–70.

26 Baehrendtz H, Einhorn N, Pettersson F et al. Paget's disease of the vulva: the Radiumhemmet series 1975–1990. *Int J Gynecol Cancer* 1994; **4**: 1–6.

27 Geisler JP, Stowell MJ, Melton ME et al. Extramammary Paget's disease of the vulva recurring in a skin graft. *Gynecol Oncol* 1995; **56**: 446–7.

28 Misas J, Larson J, Podczaski E et al. Recurrent Paget disease of the vulva in a split-thickness skin graft. *Obstet Gynecol* 1990; **76**: 543–4.

29 De Jonge ETM, Knobel J. Recurrent Paget's disease of the vulva after simple vulvectomy and skin grafting. *South Afr Med J* 1988; **73**: 46–7.

30 DiSaia PJ, Dorion GE, Cappuccini F et al. A report of two cases of recurrent Paget's disease of the vulva in a split-thickness graft and its possible pathogenesis-

labeled 'retrodissemination'. *Gynecol Oncol* 1995; **57**: 109–12.

31 Friedrich EG. Intraepithelial neoplasia of the vulva. In: Coppleson M (ed). *Gynecologic oncology: fundamental principles and clinical practice.* New York: Churchill Livingstone, 1981: 303.

32 Fetherston WC, Friedrich EG. The origin and significance of vulvar Paget's disease. *Obstet Gynecol* 1972; **39**: 735–44.

33 Hewett P. Melanosis of the labium and glands of the groin and pubes. *Lancet* 1861; **i**: 263.

34 Weinstock MA. Malignant melanoma of the vulva and vagina in the United States: patterns of incidence and population-based estimates of survival. *Am J Obstet Gynecol* 1994; **171**: 1225–30.

35 Bradgate MG, Rollason TP, McConkey CC et al. Malignant melanoma of the vulva: a clinicopathological study of 50 women. *Br J Obstet Gynaecol* 1990; **97**: 124–33.

36 Morrow CP, Rutledge FN. Melanoma of the vulva. *Obstet Gynecol* 1972; **39**: 745–52.

37 Chung AF, Woodruff JM, Lewis JL. Malignant melanoma of the vulva. *Obstet Gynecol* 1975; **45**: 638–46.

38 Pack GT. A comparative study of melanomas and epidermoid carcinomas of the vulva: A review of 44 melanoma and 58 epidermoid carcinomas (1930–1965). *Rev Surg* 1967; **24**: 305–24.

39 Yackel DB, Symmonds RE, Kempers RD. Melanoma of the vulva. *Obstet Gynecol* 1970; **35**: 625–31.

40 Podratz KC, Gaffey TA, Symmonds RE et al. Melanoma of the vulva: An update. *Gynecol Oncol* 1983; **16**: 153–68.

41 Woolcott RJ, Henry RJW, Houghton CRS. Malignant melanoma of the vulva: Australian experience. *J Reprod Med* 1988; **33**: 699–702.

42 Tasseron EWK, van der Esch EP, Hart AAM et al. A clinicopathological study of 30 melanomas of the vulva. *Gynecol Oncol* 1992; **46**: 170–5.

43 Trimble EL, Lewis JL, Williams LL et al. Management of vulvar melanoma. *Gynecol Oncol* 1992; **45**: 254–8.

44 Beller U, Demopoulos RI, Beckman EM. Vulvovaginal melanoma. *J Reprod Med* 1986; **31**: 315–19.

45 Rose PG, Piver S, Tsukada Y et al. Conservative therapy for melanoma of the vulva. *Am J Obstet Gynecol* 1988; **159**: 52–5.

46 Silvers DN, Halperin AJ. Cutaneous and vulvar melanoma: an update. *Clin Obstet Gynecol* 1978; **21**: 1117–33.

47 Lynch PJ, Edwards L. *Genital Dermatology.* New York: Churchill Livingstone, 1994.

48 Morrow CP, DiSaia PJ. Malignant melanoma of the female genitalia: a clinical analysis. *Obstet Gynecol Surv* 1976; **31**: 233–71.

49 Anderson DE. Clinical characteristics of the genetic variety of cutaneous melanoma in man. *Cancer* 1971; **28**: 721–5.

50 Kaufman RH, Faro S. Solid tumors. In: Kaufman RH, Faro S, Friedrich EG, Gardner HL (eds). *Benign diseases of the vulva and vagina.* St Louis: Mosby, 1994: 168–207.

51 Blickstein I, Feldberg E, Dgani R et al. Dysplastic vulvar nevi. *Obstet Gynecol* 1991; **78**: 968–70.

52 Rock B, Hood AF, Rock JA. Prospective study of vulva nevi. *J Am Acad Dermatal* 1990; **22**: 104–6.

53 Kraemer KH, Greene MH, Tarone R et al. Dysplastic naevi and cutaneous melanoma risk. *Lancet* 1983; **ii**: 1076–7.

54 Christensen WN. Histologic characterization of vulvar nevocellular nevi. *J Cutan Pathol* 1987; **14**: 82–91.

55 Phillips GL, Twiggs LB, Okagaki T. Vulvar melanoma: a microstaging study. *Gynecol Oncol* 1982; **14**: 80–8.

56 Jaramillo BA, Ganjei P, Averette HE et al. Malignant melanoma of the vulva. *Obstet Gynecol* 1985; **66**: 398–401.

57 Johnson TL, Kumar NB, White CD et al. Prognostic features of vulvar melanoma: A clinicopathologic analysis. *Int J Gynecol Pathol* 1986; **5**: 110–18.

58 Phillips GL, Bundy BN, Okagaki T et al. Malignant melanoma of the vulva treated by radical hemivulvectomy. *Cancer* 1994; **73**: 2626–32.

59 Scheistrøen M, Tropé C, Kœrn J et al. Malignant melanoma of the vulva. *Cancer* 1995; **75**: 72–80.

60 Bouma J, Weening JJ, Elders A. Malignant melanoma of the vulva: Report of 18 cases. *Eur J Obstet Gynecol Reprod Biol* 1982; **13**: 237–51.

61 Clark WHJ et al. The histogenesis and biologic behaviour of primary human malignant melanomas of the skin. *Cancer Res* 1969; **29**: 705–15.

62 Breslow A. Thickness, cross-sectional areas and depth of invasion in the prognosis of cutaneous melanoma. *Ann Surg* 1970; **172**: 902–8.

63 Benda JA, Platz CE, Anderson B. Malignant melanoma of the vulva: a clinical-pathologic review of 16 cases. *Int J Gynecol Pathol* 1986; **5**: 202–16.

64 Ariel IM. Malignant melanoma of the female genital system: a report of 48 patients and review of the literature. *J Surg Oncol* 1981; **16**: 371–83.

65 Look KY, Roth LM, Sutton GP. Vulvar melanoma reconsidered. *Cancer* 1993; **72**: 143–6.

66 Edington PT, Monaghan JM. Malignant melanoma of the vulva and vagina. *Br J Obstet Gynaecol* 1980; **87**: 422–4.

67 Davidson T, Kissin M, Westbury G. Vulvovaginal

melanoma – should radical surgery be abandoned? *Br J Obstet Gynaecol* 1987; **94**: 473–6.

68 AJCC. *Cancer staging manual.* Philadelphia: Lipincott-Raven, 1997.

69 Chan KK, Helm CW. Invasive vulvar cancer. In: Shingleton HM, Fowler WC, Jordan JA, Lawrence WD (eds). *Gynecologic oncology: current diagnosis and treatment.* London: WB Saunders, 1996: 264–71.

70 Symmonds RE, Pratt JH, Dockerty MB. Melanoma of the vulva. *Obstet Gynecol* 1960; **15**: 543–53.

71 Das Gupta T, D'Urso J. Melanoma of the female genitalia. *Surg Gynecol Obstet* 1964; **119**: 1074–8.

72 Aitken DR, Clausen K, Klein JP et al. The extent of primary melanoma excision – A re-evaluation – How wide is wide? *Ann Surg* 1983; **198**: 634–41.

73 Veronesi U, Cascinelle N, Adamus J et al. Thin stage I primary cutaneous malignant melanoma. Comparison of excision with margins of 1 or 3 cm. *N Engl J Med* 1988; **318**: 1159–62.

74 Bailet JW, Figge DC, Tamimi HK. Malignant melanoma of the vulva: A case report of distal recurrence in a patient with a superficially invasive primary lesion. *Obstet Gynecol* 1987; **70**: 515–17.

75 Veronesi U, Adamus J, Bandiera DC et al. Delayed regional lymph node dissection in stage I melanoma of the lower extremities. *Cancer* 1982; **49**: 2420–30.

76 Sim FH, Taylor WF, Pritchard DJ et al. Lymphadenectomy in the management of Stage I malignant melanoma: a prospective randomized study. *Mayo Clin Proc* 1986; **61**: 697–705.

77 Kirkwood JM, Strawderman MH, Ernstoff MS et al. Interferon alfa-2b adjuvant therapy of high-risk resected cutaneous melanoma: the Eastern Cooperative Oncology Group Trial EST 1684. *J Clin Oncol* 1996; **14**: 7–17.

78 Balch CM, Buzaid AC. Finally, a successful adjuvant therapy for high-risk melanoma. *J Clin Oncol* 1996; **14**: 1–3.

79 Overett TK, Shiu MH. Surgical treatment of distant metastatic melanoma: Indications and results. *Cancer* 1985; **56**: 1222–30.

80 Temesvary N. Uber ein multiples Krompecher'sches Karzinom der Vulva, mit ausgendehnter Elephantiasis. *Z Gynäkol* 1926; **50**: 1575–82.

81 Feakins RM, Lowe DG. Basal cell carcinoma of the vulva: a clinicopathologic study of 45 cases. *Int J Gynecol Pathol* 1997; **16**: 319–24.

82 Palladino VS, Duffy JL, Bures GJ. Basal cell carcinoma of the vulva. *Cancer* 1969; **24**: 460–70.

83 Breen JL, Neubecker RD, Greenwald E et al. Basal cell carcinoma of the vulva. *Obstet Gynecol* 1975; **46**: 122–9.

84 Benedet JL, Miller DM, Ehlen TG et al. Basal cell carcinoma of the vulva: clinical features and treatment results in 28 patients. *Obstet Gynecol* 1997; **90**: 765–8.

85 Simonsen E, Johnsson JE, Trope C et al. Basal cell carcinoma of the vulva. *Acta Obstet Gynecol Scand* 1985; **64**: 231–4.

86 Perrone T, Twiggs LB, Adcock LL et al. Vulvar basal cell carcinoma: an infrequently metastasizing neoplasm. *Int J Gynecol Pathol* 1987; **6**: 152–65.

87 Dudzinski MR, Askin FB, Fowler WCJ. Giant basal cell carcinoma of the vulva. *Obstet Gynecol* 1984; **63** (S3): 575–605.

88 Zerner J, Fenn ME. Basal cell carcinoma of the vulva. *Int J Gynaecol Obstet* 1979; **17**: 203–5.

89 Heaps JM, Fu YS, Montz FJ et al. Surgical-pathologic variables predictive of local recurrence in squamous cell carcinoma of the vulva. *Gynecol Oncol* 1990; **38**: 309–14.

90 Sworn MJ, Hammond GT, Buchanan R. Metastatic basal cell carcinoma of the vulva. Case Report. *Br J Obstet Gynaecol* 1986; **86**: 332–4.

91 Gleeson NC, Ruffolo EM, Hoffman MS et al. Basal cell carcinoma of the vulva with groin node metastasis. *Gynecol Oncol* 1994; **53**: 366–8.

92 Hoffman MS, Roberts WS, Ruffolo EH. Basal cell carcinoma of the vulva with inguinal lymph node metastases. *Gynecol Oncol* 1988; **29**: 113–19.

93 Winkelmann SE, Llorens AS. Metastatic basal cell carcinoma of the vulva. *Gynecol Oncol* 1990; **38**: 138–40.

94 Jimenez HT, Fenoglio CM, Richart RM. Vulvar basal cell carcinoma with metastasis: a case report. *Am J Obstet Gynecol* 1975; **121**: 285–6.

95 Mizushima J, Ohara K. Basal cell carcinoma of the vulva with lymph node and skin metastasis – report of a case and review of 20 Japanese cases. *J Dermatol* 1995; **22**: 36–42.

96 Goldberg LH, Rubin HA. Management of basal cell carcinoma. *Postgrad Med J* 1989; **85**: 57–63.

97 Safai B. Basal cell carcinoma with metastases. *Arch Pathol Lab Med* 1989; **101**: 327–31.

98 Farmer ER, Helwig EB. Metastatic basal cell carcinoma: a clinicopathologic study of seventeen cases. *Cancer* 1980; **46**: 748–57.

99 Guthrie TH. Cisplatin-based chemotherapy in advanced basal and squamous cell carcinomas of the skin: Results in 28 patients including 13 patients receiving multimodality therapy. *J Clin Oncol* 1990; **8**: 342–6.

100 Ackerman LV. Verrucous carcinoma of the oral cavity. *Surgery* 1948; 23: 670–8.

101 Goethals PL, Harrison EG, Devine KD. Verrucous squamous carcinoma of the oral cavity. *Am J Surg* 1963; **106**: 845–51.

102 Kraus FT, Perez-Mesa C. Verrucous carcinoma. *Cancer* 1966; **19**: 26–38.

103 Japaze H, Dinh TV, Woodruff JD. Verrucous carcinoma of the vulva: study of 24 cases. *Obstet Gynecol* 1982; **60**: 462–6.

104 Isaacs JH. Verrucous carcinoma of the female genital tract. *Gynecol Oncol* 1976; **4**: 259–69.

105 Kluzak TR, Kraus FT. Condylomata, papillomas and verrucous carcinomas of the vulva and vagina. In: Wilkinson EJ (ed). *Pathology of the vulva and vagina*. New York: Churchill Livingstone, 1987: 49–77.

106 Powell JL, Franklin EW, Nickerson JF et al. Verrucous carcinoma of the female genital tract. *Gynecol Oncol* 1978; **6**: 565–73.

107 Partridge EE, Murad T, Shingleton HM, et al. Verrucous lesions of the female genitalia: 2. Verrucous carcinoma. *Am J Obstet Gynecol* 1980; **137**: 419–24.

108 Rastkar G, Okagaki T, Twiggs LB et al. Early invasive and in situ warty carcinoma of the vulva: clinical, histologic, and electron microscopic study with particular reference to viral association. *Am J Obstet Gynecol* 1982; **143**: 814–20.

109 Ubben K, Krzyzek R, Ostrow R et al. Human papilloma virus DNA detected in two verrucous carcinomas. *J Invest Dermatolol* 1979; **72**: 195–8.

110 Stehman FB, Castaldo TW, Charles EW et al. Verrucous carcinoma of the vulva. *Int J Gynecol Obstet* 1980; **17**: 523–5.

111 Lucas WE, Benirschke K, Lebherz TB. Verrucous carcinoma of the female genital tract. *Am J Obstet Gynecol* 1974; **119**: 435–40.

112 Foye G, Marsh MR, Minkowitz S. Verrucous carcinoma of the vulva. *Obstet Gynecol* 1969; **34**: 484–8.

113 Gallousis S. Verrucous carcinoma. *Obstet Gynecol* 1972; **40**: 502–7.

114 Brisigotti M, Moreno A, Murcia C et al. Verrucous carcinoma of the vulva. A clinicopathologic and immunohistochemical study of five cases. *Int J Gynecol Pathol* 1989; **8**: 1–7.

115 Selim MA, Lankerani MR. Verrucous carcinoma of the vulva. *J Reprod Med* 1979; **22**: 93–6.

116 Zaaijman JD, Slabber CF. Verrucous carcinoma of the vulva. *Br J Obstet Gynaecol* 1978; **85**: 74–6.

117 Thomas G, Dembo A, DePetrillo A et al. Concurrent radiation and chemotherapy in vulvar carcinoma. *Gynecol Oncol* 1989; **34**: 263–7.

118 Wick MB, Goellner JR, Wolfe JT et al. Vulvar sweat gland carcinoma. *Arch Pathol Lab Med* 1985; **109**: 43–7.

119 Merino MJ, LiVolsi VA, Schwartz PE et al. Adenoid basal cell carcinoma of the vulva. *Int J Gynecol Pathol* 1982; **1**: 299–306.

120 Mossler JA, Woodard BH, Addison A et al. Adenocarcinoma of Bartholin's gland. *Arch Pathol Lab Med* 1980; **104**: 523–6.

121 Carlson JW, McGlennen RC, Gomez R et al. Sebaceous carcinoma of the vulva: A case report and review of the literature. *Gynecol Oncol* 1996; **60**: 489–91.

122 Taylor RN, Lacey CG, Shuman MA. Adenocarcinoma of Skene's duct associated with a systemic coagulopathy. *Gynecol Oncol* 1985; **22**: 250–6.

123 Barclay DL, Collins CG, Macey, HB. Cancer of the Bartholin gland. *Am J Obstet Gynecol* 1964; **24**: 329–36.

124 Chamlian DL, Taylor HB. Primary carcinoma of Bartholin's glands. *Obstet Gynecol* 1972; **39**: 489–94.

125 Leuchter RS, Hacker NF, Voet RL et al. Primary carcinoma of the Bartholin gland. *Obstet Gynecol* 1982; **60**: 361–8.

126 Copeland LJ, Sneige N, Gershenson DM et al. Bartholin gland carcinoma. *Obstet Gynecol* 1986; **67**: 794–801.

127 Copeland LJ, Cleary K, Sneige N et al. Neuroendocrine (Merkel cell) carcinoma of the vulva. *Gynecol Oncol* 1985; **22**: 367–78.

128 DePasquale SE, McGuinness TB, Mangan CE et al. Adenoid cystic carcinoma of Bartholin's gland: a review of the literature and report of a patient. *Gynecol Oncol* 1996; **61**: 122–5.

129 Copeland LJ, Sneige N, Gershenson DM et al. Adenoid cystic carcinoma of Bartholin gland. *Obstet Gynecol* 1986; **67**: 115–20.

130 Bernstein SG, Voet RL, Lifshitz S et al. Adenoid cystic carcinoma of Bartholin's gland. *Am J Obstet Gynecol* 1983; **147**: 385–90.

131 Rosenberg P, Simonsen E, Risberg B. Adenoid cystic carcinoma of Bartholin's gland. *Gynecol Oncol* 1989; **34**: 145–7.

132 Curtin JP, Saigo P, Slucher B et al. Soft-tissue sarcoma of the vagina and vulva: a clinicopathologic study. *Obstet Gynecol* 1995; **86**: 269–72.

133 DiSaia PF, Rutledge F, Smith PJ. Sarcoma of the vulva. *Obstet Gynecol* 1971; **38**: 180–4.

134 Davos I, Abell MR. Soft tissue sarcomas of the vulva. *Gynecol Oncol* 1976; **4**: 70–86.

135 Copeland LJ, Sneige N, Stringer CA et al. Alveolar rhabdomyosarcoma of the female genitalia. *Cancer* 1985; **56**: 849–55.

136 Brooks JJ, LiVolsi VA. Liposarcoma on the vulva. *Am J Obstet Gynecol* 1987; **156**: 73–5.

137 Barnhill DR, Boling R, Nobles W et al. Vulvar dermatofibrosarcoma protuberans. *Gynecol Oncol* 1988; **30**: 149–52.

138 Shen J-T, D'Ablaing G, Morrow CP. Alveolar soft part sarcoma of the vulva: report of first case and review of the literature. *Gynecol Oncol* 1982; **13**: 120–8.

139 Robertson AJ, McIntosh W, Lamont P et al. Malignant granular cell tumour (myoblastoma) of the vulva: report of a case and review of the literature. *Histopathology* 1981; **5**: 69–79.

140 Hall DJ, Burns JC, Goplerud DR. Kaposi's sarcoma of the vulva: a case report and brief review. *Obstet Gynecol* 1979; **54**: 478–83.

141 Steeper T, Rosai J. Aggressive angiomyxoma of the female pelvis and perineum. *Am J Surg Pathol* 1983; **7**: 463–76.

142 Bond SJ, Seibel N, Kapur S et al. Rhabdomyosarcoma of the clitoris. *Cancer* 1994; **73**: 1984–6.

143 Russo P, Brady MS, Conlon K et al. Adult urological sarcoma. *J Urol* 1995; **147**: 1032–7.

144 Conlon KC, Casper ES, Brennan MF. Primary gastrointestinal sarcomas. Analysis of prognostic variables. *Ann Surg Oncol* 1995; **2**: 26–31.

145 Tavassoli FA, Norris HJ. Smooth muscle tumors of the vulva. *Obstet Gynecol* 1979; **53:** 213–17.

146 Santoro A, Tursz T, Mourdsen H et al. Doxorubicin versus CYVADIC versus Doxorubicin plus ifosfamide in first-line treatment of advanced soft tissue sarcomas: a randomized study of the European Organization for Research and Treament of Cancer Soft Tissue and Bone Sarcoma Group. *J Clin Oncol* 1995; **13**: 1537–45.

147 Mazanet R, Antman KH. Sarcomas of soft tissue and bone. *Cancer* 1991; **68**: 463–73.

148 Tierney JF, Mosseri V, Stewart LA et al. Adjuvant chemotherapy for soft-tissue sarcoma: review and meta-analysis of the published results of randomized clinical trials. *Br J Cancer* 1995; **72**: 469–75.

149 Flamant F, Chassagne D, Cosset J et al. Embryonal rhabdomyosarcoma of the vagina in children: conservative treatment with Curietherapy and chemotherapy. *Eur J Cancer* 1979; **15**: 527–32.

150 Hays DM, Shimada H, Raney RB et al. Clinical staging and treatment results in rhabdomyosarcoma of the female genital tract among children and adolescents. *Cancer* 1988; **61**: 1893–903.

151 Talerman A. Sarcoma botryoides presenting as a polyp on the labium majus. *Cancer* 1973; **32**: 994–9.

152 Copeland LJ, Gershenson DM, Saul PB et al. Sarcoma

153 Hensley GT, Friedrich EG. Malignant fibroxanthoma: a sarcoma of the vulva. *Am J Obstet Gynaecol* 1973; **116**: 289–91.

154 Bock JE, Andreasson B, Thorn A et al. Dermatofibrosarcoma protuberans of the vulva. *Gynecol Oncol* 1985; **20**: 129–35.

155 Soltan MH. Dermatofibrosarcoma protuberans of the vulva. Case report. *Br J Obstet Gynaecol* 1981; **88**: 203–5.

156 Piver MS, Tsukada Y, Barlow J. Epithelioid sarcoma of the vulva. *Obstet Gynecol* 1972; **40**: 839–42.

157 Tan GWT, Lim-Tan SK, Salmon YM. Epithelioid sarcoma of the vulva. *Singapore Med J* 1989; **30**: 308–10.

158 Gallup DG, Abell MR, Morley GW. Epithelioid sarcoma of the vulva. *Obstet Gynecol* 1976; **48**: 14S–17S.

159 Elchalal U, Lifschitz-Mercer B, Dgani R et al. Aggressive angiomyxoma of the vulva. *Gynecol Oncol* 1992; **47**: 260–2.

160 Macasaet MA, Duerr A, Thelmo W et al. Kaposi sarcoma presenting as a vulvar mass. *Obstet Gynecol* 1995; **86**: 695–7.

161 Haverkos HW. The epidemiologic scope of Kaposi's sarcoma. *Oncology* 1996; **10**: 9S–12S.

162 Blumenfeld W, Egbert BM, Sagebiel RW. Differential diagnosis of Kaposi's sarcoma. *Arch Pathol Lab Med* 1985; **109**: 123–7.

163 Abrams DI. Current therapeutic options for Kaposi's sarcoma. *Oncology* 1996; **10**: 24–7.

164 Safai B. Clinical manifestations of Kaposi's sarcoma. *Oncology* 1996; **10**(Suppl): 13–23.

165 Olweny CL, Toya T, Katongole-Mbidde E. Treatment of Kaposi's sarcoma by combination of actinomycin-D, vincristine and imidazole carboxamide (NSC-45388:) results of a randomized clinical trial. *Int J Cancer* 1974; **14**: 649–53.

166 van Geel AN, Pastorino U, Jauch KW et al. Surgical treatment of lung metastases: the European Organization for Research and Treatment of Cancer – Soft Tissue and Bone Sarcoma Group Study of 255 patients. *Cancer* 1996; **77**: 675–82.

167 Gil-Moreno A, Garcia-Jimenez A, Gonzalez-Bosquet J et al. Merkel cell carcinoma of the vulva. *Gynecol Oncol* 1997; **64**: 526–32.

168 Tang CK, Nedwich A, Toker C et al. Unusual cutaneous carcinoma with features of small cell (oat-cell like) squamous carcinoma: a variant of Merkel cell neoplasm. *Am J Dermatopathol* 1982; **4**: 537–48.

169 Bottles K, Lacey CG, Goldberg J et al. Merkel cell

botryoides of the female genital tract. *Obstet Gynecol* 1985; **66**: 262–6.

tumour of the vulva. *Obstet Gynecol* 1984; **63**(Suppl): 61–5.

170 Chandeying V, Sutthijumroon S, Tungphaisal S. Merkel cell carcinoma of the vulva: A case report. *Asia-Oceania J Obstet Gynecol* 1989; **15**: 261–9.

171 Chen KT. Merkel's cell (neuroendocrine) carcinoma of the vulva. *Cancer* 1994; **73**: 2186–91.

172 Husseinzadeh N, Wesseler T, Newman N et al. Neuroendocrine (Merkel cell) carcinoma of the vulva. *Gynecol Oncol* 1988; **29**: 105–12.

173 Loret de Mola JR, Hudock PA, Steinetz C et al. Merkel cell carcinoma of the vulva. *Gynecol Oncol* 1993; **51**: 272–6.

174 Scurry J, Brand A, Planner R et al. Vulvar Merkel cell tumor with glandular and squamous differentiation. *Gynecol Oncol* 1996; **62**: 292–7.

175 Mercer D, Brander P, Liddell K. Merkel cell carcinoma: The clinical course. *Ann Plast Surg* 1990; **25**: 136–41.

176 Sharma D, Flora G, Grunberg SM. Chemotherapy of metastatic Merkel cell carcinoma: Case report and review of the literature. *Am J Clin Oncol* 1991; **14**: 166–70.

177 Waibel M, Richter K, von Lengerken W et al. Merkel cell carcinoma in an uncommon skin location, immunohistochemical and lectin histochemical findings. *Z Pathol* 1991; **137**: 40–50.

178 Abrams HL, Spiro R, Goldstein N. Metastases in carcinoma. *Cancer* 1950; **3**: 74–85.

179 Dehner LP. Metastatic and secondary tumours of the vulva. *Obstet Gynecol* 1973; **42**: 47–57.

180 Powell CS, Jones PA. Carcinoma of the bladder with metastasis in the clitoris. *Br J Obstet Gynaecol* 1983; **90**: 380–1.

181 Ahmed W, Beasley WH. Carcinoma of the stomach with a metastasis in the clitoris. *J Pakistan Med Assoc* 1979; **29**: 62–3.

182 Radman HM. Metastatic melanoma of the vulva. *MD Med J* 1981; **30**: 60–1.

183 Mader MH, Friedrich EGJ. Vulvar metastasis of breast carcinoma. A case report. *J Reprod Med* 1982; **27**: 169–71.

184 Egwuatu VE, Efeckam GC, Okaro JM. Burkitt's lymphoma of the vulva. *Br J Obstet Gynaecol* 1980; **87**: 827–30.

14

Vaginal intraepithelial neoplasia: characteristics, investigation and management

FH SILLMAN

Vaginal intraepithelial neoplasia (VaIN) presents the clinician with extremes in terms of outcomes, diagnoses and interventions. It is the 'best' of neoplasms, yet it can be the 'worst'; it can be easy to diagnose, yet it may also be difficult to diagnose; it can be easy to treat, but also present major therapeutic problems.

A wide range stretches between 'the best' – a patient with an intact genital tract and a readily visible single, small focus of vaginal dysplasia, which remits after a diagnostic biopsy – and 'the worst' – a patient post-hysterectomy, with VaIS (vaginal carcinoma in situ), buried in the vaginal cuff, which can occultly progress to invasion. The range of VaIN is wide because of the variety of hosts, lesions and treatments. All these variables, for this the rarest and least understood lower genital neoplasm, make it difficult to base the management of VaIN on solid scientific evidence. This chapter discusses the characteristics of VaIN and how best to apply them to investigation and management. Those characteristics that influence persistence/recurrence and progression are examined more closely. Finally, to the extent that it is possible, prevention is addressed, and most importantly, prevention of progression to invasive cancer.

CHARACTERISTICS (Table 14.1)

Age

In a study of 94 patients, spanning 15 years,[1] the mean age for developing VaIN was 51 years. This is in concert with other reports.[2–7] Immunocompromised patients had an average age 18 years younger than immunocompetent ones.[1]

Association with cervical neoplasia

There is usually an association with either preinvasive or invasive cervical neoplasia in situations when there has not been a prior hysterectomy for upper genital disease. Of 94 patients with VaIN, 26 had had a prior hysterectomy for upper genital disease.[1] Of the remaining 68 patients with a cervix, 91 per cent (62 of 68) had associated cervical neoplasia – 20 invasive and 42 intraepithelial. Ten of these 42 also had neoplasia on one or more additional anogenital sites: vulva, urethra, perineum, anus and/or intergluteal skin. One patient

Table 14.1 *Characteristics of VaIN*[1-3, 6, 7]

Characteristic	Comments
Age (years)	All = 51 (immunosuppressed = 39; immunocompetent = 57) Mild dysplasia = 39; moderate and severe = 49; in situ = 57
Associations	Other anogenital neoplasia = 67% (63/94) = 93% (63/68) of 'cervically eligible' (63 = 62 CN + 1 VIN)
Discovery	Usually = abnormal Pap Occasionally = colposcopic survey; rarely, leukoplakia
Aetiology	HPV (and other factors)
Frequency	Rare < 1% of lower genital intraepithelial neoplasia
Hysterectomy	About two-thirds; almost half not associated with CN
Time to presentation	CIN: 55% = concurrent; 45% = 67 months (5.6 years) prior Cancer of the cervix: 15% = concurrent; 85% = 100 months prior Hyst. for endometrial and ovarian cancer = 5 years prior Hyst. for benign disease = 11.6 years prior to VaIN
Location	Almost always upper third (usually only location) Occasionally, lower third, especially if associated VIN Rarely, also middle third
Multifocal	About half
Persistence/recurrence	Overall about 25% (immunosuppressed = 55%) Factors increasing risk: multifocal, associated AGN in situ (VaIN 3), immunosuppression
Prior radiation	About a quarter
Progression to invasion	All: prior in situ; inaccessible proximal vagina post-hyst. or radiation
Hidden sanctuaries	Post-hyst. cuff; RT coaptation
Superficial	0.1 mm (post-menopause or RT) to 0.3 mm (+ HPV keratosis<0.2)
Visualization	Difficult in some locations

CN, cervical neoplasia; VIN, vulvar intraepithelial neoplasia; HPV, human papillomavirus; CIN, cervical intraepithelial neoplasia; AGN, anogenital neoplasia; Hyst., hysterectomy; RT, radiotherapy.

Tables 14.1–14.4 use data from Sillman et al.[1] They are reproduced here with the permission of the publishers.

had only associated vulvar intraepithelial neoplasia (VIN) and no cervical disease. Only 7 per cent (5 of 68) of those 'cervically eligible' had no associated lower genital neoplasia.

Diagnosis

In about 90 per cent of cases, the preceding event to the diagnosis of VaIN is an abnormal Pap smear – cervical or vaginal.[1,3,6] The remaining cases of VaIN are found by colposcopic survey of high-risk patients; high risk includes those with known human papillomavirus (HPV) infection of the anogenital tract, other anogenital neoplasm or immunosuppression. Rarely, VaIN will be found macroscopically by biopsy of a leukoplakic lesion.

Aetiology

All the available evidence suggests that HPV plays a major, but not exclusive, role. This is similar to the current concepts of oncogenesis for cervical intraepithelial neoplasia (CIN) and vulvar intraepithelial neoplasia (VIN) (see Chapter 4). Vaginal epithelium appears to be less vulnerable than the cervical epithelium because it is not as metabolically active – it does normally undergo metaplastic transformation. Hence, VaIN is much rarer, with fewer than one patient with VaIN found for every 100 with CIN. There is no evidence supporting prior radiotherapy as a possible aetiological factor.

Hysterectomy

Prior hysterectomy was recorded for about two-thirds of patients in most reports.[1–4,6] In our own study,[1] 54 per cent of hysterectomies were performed for cervical neoplasia (almost half, 45%, for invasive disease and half for CIN), 14 per cent for upper genital cancers (uterine corpus and ovary) and 32 per cent for benign upper genital disease (mainly leiomyomas; rarely bleeding and pelvic inflammatory disease). Thus, in 46 per cent, hysterectomies were performed for upper genital disease, as opposed to lower genital neoplasia.

Time to presentation

When associated with CIN, VaIN was found concurrently in 55 per cent of patients.[1] In the remaining 45 per cent, the mean interval to VaIN was 5.6 years (67 months). When associated with invasive cervical cancer, VaIN was concurrently found in 15 per cent; for the other 85 per cent, there was a mean interval of 8.6 years before VaIN developed. After hysterectomy for upper genital cancer, the mean interval to VaIN was 5 years (range 1.5–14 years). The longest interval (mean 11.6 years, range 2–27) is after hysterectomy for benign disease.

Although there is no hard evidence, these data are suggestive of the vagina becoming more susceptible to carcinogenesis after the removal of the cervix, which is the preferred site for HPV-related oncogenesis in the lower genital tract.

Location

VaIN is almost always located in the upper third of the vagina[1–3,6] and this is usually the only site. Occasionally, the lower third is involved, particularly when associated with VIN. The least common location is the middle third of the vagina.

Persistence/recurrence

Persistence and/or recurrence (P/R) of disease is recognized in one quarter of patients. Multifocal neoplasia is present in half of patients.[1,3,6,7] VaIN can be hard to find in all its locations. Therefore, sometimes VaIN is not totally eradicated on initial treatment. Factors that favour P/R are listed in Table 14.2

Prior hysterectomy or radiotherapy are not significant risk factors for persistent/recurrent VaIN.

Sanctuaries

VaIN can be an easy neoplasm to treat because the vagina is the only lower genital organ without natural subsurface sanctuaries in which neoplastic epithelium can be sequestered. The cervix has crypts that can be involved by HPV and/or neoplasia. The vulva, medial to the hair line, has minor vestibular ducts which can contain VIN very superficially (< 1 mm), and the major vestibular ducts of Bartholin and Skene, into which VIN can extend more deeply. Lateral to the hair line, VIN can descend down into the hair shafts.

The only vaginal sanctuaries are iatrogenic. Ironically, in the vagina, one can create the only inaccessible site in the lower genital tract, which is the cuff that is sutured closed at the time of hysterectomy[8] or the upper vagina that undergoes co-aptation after radiotherapy. When the cuff is closed, about 1 cm of proximal, highest risk epithelium is buried therein

Table 14.2 *Relative persistence and/or progression of VaIN*

Condition	Relative risk
Multifocal lower genital tract neoplasia	6
Associated cervical dysplasia or neoplasia	3
Anogenital neoplastic syndrome (neoplasia occurring on two or more anogenital sites excepting the vagina and cervix as CIN frequently occurs in association with VaIN)	3
VaIS (VaIN 3)	2
Immunosuppression	1.5 (approximate)

(Fig. 14.1) and cannot be cytologically monitored, viewed or biopsied. After radiotherapy coaptation can close more of the vagina. In these sanctuaries, VaIN can go undetected and vaginal neoplasia is found only when invasion develops and breaks through into the accessible vagina or a rectovaginal mass is palpated.

Depth of disease

VaIN is a thin, superficial neoplasm.[1,10] In the premenopausal woman, the vaginal epithelium is 0.3 mm deep (although, with HPV, hyperkeratosis can occur and the epithelium can increase in depth to about 0.5 mm). In postmenopausal women who are not using oestrogen replacement, or post-radiation, the epithelial thickness is about 0.1 mm.

Based on these observations, treatment requires removal of only the surface neoplastic epithelium: 0.1–0.3 mm deep (or up to 0.5 mm when hyperkeratosis is present). This is in contrast to the removal of 5–7 mm for CIN and 1 mm for medial and 3 mm for lateral VIN, because of the cervical (crypts) and vulvar (adnexal) sanctuaries. The thinness of VaIN is fortunate because the underlying structures, such as the urethra, bladder, peritoneal cavity and bowel, and rectum, can be less than 5 mm from the vaginal surface. The vagina is not endowed with the more generous protective stromal 'cushions' of the cervix and vulva.

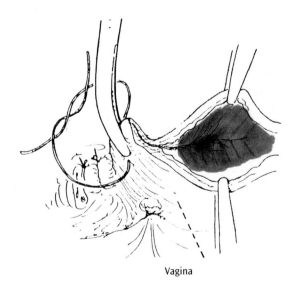

Vagina

Figure 14.1 *'Red' defines about 1 cm of vaginal epithelium that is buried when the vaginal cuff is sutured closed at hysterectomy. (Reproduced with permission from WB Saunders[9]) This figure also appears in the colour plate section.*

Visualization

Visualization of the entire vagina is not easy and finding all neoplastic foci can be exceptionally difficult. Epithelium in rugal troughs and under speculum blades can be hard to see. A successful search for all VaIN present is more likely to happen if the following are used:

- Oestrogen, when deficient. Lack of oestrogen makes acetowhiteness fainter, vascular signs less prominent, contours flatter and VaIN harder to visualize at colposcopy. Therefore, 2 weeks of vaginal oestrogen can be given to postmenopausal women before colposcopy for an abnormal Pap.
- Iodine solutions can be helpful in highlighting non-staining areas.
- The speculum should be of a proper size.
- Ring forceps can help with exposure and can flatten out rugae. An endocervical speculum can expose epithelium within vaginal angle tunnels that occur after hysterectomy.
- A fine hook can stabilize an elusive or excessively mobile biopsy target.

INVESTIGATION

Screening

The current cost-conscious consensus is not to screen after their hysterectomy women who do not have a history of CIN (i.e. not to carry out Pap smears).[11-13] As two-thirds of patients with VaIN have a hysterectomy, and almost half of these for upper genital disease, this means that approximately one-third of past patients with VaIN have had a hysterectomy for upper genital disease. Hysterectomies for upper genital disease should become relatively more frequent (versus hysterectomies for CIN) as invasive cervical cancer declines and hysterectomy becomes increasingly rare for CIN. If patients who have had a hysterectomy for upper genital disease were not to have Pap smears, then one-third or more of future patients with VaIN will not be identified. Those who progress will be discovered when they develop clinical vaginal cancer (e.g. bleeding or a rectovaginal mass). Conversely, VaIN is uncommon and many women would have to remain within a screening programme after their hysterectomies to detect the few who might develop VaIN.

There are no reliable means of predicting which women, who have had a hysterectomy for upper genital tract pathology, will develop VaIN. The author recommends that vaginal cytology be carried out 5 years after hysterectomy for upper genital disease, and at 5–10 year intervals thereafter.[1,14] For our patients with upper genital cancer, the shortest patient interval from hysterectomy to VaIN was 1.5 years and the mean interval was 5 years. For patients after a hysterectomy for benign disease, the shortest interval was 2 years and the mean time to VaIN was 11.6 years.[1] High-risk factors, such as HPV or immunosuppression, warrant initial, post-hysterectomy screening every 3 years. Not to screen at all after a hysterectomy for upper genital disease is defendable on economic grounds, but would allow a small number of women to risk the unimpeded development of vaginal cancer.

Diagnosis

Abnormal cervical or vaginal cytology, leading to colposcopy, is what commonly leads to the diagnosis of VaIN. As it is unusual for VaIN to develop in the absence of cervical dysplasia or neoplasia (unless the cervix is absent), these conditions should alert one to watch for VaIN. Scanning the upper vagina is a good practice during colposcopy (Fig. 14.2). Careful vaginal colposcopy is mandatory when cervical colposcopy does not explain a cervical smear abnormality.

A periodic colposcopic survey of the entire anogenital tract, in high-risk patients, can also lead to the diagnosis of VaIN. High-risk patients include immunosuppressed individuals or those with past or present evidence (cytological or histological) of HPV/neoplasia anywhere in the anogenital tract.

TREATMENT

A multitude of destructive (cautery, cryotherapy, 5-fluorouracil [5-FU] cream, laser) and excisional (biopsy forceps, chemosurgery, laser excision, scalpel) treatments have been used for VaIN. The depth of cautery and cryotherapy is too uncontrollable and perforations have occurred.[7] Although topical 5-FU cream achieves an 85 per cent short-term remission rate,[1,7] we discontinued its use as a sole treatment in 1977 in favour of its adjunctive use with chemosurgery because of long-term recurrences with topical 5-FU alone.

Laser is widely used but offers only one advantage over chemosurgery, which is deeper treatment of apical dysplasia at the post-hysterectomy cuff. Disadvantages of laser include the fact that vaporization does not provide tissue for examination. Although laser vaporization is precise, it is not sufficiently precise to avoid stromal injury, especially at the recommended depth of 2–4 mm.[7,10] Treatment need only remove the neoplastic epithelium, which is 0.3 (−0.5) mm deep before the menopause and about 0.1 mm deep after it.

We found that 70 per cent of patients achieved remission after their initial treatment;[1] 25 per cent went into remission after two to five treatments and 5 per cent progressed to invasion. Treatment choice is influenced by the presence of multifocal neoplasia, associated cervical neoplasia, anogenital neoplasia syndrome (AGNS), grade of disease, immunosuppression, plus lesion size, location, prior treatments and the general medical condition of the patient.

Acknowledging that there are no defining data, such as prospective, blinded, controlled trials comparing all treatments, we favour treatment by excision using biopsy forceps, chemosurgery or a scalpel (partial vaginectomy). Table 14.3 displays the results of our favoured treatments. These data are not sufficient to determine the choice of treatment, but Tables 14.3 and 14.4 offer some guidance in comparing and considering treatments.

Colposcopic biopsies or excision

Diagnostic biopsy or biopsy-excision using colposcopic control produced remission in 87 per cent ([21+6]/[22+9] = 27/31) of such treatments (*see* Table 14.3). This reflects the relatively low risk of these patients – only one had an AGNS, one was immunosuppressed and only 26 per cent had multiple foci. Excision was successful in five of six patients (83 per cent) as initial treatment, and in one of three (33 per cent) when used for recurrent VaIN. So, for initial treatment, biopsy and excision produced remission in

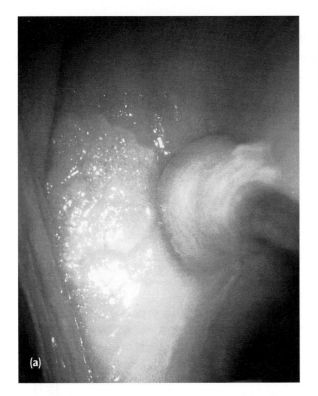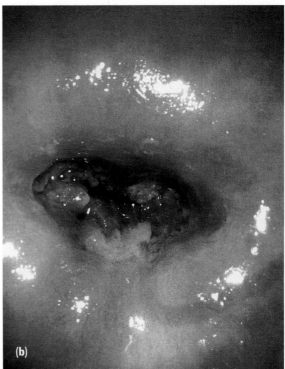

Figure 14.2 (a) Colposcopic scanning of the upper vagina led to the discovery of the larger area of severe dysplasia in the right vaginal fornix. (b) A small focus of moderate dysplasia at 6 o'clock on the cervix.

93 per cent ($[21+5]/[22+6] = 26/28$) of such patients. Biopsy and excision are excellent modalities for treating initial, small, focal lesions in low-risk patients (*see* Table 14.4).

Chemosurgery

Chemosurgery means the preoperative use of topical 5-FU for 5 nights before surgery.[1,7,15,16] The 5-FU disables DNA and RNA, which control protein synthesis.

Table 14.3 *Outcome in relation to recommended treatments and risk factors[1]*

Treatment	Risk factors of treated patients[a] (%)					Outcome[a] (%)		
	AGNS	CIN	Immunos-suppressed	Multifocal	VaIS	Remission	Persistence/recurrence	Invasion[b]
Biopsy (n = 22)		68 (15)		27 (6)	14 (3)	95 (21)	4.5 (1)	
Excision (n = 9)	11 (1)	56 (5)	11 (1)	22 (2)	67 (6)	67 (6)	22 (2)	11 (1)
Chemosurgery (n = 45)	29 (13)	73 (33)	29 (13)	71 (32)	31 (14)	73 (33)	20 (9)	7 (3)
Partial vaginectomy (n = 18)	22 (4)	72 (13)	6 (1)	72 (13)	83 (15)	39 (7)	56 (10)	6 (1)

[a] Numbers in parentheses are the actual numbers.
[b] Invasion listed in row of treatment immediately prior to diagnosis of invasion.
AGNS, anogenital neoplasia syndrome.
VaIS, vaginal carcinoma in situ

Table 14.4 *Guidelines for the initial treatment of VaIN*

Disease description	Treatment	Comments
Mild dysplasia (VaIN 1)	Biopsy and observe	Treat large, persistent lesions in high-risk patients
Small, focal lesions	Biopsy/excision	Best as initial treatment in low-risk patients
VaIN 3 at vaginal apex after hysterectomy	Partial vaginectomy or radiotherapy	VaIN 2, possible chemosurgery or laser
Other	Chemosurgery	Chemosurgery is also a choice for immunosuppressed, AGNS, persistence/recurrence

AGNS, anogenital neoplasia syndrome.

Hence, basal cell pseudopodial attachments to the underlying stroma are weakened, resulting in a partial epidermolysis. Epidermolysis is completed with low-power electrosurgical energy (Fig. 14.3). We use a flat blade attached to a 'loop'-type generator at a setting of about 10 watts. The resulting chemo-electro-epidermolysis allows one to remove just the neoplastic epithelium (Fig. 14.4c), leaving the underlying stroma intact (Figs 14.3b, 14.4b, 14.5b and 14.6b, c). The procedure is analogous to shovelling a thin coat of snow (neoplastic epithelium) off a road (stroma), because the plane of dissection at the epidermal depth of 0.1 or 0.3 mm has been predetermined by the preoperative 5-FU epidermolysis (Fig. 14.6a, b). Chemosurgery is the only type of surgery that does not injure the stroma. All surgery, except chemosurgery, goes deeper than the required epithelial depth, injures stroma, produces scarring and may injure subepithelial structures (urethra, bladder, peritoneal cavity, rectum). Stromal damage is particularly problematic for patients with large and multifocal lesions, and for those with persistent or recurrent VaIN. Repeated other surgery, with cumulative stromal damage and scarring, can compromise sexual and reproductive function.

Chemosurgery offers the added advantages of highlighting foci (5-FU enhances acetowhitening) (Figs 14.4a, 14.5a and 14.6a) of VaIN that might otherwise be colposcopically occult. Another potential advantage is that 5-FU provides regional HPV/neoplastic suppression pre-operatively. If 5-FU is used once or twice every month postoperatively (after chemosurgery or other surgery), as maintenance therapy in high-risk patients, there appear to be fewer recurrences.

Chemosurgery is particularly useful in patients who have extensive, multifocal or persistent/recurrent lesions, have an AGNS or are immunosuppressed. Chemosurgery can be repeated, if necessary, without the cumulative morbidity of other surgery. It can also

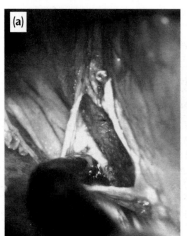 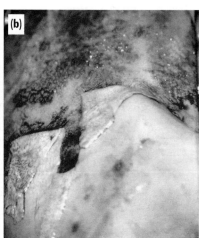 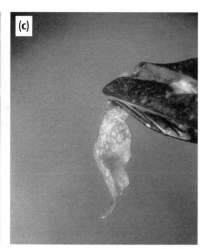

Figure 14.3 *A patient with moderate vaginal dysplasia covering much of the upper two-thirds of her vagina. (a) Starting chemosurgery in the left anterior fornix, with an electrosurgical instrument completing the separation of the dysplastic epithelium pre-treated with 5-fluorouracil from the underlying stroma. (b) The anterior vaginal fornix, showing bare, but undamaged, stroma. (c) A strip of removed dysplasia.*

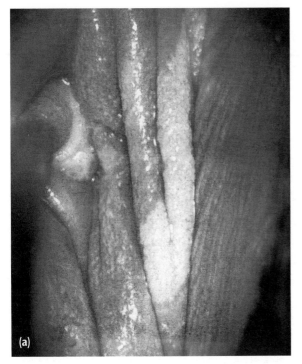

(a)

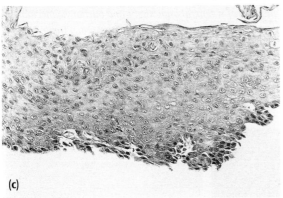

(c)

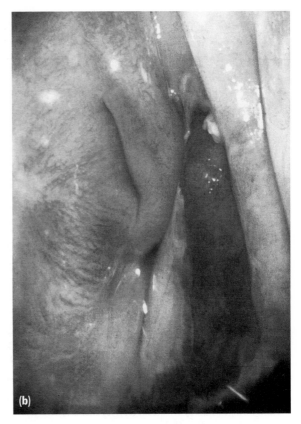

(b)

Figure 14.4 *(a) A 'hockey stick'-shaped lesion of severe dysplasia in the left vaginal apex, after a hysterectomy for cervical in situ. (b) Bare stroma after chemosurgical excision. (c) Histology of dysplasia removed; thickness = 0.25 mm. Note the margin is along the basal epithelial border, where there is evidence of epidermolysis in the deepest basal cell layer, as a result of presurgical 5-fluorouracil. (Reproduced with permission from Williams and Wilkins[7])*

be done as an outpatient procedure and is not expensive. In susceptible individuals, the discomfort from 5-FU-induced chemoinflammation can be particularly bothersome for 1 week postoperatively. Postoperatively, maintenance 5-FU (once or twice a month) is well tolerated.

As chemosurgery is the most superficial surgery, it should not be used for VaIS at the post-hysterectomy cuff. This technique cannot reliably remove in situ that is buried in the vaginal vault scar. The technique is effective in patients who have not had a hysterectomy, and may be used for VaIS when there is a visible free margin from the post-hysterectomy cuff (although this does not rule out another focus in the buried

cuff). For extensive, multifocal VaIS, chemosurgery can be used for all but the most proximal disease, where partial vaginectomy can complete and complement the chemosurgical excisions.

Partial vaginectomy

This procedure is the treatment of choice for proximal post-hysterectomy VaIS.[1,4,5,8] The technique offers the deepest, best specimens to assess pathology, including margins and whether or not there is invasion. However, to remove the entire vaginal cuff safely, an abdominal-vaginal approach might be required.[5,8]

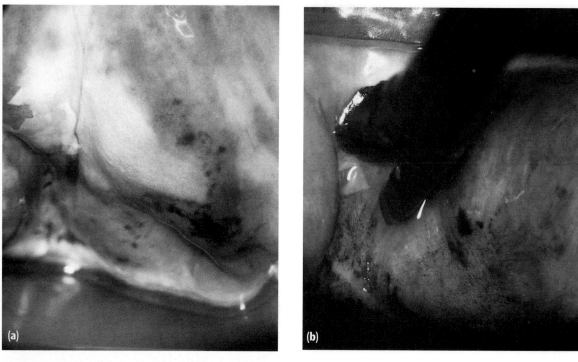

Figure 14.5 *A 66-year-old with severe cardiac disease, which precluded use of a general anaesthetic and partial vaginectomy for her vaginal carcinoma in situ (VaIS) at the apex, 22 years after hysterectomy for leiomyomas. (a) 5-Fluorouracil-treated VaIS (0.1mm thick) at start of chemosurgery. (b) Last piece of loose VaIS being grasped; note unharmed stroma. The mystery of what lies buried in the cuff proximal to the visible apex would be of concern in a younger, healthier patient.*

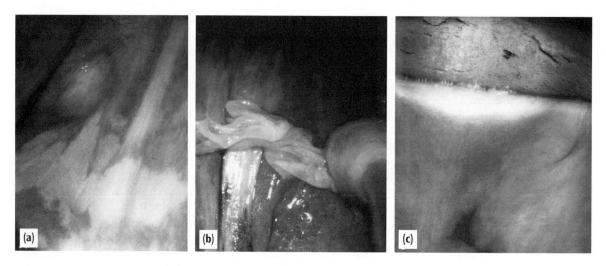

Figure 14.6 *A patient who had a radical hysterectomy and then developed recurrent severe dysplasia at the vaginal apex, which had previously been excised. (a) Severe dysplasia highlighted by acetowhitening after presurgical 5-fluorouracil. (b) Dysplasia separated from the underlying stroma during chemosurgery. (c) Rapid healing of vaginal apex 8 weeks after surgery, with only a small area still to re-epithelialize. There was no additional scarring in this previously twice-operated field because the chemosurgery did not damage the stroma. (Reproduced with permission from Williams and Wilkins.[8])*

This is rarely done, and resuturing can again bury epithelium. Any buried vaginal epithelium is potentially dangerous.

Ireland and Monaghan,[5] and Hoffman and colleagues[4] describe upper vaginectomies, for VaIS, in 63 patients who had previously undergone hysterectomy. (Included were a few patients who had total vaginectomy, which is almost never indicated and provides no benefit beyond removal of all foci of VaIN.[1]) Occult invasion was found in 29 per cent. The authors emphasize that a destructive procedure, such as laser vaporization, would have missed the invasion.

When pathology specimens from partial vaginectomy reveal no invasion, and the margins are free, the prognosis is good, but not certain. Hoffman and colleagues[4] found that 19 of 22 (86 per cent) of patients with free margins remained in remission. Two patients on whom we reported,[1] who had partial vaginectomy twice and still developed invasion, illustrate that free margins do not mean certain cure in a disease that is multifocal half of the time. One of these patients particularly illustrates how difficult it can be to prevent invasion. She had an upper vaginectomy for VaIS 7 years after a hysterectomy for leiomyomas. Eighteen months later, she had chemosurgery for a recurrence; 2 years after chemosurgery she was found to have VaIS in her left apical tunnel. Her left upper vagina and tunnel were resected (second partial vaginectomy) and her specimen closely resembles Fig. 14.7 (a patient who also developed invasion), with free wide and deep margins. Sixteen months later, a left 'supra-vaginal' mass was palpated rectovaginally. Laparotomy revealed no spread of this previously occult invasive cancer and she is currently free of disease 7 years after radiotherapy.

Vaginal dysplasia (VaIN 1 and 2) after hysterectomy has not yet been shown to require partial vaginectomy. Therefore, we do not use partial vaginectomy for low-grade disease. The operation is a major procedure requiring general anaesthesia and is not without morbidity. The remission rate (see Table 14.3) does not compare favourably with other surgery, but patients treated by partial vaginectomy had more VaIS in more inaccessible locations. Although it is theoretically possible that a patient could have colposcopically overt dysplasia, while occultly developing invasion in the buried vaginal cuff, we know of no reported patient progressing directly from vaginal dysplasia to invasive cancer. All patients diagnosed with VaIN, and progressing to invasion, had prior biopsies of VaIS (VaIN 3).

Moderate-severe dysplasia (VaIN 2) at the post-hysterectomy apex is the one instance in which we sometimes use laser to go deeper into the cuff. We, and some pathologists, believe that the term VaIN 3 should be reserved for VaIS; thus, VaIN 2 should encompass moderate-severe dysplasia. This is clinically logical, since moderate and severe dysplasia are treated the same way. In situ is finely, but clinically, distinct in all parts of the anogenital tract (e.g. see above re progression to invasion; atypical vessels are not seen with dysplasia, but with 3 per cent of cervical in situs; occult invasion is present in 10 per cent of cervical in situs; in situ is more persistent than dysplasia; etc.) and warrants different therapeutic consideration and respect.

Mild dysplasia (VaIN 1) can usually be followed, as is often done on other anogenital sites. Treatment should be considered for large, persistent lesions, especially with high-risk virus types, in high-risk patients.

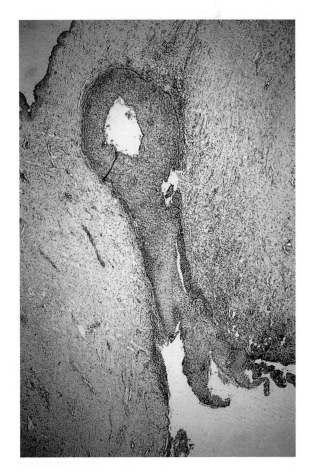

Figure 14.7 *Histology of left upper vaginectomy specimen; in situ it extends into the left vaginal 'tunnel'. The wide and deep margins are free. (Reproduced with permission from CV Mosby[7])*

Radiotherapy

There are theoretical advantages to using radiotherapy to treat VaIS at the post-hysterectomy cuff because radiation can penetrate the occult proximal extent of the closed cuff.[9,17] Radiotherapy for VaIN was abandoned in most clinics two decades ago because of atrophy, scarring, stenosis, dyspareunia, coaptation and the same P/R rates as less morbid alternatives. Also, from cervical radiation studies, there was the unproven suggestion that in situ is less radiosensitive than invasive cancer. There may be a role for radiotherapy in patients with VaIS in the post-hysterectomy cuff, for whom vaginectomy of any type would pose a high surgical risk.

PREVENTION OF PROGRESSION TO INVASION

Although most patients with VaIN respond to initial treatment, even as simple as diagnostic biopsy, and most others respond to more extensive treatment, about 5 per cent[1,3,6] progress to invasive cancer. Their common denominator is having (VaIS) in the most proximal vagina, rendered inaccessible by burial at hysterectomy or by radiotherapy. These patients are challenging and frustrating because they progress silently to invasion, despite careful recommended monitoring.

Prevention should be the primary objective. The following are suggestions about how this might be achieved:

- Hysterectomy for cervical in situ should be limited to those for whom there is no other reasonable alternative.
- Colposcopy of the upper vagina should be performed before hysterectomy for cervical neoplasia to identify any VaIN present.[5,7,18]
- At hysterectomy, the cuff can be left open[1,2,18] or the exposed vaginal edge (which would normally be buried) of the cuff (red in Fig. 14.1) can be de-epithelialized with electrosurgery or laser before closing. This should be done for all patients with cervical neoplasia, but can be considered for others in whom HPV could have silently initiated a process that might ultimately lead to vaginal cancer.
- Supracervical hysterectomy does not bury proximal vaginal epithelium. It can be considered in patients with benign upper genital disease.
- After radiation, total vaginal patency should be maintained.

CONCLUSIONS

VaIN is a rare disease for which the current consensus is not to screen patients after hysterectomy for upper genital diseases even though one-third of patients who develop VaIN will be in this cohort. As populations become more effectively screened for CIN, one might hope that the number of women having 'benign hysterectomies' who have not been thoroughly screened beforehand will be small and thus the risk of subsequent VaIN will lessen. At present, there are no definitive data to support or refute screening after hysterectomy for upper genital diseases.

When VaIN is diagnosed in a timely fashion, it usually responds to treatment, particularly if the lesion is focal and the patient at low risk. However, certain patients (with associated anogenital neoplasia and/or immunosuppression), and certain lesions (multifocal and/or in situ) are at higher risk for recurrence. After hysterectomy or radiotherapy, patients diagnosed with VaIS at the vaginal cuff are at risk of occult invasion. Careful attention to prevention, screening, diagnosis, treatment and follow-up, taking into account patient and lesion characteristics, can significantly reduce, but not eliminate, recurrence and progression to invasion.

ACKNOWLEDGEMENTS

Pervading this chapter, more than referenced, are the thoughts and inspirations of my long-time mentors, colleagues and friends: Alexander Sedlis MD, Christopher Crum MD and Ellen McTigue RN.

REFERENCES

1 Sillman FH, Fruchter RG, Chen YS, Camilien L, Sedlis A, McTigue E. Vaginal intraepithelial neoplasia: Risk factors for persistence, recurrence, and invasion and its management. *Am J Obstet Gynecol* 1997; **176**: 93–9.
2 Audet-LaPointe P, Body G, Vauclair R, Drouim P, Ayoub J. Vaginal intraepithelial neoplasia. *Gynecol Oncol* 1990; **36**: 232–9.
3 Benedet JL, Sanders BH. Carcinoma in situ of the vagina. *Am J Obstet Gynecol* 1984; **148**: 695–700.
4 Hoffman MS, DeCesare SL, Roberts WS, Fiorica JV, Finan MA, Cavanagh D. Upper vaginectomy for in situ and occult, superficially invasive carcinoma of the vagina. *Am J Obstet Gynecol* 1992; **166**: 30–3.

5   Ireland D, Monaghan JM. The management of the patient with abnormal vaginal cytology following hysterectomy. *Br J Obstet Gynaecol* 1988; **95**: 973–5.

6   Lenehan PM, Meffe F, Lickrish GM. Vaginal intraepithelial neoplasia: biologic aspects and management. *Obstet Gynecol* 1986; **68**: 333–7.

7   Sillman FH, Sedlis A, Boyce J. A review of lower genital intraepithelial neoplasia and the use of topical 5-fluorouracil. *Obstet Gynecol Surv* 1985; **40**: 190–220.

8   Soutter WP. The treatment of vaginal intraepithelial neoplasia after hysterectomy. *Br J Obstet Gynaecol* 1988; **95**: 961–2.

9   Parsons L, Ulfelder H. *An atlas of pelvic operations* (illustrations by MB Codding). Philadelphia: WB Saunders, 1968: 33.

10 Benedet JL, Wilson PS, Matisic JP. Epidermal thickness measurements in vaginal intraepithelial neoplasia. *J Reprod Med* 1992; **37**: 809–12.

11 Fetters MD, Fischer G, Reed BD. Effectiveness of vaginal Papanicolaou smear screening after total hysterectomy for benign disease. *JAMA* 1996; **275**: 940–7.

12 Noller KL. Screening of vaginal cancer. *N Engl J Med* 1996; **335**: 1599–600.

13 Pearce KF, Haefner HK, Sarwar SF, Nolan TE. Cytopathological findings on vaginal Papanicolaou smears after hysterectomy for benign gynecologic disease. *N Engl J Med* 1996; **335**: 1559–62.

14 Piscitelli JT, Bastian LA, Wilkes A, Simel DL. Cytologic screening after hysterectomy for benign disease. *Am J Obstet Gynecol* 1995; **173**: 424–32.

15 Sillman FH, Boyce J, Macasaet M, Nicastri A. 5-Fluorouracil/chemosurgery in the treatment of intraepithelial neoplasia of the lower genital tract. *Obstet Gynecol* 1981; **58**: 356–60.

16 Sillman FH, Sedlis A, Boyce J. 5-FU/chemosurgery for difficult lower genital intraepithelial neoplasia. *Contemp Obstet Gynecol* 1985; **27**: 79–101.

17 MacLeod C, Fowler A, Dalrymple C, Atkinson K, Elliott P, Carter J. High dose-rate brachytherapy in the management of high grade intraepithelial neoplasia of the vagina. *Gynecol Oncol* 1997; **65**: 74–7.

18 Woodman CBJ, Mould JJ, Jordan JA. Radiotherapy in the management of vaginal intraepithelial neoplasia after hysterectomy. *Br J Obstet Gynaecol* 1988; **95**: 976–9.

Vaginal cancer

GC DU TOIT

Primary cancer of the vagina remains a rare neoplasm of the female genital tract. It occurs in 1.5–3.1 per cent of all genital malignancies.[1] The close proximity of the rectum and bladder to the vagina results in disease-associated and treatment-related morbidity and complications. Screening for the disease is not cost-effective.[2] Most vaginal malignancies are metastatic in nature. Primary cervical, vulvar, rectal and bladder tumours may invade the vagina in continuity with the primary tumour. Endometrial carcinoma, choriocarcinoma and gastrointestinal malignancies may present with vaginal metastases.

LYMPHATIC DRAINAGE OF THE VAGINA

Vaginal carcinoma spreads by direct invasion and via lymphatic channels to the regional lymph nodes. A fine lymphatic network begins in the epithelium and subepithelial tissue of the vagina. This network communicates with a more coarse lymphatic system in the subepithelial and muscularis layers via irregular anastomoses. Both systems drain to the lateral vaginal lymphatic trunks which, in turn, drain to the regional lymph nodes.

The upper third of the vagina usually drains to the common iliac and internal iliac node groups. The distal third of the vagina drains to the inguinofemoral nodes. The anterior aspect of the middle third drains to the lateral pelvic nodes (external iliac) and vesical nodes. The posterior aspect of the middle third drains to the deep pelvic nodes (presacral)[3] (Fig. 15.1).

As a result of the complexity of the lymphatic system, the course and destination of lymphatics from a specific vaginal region are not consistent. Embolization of tumour cells in the lymphatics results in obstruction of lymph channels and altered drainage. All pelvic lymph nodes may therefore serve as primary drainage sites.

The site of carcinoma in the vagina serves as an indicator of which regional nodes would be involved in metastases. Treatment of the disease should include therapy to the regional lymph nodes, as indicated by the site of the tumour in the vagina.

SQUAMOUS CARCINOMA

Aetiology

Epidemiological factors that have been associated with vaginal squamous carcinoma include previous pelvic radiotherapy, sexually transmitted disease and previous cervical disease. Although long-term pessary use has been cited as a cause in the past, the evidence for this is weak. In a case-controlled study of 41 patients, 19 with vaginal carcinoma in situ and 22 with invasive carcinoma, Brinton and colleagues[4] identified low

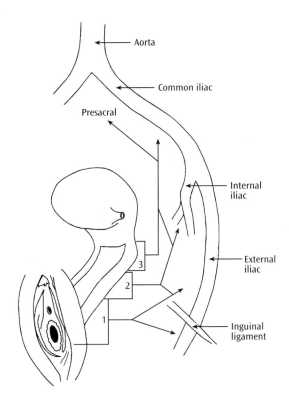

Figure 15.1 *Regional lymph nodes of vagina. (Modified from Plentl and Friedman.)*

educational level and low family income as risk factors for the disease. Sexual behaviour, a history of genital warts and smoking were not found to be statistically significant risk factors.[4] Sexually transmitted agents (human papillomavirus [HPV] type 16, herpes simplex virus [HSV] type 2 and *Chlamydia trachomatis*) may play a role in the aetiology of the disease. In another case-controlled study, Hildesheim and colleagues[5] illustrated a strong association between the above-mentioned micro-organisms and the risk of vaginal carcinoma. Seropositivity for all of those agents was associated with a statistically significant risk for vaginal carcinoma (relative risk, RR = 17) in comparison with the control group.[5] Previous pelvic radiotherapy as a potential causative agent has been challenged by Perez and colleagues.[6] Ireland and Monaghan[7] showed a high risk of invasive carcinoma developing in patients who had persistent abnormal vaginal cytology after hysterectomy. Brinton and colleagues[4] indicated a clear increased risk associated with previous abnormal cervical cytology (RR = 3.8; 95% confidence interval, 95%CI = 1.6–9.0). A field effect of premalignancy and

malignancies is demonstrated by 2.5 per cent concurrent vaginal intraepithelial neoplasia (VaIN) in patients with confirmed cervical intraepithelial neoplasia (CIN) lesions. The reported frequency of VaIN in patients with a previous history of CIN ranges from 0.9 per cent to 6.8 per cent.[8,9] Aho and colleagues[10] describe the natural history of VaIN in 23 untreated women. Invasive carcinoma developed in two women (9 per cent), although in three (13 per cent) persistent disease could be documented with a 3-year follow-up. In most women (87 per cent), the VaIN lesion underwent spontaneous regression.[10] For further details regarding VaIN, the reader is referred to Chapter 14.

Clinical presentation

Squamous cell vaginal carcinoma mainly presents in women in their 50s and 60s. Occasionally, the disease occurs in younger women in their 20s and 30s.

Common presenting symptoms include painless abnormal vaginal bleeding and vaginal discharge.[11] Bladder and rectal symptoms occur as a result of the close proximity of the vagina. Pain as the presenting feature is uncommon and the diagnosis is often made incidentally during a routine examination. Symptoms vary from frequency to incontinence of faeces and/or urine secondary to fistula formation. A delay from the time of first presentation to eventual diagnosis has been reported.[12]

Signs

Vaginal carcinoma presents as an endophytic or fungating tumour in the vagina. The suspicion of tumour beneath intact vaginal epithelium should alert the clinician to the possibility of metastatic rather than primary disease.

The most frequent site of involvement is the upper third of the vagina (56 per cent). The lesion is present in the middle third and lower third in 13 per cent and 31 per cent, respectively.[1]

Management

STAGING AND PRE-TREATMENT ASSESSMENTS

Subsequent to histological confirmation of malignancy, patients are staged according to the current International Federation of Gynaecologists and Obstetricians (FIGO) guidelines (Table 15.1).[13] This staging requires that a tumour extending to the external os of the cervix be regarded as primary cervical carcinoma and, in cases with a colposcopically normal cervix, random biopsies may be indicated to exclude invasion. Tumours invading the lower third of the vagina and vulva are classified as vulvar carcinomas. Individualized treatment of women with vaginal carcinoma requires considerable skill and experience. Examination under anaesthesia with cystoscopy and proctosigmoidoscopy allows the extent of the disease to be determined. Computed tomography (CT) may be used to identify possible intra-abdominal lymph node metastasis, although this is not a part of formal FIGO staging. Fine needle aspiration is indicated if suspicious nodes are identified. Particular attention should be paid to the inguinal nodes.

Treatment

In most cases of vaginal carcinoma, an individualized approach to treatment is required. The close proximity of the bladder, rectum and urethra limits the amount of radiation and also imposes limitations on surgical resection. Psychological considerations and maintenance of a functional vagina should be prioritized in decision-making.

RADIOTHERAPY

The mainstay of treatment remains radiotherapy. Good functional results are obtained with concurrent tumour control. Radiotherapeutic doses must be applied to the primary tumour and to possible sites of regional spread. The pelvic nodes should be included in cases where lesions involve the middle and upper third, whereas inguinal nodes must be included when tumours involve the lower third of the vagina. A combination of teletherapy, brachytherapy and/or interstitial therapy should be applied on an individual basis.

Table 15.1 *FIGO staging of vaginal cancer*

Stage	Spread
I	Carcinoma limited to the vaginal wall
II	Carcinoma has involved the subvaginal tissue but has not extended to the pelvic wall
III	Carcinoma has extended onto the pelvic wall
IVa	Spread of the tumour to adjacent organs and/or direct extension beyond the true pelvis
IVb	Spread to distant organs

Radiotherapy for stage I disease

Vaginal lesions of less than 2 cm in diameter and less than 3 mm invasion can be treated with 60–70 Gy as intracavitary or interstitial therapy. Interstitial implants with a Syed–Neblett applicator allow for higher doses than intracavitary therapy with cylinders (Fig. 15.2).[14]

Adverse tumour factors such as lesions larger than 2 cm in diameter, with lymphovascular space invasion, and/or grade 3 tumours require external beam therapy to the regional lymph nodes. In cases of upper and middle third tumours, 40–50 Gy to the pelvis, including the entire paracolpium, is indicated. Disease in the lower third of the vagina requires radiotherapy to the inguinal nodes.[15]

Radiotherapy for stage II disease

The primary tumour is treated with intracavitary and/or interstitial therapy to a dose of 45–55 Gy. Fletcher Suit applications can be utilized in patients with upper third lesions and the uterus in situ. External beam pelvic radiotherapy of 40–50 Gy is indicated in upper and middle third lesions. Inguinal node therapy is indicated in distal third lesions.

Radiotherapy for stage III/IVa disease

In cases with bulky tumours, external radiotherapy will cause tumour shrinkage, which can be followed by intracavitary and/or interstitial radiation to the primary tumour as indicated. The recommended total dose to the tumour is 75–80 Gy and 55–60 Gy to the pelvic side wall.[16]

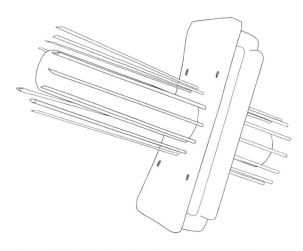

Figure 15.2 *Syed–Neblett applicator for interstitial radiation delivery.*

Radiotherapy for stage IVb disease

Palliative radiotherapy to the primary tumour to control bleeding and pain may be indicated; an individualized approach is necessary. Bony metastases benefit from local radiotherapy for pain control.

Radiotherapy complications

As the result of close proximity, the rectum, bladder and bowel are predisposed to radiation-induced side effects. Acute side effects include cystitis, proctitis, vaginitis, and desquamation of the vulvar and inguinal skin areas. Long-term side effects may present with fistula formation, rectal ulceration or stricture formation of the rectum and urethra. This can cause debilitating urinary and faecal incontinence. Vaginal stenosis subsequent to radiation-induced fibrosis will lead to dyspareunia. Radiation-induced side effects occur in 5–15 per cent of cases.[15]

SURGERY

The role of surgery in the management of vaginal carcinoma includes primary therapy, reconstructive procedures, secondary therapy in cases of recurrence and management of complications such as rectovaginal fistulae.

Primary surgery

Early lesions can be treated with wide local excision. Thus, a conservative surgical approach may be sufficient for lesions with a depth of invasion of less than 3 mm.[17] Surgical management of stage I lesions in the upper and middle third requires radical vaginectomy and pelvic node dissection. In the presence of a uterus, a radical hysterectomy is mandatory. Involvement of the distal third of the vagina is surgically treated by vaginectomy with concurrent vulvar excision and inguinal node dissection. In selected cases of stage II disease without parametrial involvement, a surgical approach is possible. Cases presenting with stage IVa disease without extensive parametrial involvement can be managed surgically with anterior, posterior or total exenteration. Exenteration offers a treatment option in cases of vaginal carcinoma after previous irradiation as well as in cases with recurrence of disease subsequent to primary radiotherapy.[18]

Complications of primary surgery

Complications of radical hysterectomy and radical vulvar surgery with groin dissection are well described. They include acute problems associated with anaesthesia and intraoperative complications.

Long-term sequelae such as lymphoedema, bladder and rectal dysfunction, as well as fistula formation, seriously impact on quality of life.[19] Radical vulvectomy and vaginectomy lead to special physical and psychosexual problems.[20]

Choice of primary treatment

In the absence of randomized trials comparing radiotherapy and surgery as primary treatment, a highly individualized approach in the management of patients is required. Adequate patient counselling before therapy results in improved compliance if complications occur. Based on the current literature, surgery in patients with stage I lesions confined to the upper third of the vagina includes radical hysterectomy and a partial vaginectomy with pelvic node dissection. In patients with lesions in the distal third of the vagina, the preferred surgical option is a vaginectomy with modified vulvectomy and groin node dissection. In selected patients with rectovaginal and vesicovaginal fistulae, primary pelvic exenteration offers a suitable treatment option. Exenteration remains the only curative treatment option in patients with central recurrence after radiotherapy. The role of groin node dissection is controversial. The distal third of the vagina drains to the inguinal nodes. In patients with vulvar carcinoma, primary radiotherapy to the groin nodes results in poor control.[21] Recurrence of a vulvar carcinoma in the undissected groin has a high mortality.[22] As the lymphatic drainage of the distal third of the vagina correlates with vulvar drainage, a strong case for groin node dissection as a diagnostic and a therapeutic procedure could be made in cases with carcinoma in the distal third. As a result of limited reported series in vaginal carcinoma, this approach remains controversial.

Both surgery and radiotherapy as primary treatment modalities are associated with complications. Surgical complications occur on a short-term basis whereas radiotherapy complications may appear over a period of time.

Stock and colleagues[23] report superior survival rates in patients with stage II disease treated with surgery in comparison to radiotherapy ($p = 0.00004$).[22] This is an isolated report, and bias in treatment selection may explain the superior results.

Surgery therefore has a limited role in the primary treatment of patients, and the majority should be managed with primary radiotherapy.

Survival

A combination of surgery and radiotherapy as treatment modalities has been reported in several series. Follow-up periods and survival figures vary (Table 15.2). The reported series include both squamous and adenocarcinomas. The outcomes of the larger series relate mainly to treatment with radiotherapy.

Reconstructive surgery

Radical surgery results in a significant or total loss of vaginal function. The same impairment may occur after vaginal fibrosis as a result of radiation. Vaginal reconstruction should form an integral part of the management of sexually active patients with vaginal carcinoma.

Preoperative counselling is of paramount importance in decision-making regarding vaginal reconstruction and should include specific counselling for psychosexual dysfunction, which may require additional attention. Grafts used in vaginal reconstruction procedures include skin grafts, myocutaneous grafts and intestinal grafts.

SKIN GRAFTS

For the new reconstruction of a vagina, full-thickness or split-thickness grafts may be used. Harvesting sites include the buttock, anterior thigh and medial thigh. The split-thickness skin graft is placed over a suitable stent, e.g. Heyer–Schulte, and inserted into the void space left after vaginectomy. In cases of exenteration, omental mobilization on the gastroepiploic arteries allows for an omental pocket to be created for the new vagina.[44]

MYOCUTANEOUS GRAFTS

The most frequently used myocutaneous grafts include gracilis myocutaneous and rectus abdominis grafts. The rectus abdominis myocutaneous graft is harvested from the ventral abdominal wall. The upper abdominal part of the muscle is supplied by the superior epigastric artery. The inferior epigastric artery supplies the distal part of the muscle and serves as a vascular pedicle for the graft. A myocutaneous graft is created by mobilizing the skin and underlying fascia after appropriate skin incisions. Incision of the skin is followed by incision of the underlying rectus sheath, by transecting the muscle at the costal level and ligat-

ing the superior epigastric artery. The entire myocutaneous graft can be lifted from the posterior rectus sheath by serial ligation of the segmental perforating neurovascular pedicles. The vaginal pouch is fashioned by inversion of the skin, which is transferred to the pelvis and sutured to the perineum. The procedure introduces bulk into the pelvis which is of particular value in cases of exenteration. Filling the residual pelvic space excludes bowel from the pelvis. The graft provides neovascularization in a previously irradiated pelvis (Fig. 15.3).[45]

The gracilis muscle located at the medial aspect of the thigh serves as an alternative option. The medial femoral circumflex artery supplies the muscle with cutaneous perforators supplying the overlying skin. The anterior aspect of the muscle is identified by surface markers, consisting of a line between the medial epicondyle and the pubic tubercle. Skin incision over the anterior aspect of the muscle is followed by appropriate skin incisions to harvest a graft of approximately 6 × 12 cm. After transecting the muscle insertion, the graft is mobilized from the underlying tissue. The proximal vascular pedicle should be preserved. Broad subcutaneous tunnels are created over the muscular origin below the labia majora. The grafts are passed through these tunnels. The two grafts are sutured to create a neovaginal pouch that is introduced into the pelvis. Suspension of the cranial end of the new vagina to the sacrum prevents prolapse[46,47] (Fig. 15.4).

INTESTINAL SEGMENTS

Small bowel and colon segments transposed on mesenteric vascular supplies can serve as a basis for vaginal reconstruction.[48] The rectosigmoid area has a dual vascular supply from the inferior mesenteric artery and the superior haemorrhoidal artery. The marginal artery of Drummond supplies the descending colon. Mobilizing the rectosigmoid on the inferior mesenteric artery allows for the identification of an appropriate segment of colon. Transillumination of the bowel mesentery makes identification of mesenteric vascular structures possible. The proximal and distal blood supply to the colon segment should be temporarily occluded to ascertain whether the selected arterial supply is sufficient to support the segment. The bowel is transected proximally and distally, and the vascularized colon segment can be introduced into the pelvis and sutured to the introitus. The mobility of the colon to reach the introitus should be assessed

Table 15.2 *Vaginal carcinoma: stage distribution and survival rate*

Reference	Stage I Number	Stage I Survival rate (%)	Stage II Number	Stage II Survival rate (%)	Stage III Number	Stage III Survival rate (%)	Stage IV Number	Stage IV Survival rate (%)	Follow-up (years)
Prempree et al.[24]	6	83	20/11	65/64[a]	20	40	7	0	5
Pride et al.[25]	9	66	6/16[a]	66/31[a]	4	25	8	0	5
Al-Kurdi and Monaghan[11]	14	71	34	29	8	25	9	22	5
Ball and Berman[26]	27	76	18	37	6	17	5	0	5
Prempree et al.[27]	9	88	23/14[a]	78/50[a]	26	42	8	0	5
Benedet et al.[28]	32	75	31	68	16	42	18	21	2
Puthavala et al.[14]	1	100	7/9[a]	86/67[a]	9	22	1	0	4
Rubin et al.[29]	14	75	35	48	14	54	12	0	5
MacNaught et al.[30]	14	68	22	34	18	29	7	14	5
Shimm and Ropar[31]	4	71	7	29	6	48	5	52	5
Gallup et al.[32]	4	100	12	75	4	0	8	25	2
Reddy et al.[33]	8	100	18	72	5	0	1	0	2
Perez et al.[15]	50	75	49/26[a]	55/43[a]	16	32	8	0	5
Andersen[16]	12	58	7	43	6	30	4	0	5
Spirtos et al.[34]	18	94	5	80	10	50	5	0	3
Manetta et al.[35]	19	87	20	70	7	71	7	17	2
Davis et al.[36]	44	88	45	53	15	53	11	25	4
Eddy et al.[37]	25	73	39	39	15	39			<2
Kucera and Vavra[38]	73	77	110	45	174	31	77	18	5
Dixit et al.[39]	8	100	10	70	42	19	10	0	2
Leminen et al.[40]	21	47	10	50	4	25	8	0	5
Stock et al.[23]	23	67	58	53	9	0	10	15	11
Ali et al.[41]	13	53	21	22	3	0	3	37	5
Chyle et al.[42]	65	49	122	38	60	29	17	23	13
Urbanski et al.[43]	33	73	37	54	40	23	15	0	5

[a] Subdivision into stage IIa and IIb.

before division of vascular structures. An adequate portion of colon can be obtained by mobilizing the descending colon up to the splenic flexure. The colon is transected at the splenic flexure, and the descending part is further mobilized to isolate the mesenteric pedicle, consisting of the inferior mesenteric artery and veins. The distal end of the colon is transected at the rectum. The graft thus created is rotated through 180°. The splenic flexure of the colon is therefore rotated into the pelvis with adequate length to reach the introitus. The colon is sutured to the introitus to form the neovagina. To prevent prolapse, the mobilized segment is fixed to the sacrum)[49] (Fig. 15.5).

SMALL BOWEL

A neovagina can also be created using small bowel. A segment of small bowel with at least two vascular arcades is isolated by transection of the bowel. The vascularized small bowel segment should be in close proximity to the ileocolic junction. The anti-mesenteric aspect of the isolated small bowel segment is incised, and a pouch is created by suturing opposing bowel edges together. The pouch thus created serves as a neovagina and is introduced into the pelvis and sutured to the introitus[50] (Fig. 15.6).

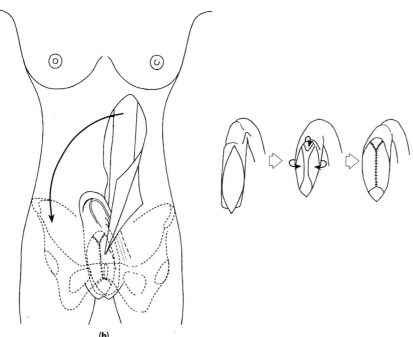

(a)

(b)

Figure 15.3 (a) Preparing rectus abdominis myocutaneous graft. (b) Placing rectus abdominis graft in the pelvis.

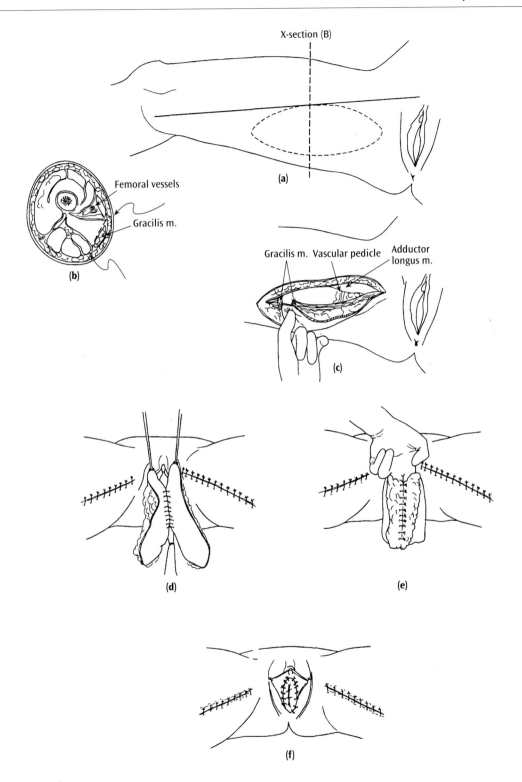

Figure 15.4 *(a–e) Preparing gracilis myocutaneous graft. (f) Placing gracilis myocutaneous graft.*

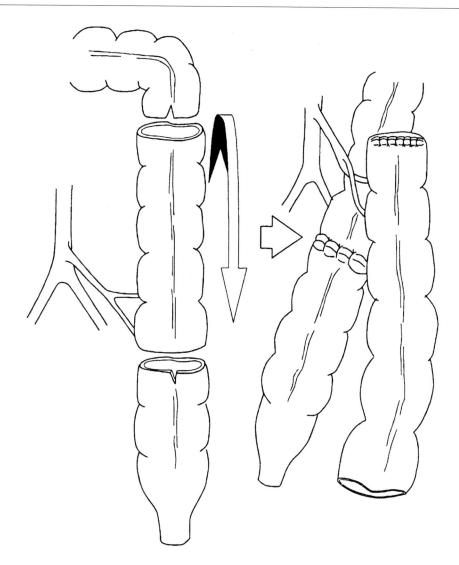

Figure 15.5 *Vaginal reconstruction using a colon segment.*

COMPLICATIONS OF RECONSTRUCTIVE PROCEDURES

Immediate complications attributable to reconstructive procedures include primary embolism, necrosis of the myocutaneous graft and infection. The long-term sequelae include vault contraction.[46–48] The regular use of dilators in selected cases may avoid this. Prolapse of the neovagina can be prevented by securing the neovagina to the sacrum during the initial procedure. The complication of mucus discharge occurs when intestinal grafts are employed in the reconstruction. Small bowel grafts are associated with a worse degree of discharge than colonic grafts and may also be associated with periumbilical pain during coitus.[50] After

bowel reconnection, patients should be monitored for leaks and breakdown of the anastomosis in the postoperative period. Long-term psychosexual consequences after vaginal reconstruction are well described.[51,52] Despite an anatomically functional result, psychosexual dysfunction may develop. Psychological distress is further aggravated should physical complications, such as contracture of the neovagina, occur. In a prospective study of 44 patients, Ratliff and colleagues[53] assessed sexual adjustment subsequent to exenteration and myocutaneous vaginal reconstruction. Despite the presence of a functional vagina in 70.4 per cent of cases, as assessed by the attending medical practitioner, only 19 of 44 patients (43 per cent) resumed sexual activity. This means that in spite

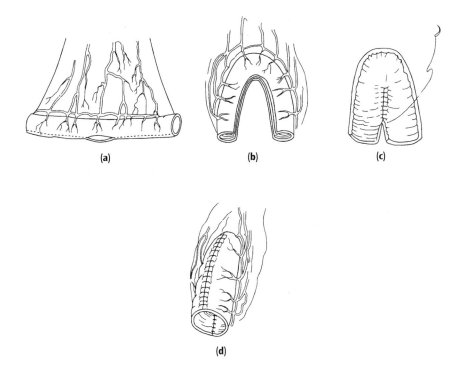

Figure 15.6 *(a–d) Vaginal reconstruction using small bowel.*

of anatomically satisfactory results, psychosexual dysfunction after reconstruction may lead to abstinence in a significant number of cases. It is clearly important that realistic preoperative patient counselling with postoperative psychological support is required. Counselling about sexual adjustment postoperatively should address the realistic problems of self-conciousness as a result of urostomy and colostomy. Vaginal dryness and vaginal discharge should be appropriately managed.

Recurrence

Over a 5- to 15-year period, a recurrence rate of 23–26 per cent has been reported.[36] Surgery offers the only curative treatment modality in patients with recurrence after irradiation. Patient selection for exenteration surgery is based on well-described criteria.[39]

NON-SQUAMOUS CARCINOMAS

Adenocarcinoma

Primary adenocarcinoma of the vagina affects predominantly younger patients. In the presence of histologically proven adenocarcinoma, the possibility of metastatic disease should be contemplated. Exclusion of a primary gastrointestinal, breast, ovarian and endometrial carcinoma should be done utilizing appropriate examinations, e.g. gastroscopy, colonoscopy and endometrial biopsy. Primary adenocarcinoma can arise in the periurethral glands and possibly in wolffian remnants. Areas of vaginal adenosis, particularly associated with *in utero* diethylstilboestrol (DES) exposure, can give rise to adenocarcinoma. Herbst and Sculley[54] documented the transplacental effect of DES on women. A subsequent retrospective epidemiological study revealed DES exposure in the first trimester in seven of eight mothers of afflicted women. A registry for research on hormonal transplacental carcinogenesis was established in 1971.[55] DES acts as a teratogen and is not a carcinogen. Vaginal adenosis is reported in 45 per cent of patients after

DES exposure *in utero* and 25 per cent of patients have structural abnormalities of the genital tract. The risk of clear-cell carcinoma in exposed individuals is 1:1000. The highest risk exists if hormone exposure occurred before 12 weeks. DES-associated clear-cell adenocarcinoma is predominantly seen in young patients with a peak incidence at the age of 19.[56] This type of carcinoma rarely occurs beyond 30 years of age. Patients identified with *in utero* exposure to DES should be assessed at menarche. Careful evaluation of the areas of adenosis by palpation and cytological smears is indicated. The patient's genital tract should also be assessed for concurrent structural abnormalities. Clear-cell adenocarcinomas arise commonly in the anterior vaginal wall and most are at an early stage. Herbst and colleagues reported stages to be as follows: stage I = 59 per cent, stage II = 33 per cent, stage III = 7 per cent and stage IV = 1 per cent.[57] Vaginal adenosis undergoes metaplasia to be replaced by squamous epithelium. DES-exposed women have an unexplained increased incidence of CIN and VaIN, so appropriate cytology is indicated. Clear-cell adenocarcinoma of the vagina unrelated to prenatal DES exposure accounts for 20 per cent of cases in reported series. A bimodal age distribution occurs with a peak at a young age (26 years) and another peak at a mean age of 71 years.[58]

Diethylstilboestrol-exposed clear-cell adenocarcinoma has a significantly better prognosis than carcinomas with no DES exposure.

Positive pelvic node involvement occurred in 1.2 per cent of DES-exposed patients, compared with 8.6 per cent in cases not exposed to DES ($p = 0.0041$). The probability of survival at 5 and 10 years for DES-exposed cases was 84 per cent and 78 per cent, respectively, compared with 69 per cent and 60 per cent, respectively, in cases not exposed to DES (5 years, $p = 0.0007$ and 10 years, $p = 0.0008$).[59]

A particularly high incidence of nodal spread occurs even in stage I clear-cell adenocarcinoma. Reported figures of nodal involvement of stages I and II are 16 per cent and 30 per cent, respectively. When managing these cases, cognizance of the patient's age should be taken in the planning of treatment. Upper vaginal, early stage disease is treated with radical hysterectomy, vaginectomy and lymph node dissection, with concurrent vaginal reconstruction. Less radical treatment consists of wide local excision and lymph node dissection and, in selected cases, radiotherapy may be employed. Preservation of vaginal and ovarian function should be considered. If primary radiother-

apy treatment is employed, pre-treatment laparotomy with ovarian transposition may be indicated. The role of pre-treatment lymph node dissection in advanced disease may yield prognostic factors. The survival rate in stage I disease is reported to be 90 per cent. Five-year survival rates for stages II, III and IV disease are, respectively, 76 per cent, 30 per cent and 0 per cent. Distant recurrence involving the lungs and supraclavicular nodes has a tendency to occur late.[57]

Verrucous carcinoma

These tumours are rare and present as large exophytic tumours. They are locally aggressive and lymph nodes metastases are rare. Histologically, the appearance of the tumour has an infiltrating border. Surgical excision of the tumour is the basis of treatment.

Most authors are of the opinion that radiotherapy induces anaplastic transformation of verrucous carcinoma. Reinecke and colleagues[60] challenged this opinion when reviewing 16 cases of verrucous carcinoma of the vagina and concluded that radiotherapy could be utilized.

Melanoma

Melanomas of the vulva and vagina comprise less than 2 per cent of melanomas in women. Surgery remains the primary treatment modality and staging incorporates the criteria of Breslow and Clarke. Adverse prognostic factors include advanced age at diagnosis, capillary–lymphatic space involvement, high mitotic count and aneuploidy. Patients with vaginal melanoma have a 15–19 per cent chance of 5-year survival.[61–63]

Embryonal rhabdomyosarcoma

This tumour occurs in infancy. Treatment should aim to preserve rectal and bladder function. Preoperative chemotherapy and radiotherapy will cause tumour shrinkage and even complete remission, with less reliance on radical surgery. A survival rate of 30 per cent is reported.[64]

Endodermal sinus tumours

This carcinoma occurs in infants with an average age of 3 years. Combination therapy with primary chemotherapy, followed by surgery and/or radiotherapy, is the treatment of choice.[65]

REFERENCES

1 DiSaia PJ, Creaseman WT. Invasive cancer of the vagina and urethra. In: DiSaia JP, Creaseman WT (eds). *Clinical gynecologic oncology*. St Louis, MI: CV Mosby, 1959: 273–91.

2 Noller KL. Screening for vaginal cancer. *N Engl J Med* 1996; **21**: 1559–62.

3 Plentl AA, Friedman EA. *Lymphatic system of the female genitalia*. Philadelphia: WB Saunders, 1971.

4 Brinton LA, Nasca PC, Mallin K. Case control study of in situ and invasive carcinoma of the vagina. *Gynecol Oncol* 1990; **38**: 49–54.

5 Hildesheim A, Han C, Brinton LA et al. Sexually transmitted agents and risk of carcinoma of the vagina. *Int J Gynecol Cancer* 1997; **7**: 251–5.

6 Perez CA, Arneson AN, Galaktos A, Samouth HK. Management of tumours of the vagina. *Cancer* 1973; **31**: 36.

7 Ireland D, Monaghan JM. The management of the patient with abnormal vaginal cytology following hysterectomy. *Br J Obstet Gynaecol* 1988; **95**: 973.

8 Lenehan PM, Meffe F, Lickrish GM. Vaginal intraepithelial neoplasia: biological aspects and management. *Obstet Gynecol* 1986; **66**: 333–5.

9 Nwabeni NJ, Monaghan JM. Vaginal epithelial abnormalities in patients with CIN: clinical and pathological features and management. *Br J Obstet Gynaecol* 1991; **98**: 25.

10 Aho M, Vestermen E, Meyer B. Natural history of vaginal intraepithelial neoplasia. *Cancer* 1991; **68**: 195.

11 Al-Kurdi M, Monaghan JM. Thirty-two years experience in management of primary tumours of the vagina. *Br J Obstet Gynaecol* 1981; **88**: 1145–50.

12 Manetta A, Pinto JL, Larson JE. Primary invasive carcinoma of the vagina. *Obstet Gynecol* 1988; **72**: 77–81.

13 Petterson F. *Annual report of the results of treatment in gynaecological cancer*, Vol 22. Stockholm, Sweden: FIGO. 1994; 46–7.

14 Puthavala A, Syed AMN, Nalick R. Integrated external and interstitial radiotherapy for primary carcinoma of the vagina. *Obstet Gynecol* 1983; **62**: 367–72.

15 Perez CA, Camel HM, Galakatos AE. Definitive irradiation in carcinoma of the vagina: long-term evaluation of results. *Int J Radiat Oncol Biol Phys* 1988; **15**: 1283–90.

16 Andersen ES. Primary carcinoma of the vagina. A study of 29 cases. *Gynecol Oncol* 1989; **33**: 317–20.

17 Peters WA, Kuma MB, Morley GW. Microinvasive carcinoma of the vagina. A distinct clinical entity? *Am J Obstet Gynecol* 1985; **153**: 505–7.

18 Lindeque BG. The role of surgery in the management of carcinoma of the vagina. *Baillieres Clin Obstet Gynaecol* 1987; **1**: 319–29.

19 Shingleton HM, Orr JW Jr. Primary surgical treatment of invasive cancer. In: Shingleton HM, Orr JW Jr eds. *Cancer of the cervix*. Philadelphia: JP Lippincott, 1995: 123–54.

20 Helm CW, Shingleton HM. The management of squamous cell carcinoma of the vulva. *Curr Obstet Gynecol* 1992; **2**: 31–7.

21 Stehman FB, Bundy BN, Bell J et al. Groin dissection versus groin radiation in carcinoma of the vulva: A Gynaecological Oncology Group study. *Int J Radiat Oncol Biol Phys* 1992; **24**: 389.

22 Stehman FB, Bundy BN, Droretsky PH, Creasman WT. Early stage I carcinoma of the vulva treated with bilateral inguinal lymphadenectomy and modified radical hemivulvectomy: A prospective study of the Gynecologic Oncology Group. *Obstet Gynecol* 1992; **79**: 490.

23 Stock RG, Chen AS, Seski J. A 30-year experience in the management of primary carcinoma of the vagina: analysis of prognostic factors and treatment modalities. *Gynecol Oncol* 1995; **56**: 45–52.

24 Prempree T, Viravathana T, Slawson RG, Wizenberg NJ, Cuccia CA. Radiation management of primary carcinoma of the vagina. *Cancer* 1977; **40**: 109.

25 Pride GL, Schultz AE, Chuprevich TW, Buchler DA. Primary invasive carcinoma of the vagina. *Obstet Gynecol* 1979; **53**: 218.

26 Ball HG, Berman ML. Management of primary vaginal carcinoma. *Gynecol Oncol* 1982; **14**: 154–63.

27 Prempree T, Viravathana T, Slawson RG. Role of radiation therapy in management of primary carcinoma of the vagina. *Acta Radiat Oncol* 1982; **21**: 195–201.

28 Benedet JL, Murphy KJ, Fairey RN, Booyes DA. Primary invasive carcinoma of the vagina. *Obstet Gynaecol* 1983; **62**: 715–19.

29 Rubin SC, Young J, Mikuta JJ. Squamous carcinoma of the vagina. *Gynecol Oncol* 1985; **20**: 346–53.

30 MacNaught R, Symonds RP, Hole D, Watson ER. Improved control of primary vaginal tumours by combined external beam and interstitial radiotherapy. *Clin Radiol* 1986; **37**: 29–32.

31 Shimm DS, Ropar RM. Radiation therapy of carcinoma of the vagina. *Acta Obstet Gynecol Scand* 1986; **65**: 449–52.

32 Gallup DJ, Talledo OE, Shah KJ, Hayes C. Invasive squamous cell carcinoma of the vagina. *Obstet Gynecol* 1987; **69**: 782–5.

33 Reddy S, Lee MS, Graham JE et al. Radiation therapy in primary carcinoma of the vagina. *Gynecol Oncol* 1987; **26**: 19–24.

34 Spirtos NM, Doshi BP, Kapp DS, Teng N. Radiation therapy for primary squamous cell carcinoma of the vagina: Stanford University experience. *Gynecol Oncol* 1989; **35**: 20–6.

35 Manetta A, Gutrecht EL, Berman ML. Primary invasive carcinoma of the vagina. *Obstet Gynecol* 1990; **76**: 639–42.

36 Davis KP, Stanhope CR, Garton GR. Invasive vaginal carcinoma: analysis of early-stage disease. *Gynecol Oncol* 1991; **42**: 131–6.

37 Eddy GL, Marks RD, Miller MC, Underwood PB. Primary invasive vaginal carcinoma. *Am J Obstet Gynecol* 1991; **165**: 292–8.

38 Kucera H, Vavra N. Radiation management of primary carcinoma of the vagina: clinical and histopathological variables associated with survival. *Gynecol Oncol* 1991; **40**: 12–16.

39 Dixit S, Singhal S, Baboo HA. Squamous cell carcinoma of the vagina: a review of 70 cases. *Gynecol Oncol* 1993; **48**: 80–7.

40 Leminen A, Forss SM, Lehtovirta P. Therapeutic and prognostic considerations in primary carcinoma of the vagina. *Acta Obstet Gynecol Scand* 1995; **74**: 379–83.

41 Ali MM, Huang DT, Gopelrud DR, Howess R, Lu JD. Radiation alone for carcinoma of the vagina. Variation and response related to the location of the tumor. *Cancer* 1996; **77**: 1934–9.

42 Chyle V, Zagars GK, Wheeler JA, Wharton JT, Delclos L. Definitive radiotherapy of carcinoma of the vagina: outcome and prognostic factors. *Int J Radiat Oncol Biol Phys* 1996; **35**: 891–905.

43 Urbanski K, Kojs Z, Reinfuss M, Fabisiak W. Primary invasive vagina carcinoma treated with radiotherapy: analysis of prognostic factors. *Gynecol Oncol* 1996; **60**: 16–21.

44 Kusiak JA, Rosenblum NG. Neovaginal reconstruction after exenteration using an omental flap and split thickness skin graft. *Plast Reconstr Surg* 1996; **97**: 775–81.

45 Tobin GR. Pelvic, vaginal and perineal reconstruction in pelvic surgery. *Surg Oncol Clin North Am* 1994; **3**: 397–412.

46 Berek JS, Hacker NF, Lagasse LD. Vaginal reconstruction performed simultaneously with pelvic exenteration. *Obstet Gynecol* 1984; **63**: 318–23.

47 Copeland LJ, Hancock KC, Gershenson DM, Stringer CA, Atkinson EN, Edwards CL. Gracilis myocutaneous vaginal reconstruction concurrent with total pelvic exenteration. *Am J Obstet Gynecol* 1989; **116**: 1095–101.

48 Goligher JC. The use of the pedicled transplant of sigmoid or other parts of the intestinal tract for vaginal construction. *Ann R Coll Surg* 1983; **65**: 353–5.

49 Pratt JH, Smith GR. Vaginal reconstruction with a sigmoid loop. *Am J Obstet Gynecol* 1966; **96**: 31–40.

50 Baldwin JF. The formation of an artificial vagina by intestinal transplantation. *Ann Surg* 1904; **40**: 398.

51 Gleeson N, Bailey W, Roberts WS et al. Surgical and psychological outcome following vaginal reconstruction with pelvic exenteration. *Eur J Gynaecol Oncol* 1994; **15**: 89–95.

52 Morley GW, Lindenauer SM, Young SD. Vaginal reconstruction following pelvic exenteration: surgical and psychological considerations. *Am J Obstet Gynecol* 1973; **116**: 996–1002.

53 Ratliff CR, Gershenson DM, Morris M et al. Sexual adjustment of patients undergoing gracilis myocutaneous flap vaginal reconstruction in conjunction with pelvic exenteration. *Cancer* 1996; **78**: 2229–35.

54 Herbst HZ, Sculley RE. Adenocarcinoma of the vagina in adolescense. *Cancer* 1970; **25**: 745.

55 Robboy SJ, Herbst HL, Sculley RE. Clear cell adenocarcinoma of the vagina and cervix in young females: Analysis of 37 tumours that persisted or recurred after primary therapy. *Cancer* 1974; **34**: 606–14.

56 Melnick S, Cole P, Anderson D, Herbst AL. Rates and risks of diethylstilbestrol-related clear cell adenocarcinoma of the vagina and cervix. *N Engl J Med* 1987; **316**: 514–16.

57 Herbst AL, Norussis MJ, Rossouw PJ et al. An analysis of 346 cases of clear cell adenocarcinoma of the vagina and cervix with emphasis on recurrence and survival. *Gynecol Oncol* 1979; **7**: 111–22.

58 Hanselaar A, van Loosbroek M, Schuurbiers O, Helmerhorst T, Bulten J, Bernhelm J. Clear cell adenocarcinoma of the vagina and cervix. An update of the central Netherlands registry showing twin age incidence peaks. *Cancer* 1997; **79**: 2229–36.

59 Waggoner SE, Mitterndorf R, Biney N, Anderson D, Herbst AL. Influence of in-utero diethylstilbestrol exposure on the prognosis and biological behaviour of

clear cell adenocarcinoma. *Gynecol Oncol* 1994; **55**: 238–44.

60 Reinecke L, Thonley AL. Case report: Radiotherapy – an effective treatment for vaginal verrucous carcinoma. *Br J Radiol* 1993; **66**: 375–8.

61 Giesler JP, Look KY, Moore DA, Sutton GP. Pelvic exenteration for malignant melanomas of the vagina or urethra with over 3 mm of invasion. *Gynecol Oncol* 1995; **59**: 338–41.

62 Weinstock MA. Malignant melanoma of the vulva and vagina in the United States: Patterns of incidence and population-based estimates of survival. *Am J Obstet Gynecol* 1994; **171**: 1225–30.

63 Trimble EL. Melanomas of the vulva and vagina. *Oncology (Huntingt)* 1996; **10**: 1017–23.

64 Chavimi F, Herr H, Exelby PR. Treatment of genitourinary rhabdomyosarcoma in children. *J Oncol* 1984; 132–313.

65 Leverger G, Flamant F, Gerbaulet A. Tumours of vitelline sac located in the vagina in children. *Arch F Pediatr* 1983; **40**: 85.

Sexuality and quality of life for women with vulvar cancer

BL ANDERSEN

Sexuality is the major life area most vulnerable to quality of life morbidity for the sexually active survivor of gynaecological cancer. Difficulties often begin with the signs/symptoms of the disease and continue, although with a different clinical picture, as the attempt is made to resume sexual activity after treatment. For some, the genital changes are too difficult to overcome or the emotional sequelae so disruptive that all sexual activity – individual and partner shared – ceases. Far from being a limited source of difficulty, other data suggest that sexual difficulties of this sort have a 'ripple effect', with women feeling negative about their self-confidence, their sexual self-esteem, and their view of themselves as women. Whether or not women have sexual relationships with partners, the latter problems are important for all women,[1] but these problems can be especially traumatic for the woman treated for vulvar cancer.

Although the focus of this discussion is sexual morbidity, it is considered within the context of other aspects of life. Sexuality is affected by other life areas, such as mood and interpersonal adjustment, among others. But it is important to note that, when data on major life areas (e.g. mood, marital adjustment, social adjustment, employment status) have been obtained

from women with gynaecological cancer, sexual functioning is the life area with the most severe and long-lasting morbidity. The importance of sexuality for the individual woman may vary and some who are not sexually active, for example, may be less concerned about permanent disruption, although this is not uniformly the case. If women are asked about the availability of information on sexual outcomes, the need for assistance in managing sexual difficulties or related topics, their importance is frequently noted by vulvar cancer patients.[2–4] In combination, these factors urge special consideration of issues of sexuality.

CENTRAL ASPECTS OF FEMALE SEXUALITY

Sexual self-concept (sexual self-schema)

Perhaps the most important aspect of one's sexuality is the aspect that is rarely considered, namely, one's own personal view of the sexual self. A person has many self-views, for example 'I am intelligent, kind, hardworking, a good mother, etc.'. However, how does a woman view herself as a sexual person? Would she describe herself as arousable, loving, open or uninhibited, or would words such as nervous, tense, prudent or conservative be more descriptive?

Our research indicates that there are individual differences among women in their view of themselves as sexual people. This personal view of one's sexuality 'sexual self-view or sexual schema' has been defined as one's cognitions or thoughts about sexual aspects of the self.[5] A woman's view of her sexuality is derived from her past sexual experiences and her current experiences, and it appears to be an important determinant for her future sexuality, i.e. a woman is guided in the processing and interpreting of sexually relevant information, and it guides her future sexual behaviour.

Although more than the sum of the parts, a woman's view of herself as a sexual person includes two positive aspects – an inclination to experience romantic/passionate emotions and a behavioural openness to sexual experience – and one negative one – embarrassment or conservatism, which may be a deterrent to sexual/romantic feelings and sexual activity. Women who differ in their views of their own sexuality 'positive versus negative self-views' evidence very different sexual selves. Women with a positive sexual schema view themselves as emotionally romantic or passionate, and as women who are behaviourally open to romantic and sexual relationships and experiences. These women tend to be liberal in their sexual attitudes, and are generally free of self-consciousness or embarrassment when they are in a sexual situation. Positive schema women, for example, tend to evaluate various sexual behaviours more positively, report higher levels of arousability across sexual experiences, and are more willing to engage in sexual relationships. These positive schema women also anticipate a more active and fulfilling future sexual life.

Conversely, women holding negative self-views of their sexuality tend to describe themselves as emotionally cold or unromantic and, by their own admission, they are behaviourally inhibited in their sexual and romantic relationships. These women tend to espouse conservative and, at times, negative attitudes and values about sexual matters, and may describe themselves as self-conscious, embarrassed or not confident in a variety of social and sexual contexts. Finally, there may be some potential vulnerability for negative women because their self-view can be significantly moderated by external circumstances (e.g. their sexual self-esteem waivers when a sexual relationship ends), whereas this does not appear to be the case for the positively schematic women.

Many have noted that, in addition to the disruption in sexual activity (usually intercourse) that may occur for vulvar treatments, women often report declines in feeling attractive[6] or in their self-view.[7] It would appear that women with initially positive views of their sexuality would be more resilient to the disruptive effects of gynaecological cancer and/or better able to cope with sexual difficulties than women whose sexual self-view is negative.

Data indicate that these important self-views do, indeed, predict sexual morbidity for gynaecological cancer survivors.[8] We tested the schema construct with a cancer sample in the prediction of two different sexual outcomes 'sexual responsiveness' (e.g. desire, excitement, orgasm and resolution) and sexual behaviour. Forty women previously treated for gynaecological disease participated. A marker of pre-treatment sexuality (frequency of intercourse), extent of disease/treatment and menopausal symptomatology were selected for control in the analyses, in view of their general relevance to sexuality and their proposed relevance to predicting outcomes for cancer survivors.[9] Of note in the control analyses was the contribution of the extent of disease/treatment, analysed with a contrast of women receiving 'limited' (e.g. modified radical vulvectomy) versus 'extensive' surgery (e.g. radical vulvectomy). In the prediction of sexual behaviour after treatment, extent of disease/treatment accounted for 9 per cent of the total variance, but only 3 per cent of the variance in the prediction of sexual responsiveness, such as sexual arousal. More importantly, sexual self-schema accounted for a significant and much larger portion of the variance in the prediction of both outcomes. Schema accounted for a significant 6 per cent of the variance in the prediction of sexual behaviour; with the additional control variables, 48 per cent of the total variance was accounted for. Schema accounted for 28 per cent in the prediction of current sexual responsiveness; with the other components of the model, 42 per cent of the total variance was accounted for. These data indicate that although extent of disease and surgical treatment will be important predictors of sexual morbidity for women with gynaecological cancer, a woman's sense of her sexuality – 'her sexual-self-schema' – is a more important determinant.

Sexual behaviour

Partnered sexual behaviour among heterosexual females falls within the following groupings: preliminary foreplay (e.g. kissing, embracing, undressing), intimate foreplay (e.g. manual/oral genital stimulation), intercourse, anal stimulation and masturbation. Such a broad view of sexual behaviour is rarely assessed; instead, a report of intercourse is documented. If such an assessment is attempted, rather than obtain judgements of an 'increase', 'decrease' or 'no change' in intercourse frequency, a more reliable strategy is to obtain an estimate of intercourse frequency (e.g. times per week or per month), even though validated behavioural inventories are available.[10]

Sexual response cycle and sexual dysfunctions

In addition to changes in behaviour, it is important to consider that the disruption of sexual responses (desire, excitement, orgasm and resolution) and the occurrence of specific sexual dysfunctions (sexual aversion, vaginismus and dyspareunia) can appear after treatment for gynaecological cancer. In Table 16.1, we provide the clinical characteristics of such difficulties. It is important to understand the broad impact that the vulvar disease/treatments may have on sexuality, rather than focusing only on disruption of specific activities, such as intercourse.

REVIEW OF THE LITERATURE

Despite the morbidity of vulvar surgery, attention to the sexual or psychological outcomes for women is recent, with the first substantive reports not appearing until 1983. As with pelvic exenteration, vulvar treatments can have a dramatic impact on sexuality as well as other life areas. Following early observations on the benefits of conservative therapy,[16] individualized approaches for the treatment of the vulva have been advocated (see Chapter 9), and comparison of conservative procedures with radical ones can indicate significant reductions in operative morbidity with no compromise in survival.[17]

Vulvar intraepithelial neoplasia

Andersen and colleagues[2] provided data on the sexual outcomes for women treated with wide local excision and related treatments for in situ disease. Patients with in situ disease are more likely be sexually inactive at follow-up, whether or not they have available sexual partners, than age-matched healthy counterparts. However, if the women have a sexual relationship, the rates of sexual dysfunction appear to be only slightly higher than those for healthy women. Additional analyses contrasting treatment methods (e.g. surgery

Table 16.1 *Summary of retrospective studies of sexual outcome (percentage of sample with significant sexual behaviour changes or sexual difficulties) following in situ or invasive vulvar cancer*

| Disease type/ Reference | Country | Year | No. | Sexual behaviour | | Sexual dysfunction | | | |
				Not active (%)	Decreased frequency (%)	Desire (%)	Excitement (%)	Orgasm (%)	Dyspareunia
In situ									
Andersen[10]	USA	1988	42	33	–	15	36	28	8
BL Andersen			42[a]			(21)	(12)	(10)	(0)
(unpublished)	USA		127	46	–	35	14	17	0
			57[a]			(27)	(12)	(10)	(0)
Invasive									
Andersen[11]	USA	1983	15	60	100	–	–	–	–
Stellman[12]	USA	1984	9	100	100	–	–	–	–
Corney[7]	UK	1993	9	44	–	–	–	–	–
Moth[4]	Denmark	1983	15	47	–	70	62	67	70
Andeasson[13]	Denmark	1986	25	40	–	68	63	57	41
Weijmar Schultz[14]	Netherlands	1986	10	30	30	–	–	44	–
Tamburini[15]	Italy	1986	21	52	76	–	–	–	–

[a] Denotes inclusion of data for age-matched comparison group of healthy women.

versus laser versus combined treatment) found no significant differences; however, this may be the result of the small sample sizes in the subgroup comparison.

Invasive disease

The outcomes above contrast markedly with those for women with invasive disease, many of whom are treated with radical vulvectomy, with or without groin dissection. Although these reports are limited by their small sample sizes (ranging from 9 to 25), and they are primarily retrospective evaluations, the trends are consistent: at least 30–50 per cent of patients become sexually inactive and, of the women remaining active, 60–70 per cent have multiple sexual dysfunctions. For the women who become sexually inactive, reasons have included negative feelings (by the woman or her partner) about the physical changes to her body, and for others it may be caused by severe dyspareunia, such as may occur with a narrowed introitus. Rather than being resigned to an end to their sexual life, most women would have preferred to remain sexually active.[11]

The data in Table 16.1 summarize the difficult sexual sequelae from vulvar cancer and reveal the consistency in the international literature. The shift to lesser surgical therapies may improve these outcomes, although confirmatory data will need to be gathered. Some have suggested that outcomes such as these are less problematic because, as a group, women with vulvar cancer are older, often in their 60s, 70s or 80s, and they may already have stopped sexual activity. There is a natural decline in the frequency of sexual behaviour with age for women and men alike, but the presence of a healthy and interested partner, rather than one's age, is more important to the maintenance of sexual activity. Thus, the data do not suggest that these women will be either less distressed by their genital distortion and sexual dysfunctions or content to have their sexual life end.

The single prospective study is that concerning the outcomes for 10 women treated for vulvar cancer.[18] There was a 77 per cent participation rate; however, 2-year follow-up data are only available for 70 per cent ($n = 7$) of the participants. In addition to the pretreatment assessment, follow-ups were conducted 6, 12 and 24 months post-treatment. A comparison group of 24 healthy women was assessed on one occasion. There were reductions in the frequency of sexual behaviour and disruption of sexual desire and arousal

at 6 months, but with some improvement by 12 months, and the gains remained stable over the next 12 months. All women remained sexually active despite a 50 per cent increase in negative sensations during sexual arousal. These results are more favourable than the outcomes reported in the retrospective studies of vulvectomy patients, and may be the result of the selected samples participating in each (i.e. more dysfunctional patients in the retrospective studies and more 'adjusted' patients continuing in this prospective report).

SEXUALITY IN THE QUALITY OF LIFE CONTEXT FOR THE SURVIVOR

Despite the emotional trauma of a cancer diagnosis and the ensuing difficult treatments, the majority of individuals cope and resume their life patterns if they remain disease free.[19–21] A caveat to this generally positive prognosis for cancer survivors is the occurrence of 'islands' of life disruption. Some of the areas of difficulty relate to the direct effects of the disease and/or treatments, specifically continuing or late physiological effects and oncological events, such as recurrence or second malignancies. These physical sequelae can, in turn, produce disruptive indirect effects, for example, psychological and behavioural sequelae, such as increased psychological distress or decrements in cognitive functioning. Also, there is some suggestion that, even when adverse physiological effects do not occur, many cancer patients remained worried, and a few traumatically so, about their health. These concerns range from nagging health worries to anxiety about death. In addition to the physiological effects, scholars have focused on independent psychological and behavioural sequelae, including emotional distress (i.e. mood disturbance, traumatic stress), disrupted interpersonal relationships, and fertility and sexuality concerns.[22] Finally, economic or health benefit hardships may befall the cancer patient, including discriminatory employment practices, occupational difficulties[21,23] or restriction of health insurance coverage in those countries without nationalized health plans.[24]

Although many of the studies reviewed here did not include other dimensions of quality of life along with the sexuality measures, those that did include a comprehensive assessment usually found that, from a psychological perspective, survival after gynaecological cancer is, in general, positive.[8,25] This conclusion is tempered by factors that appear to be important moderators of outcome.[26] For example, the magnitude of treatment that women undergo correlates with adjustment, such that women who receive conservative therapies will, in general, report better psychological outcomes (*see* Table 16.1) than those who undergo radical therapies. Similarly, 'older' women report less distress than 'younger' women.[27]

Thus, it is within the context of generally positive adjustment for the 'average' gynaecological survivor that sexual disruption will occur for most. Although the positive adjustment in other life areas, mood, social relationships, etc., may provide a significant buffer for women in adjusting to any sexual problems that arise, it is clear that they cannot prevent most of the significant sexual problems.

CONCLUSION

The frequency of women abandoning sexual activity after vulvar cancer treatment is higher than the 'normal' base rate for healthy women. Moreover, even if intercourse is maintained, the post-treatment decline is more precipitous and reaches a significantly lower level than the decline that occurs with advancing age. Frequency of intercourse is an important 'barometer' of the sexual health of intimate relationships. Thus, any decline that is noticeable and extends in time will, necessarily, burden a woman, and possibly threaten the stability and satisfaction of her intimate sexual relationships.

Sexual morbidity is directly correlated with the extent of treatment, such that genital-preserving treatments will, necessarily, be more preserving of sexual functioning. Continued efforts to examine empirically the suitability of conservative, vulva-preserving therapies is one important effort that can be made by gynaecological oncologists to reduce sexual morbidity directly.

Regarding specific sexual difficulties, arousal (excitement) deficits play a central role in influencing the incidence and severity of other responses, such as desire and orgasm. Dyspareunia is also an important moderator of arousal. To the extent that medical interventions can directly address the problems of dyspareunia, rates of sexual dysfunction can be significantly lowered. Vigorous medical efforts to treat dyspareunia are needed; for example, encouragement to use vaginal dilators, lubricants and oestrogen therapy can be important.

In addition to the nature of the medical treatments, it is also clear that psychological factors, such as a woman's view of herself as a sexual person, is important in determining post-treatment adjustment. Women with negative sexual views will probably find that vulvar cancer treatment ends their sexual life; such women are not resilient to the multiple challenges that genital change brings. Identification of this risk factor can provide an opportunity to target rehabilitative services to such women.

REFERENCES

1 Andersen BL, van der Does J. Sexual morbidity following gynecologic cancer: An international problem. *Int J Gynecol Cancer* 1994; **4**: 225–40.

2 Andersen BL, Turnquist D, LaPolla J, Turner D. Sexual functioning after treatment of in-situ vulvar cancer: Preliminary report. *Obstet Gynecol* 1988; **71**: 15–19.

3 Weijmar Schultz WCM, Van de Wiel HBM, Bouma J. Psychosexual functioning after treatment for cancer of the cervix: A comparative and longitudinal study. *Int J Gynecol Cancer* 1991; **1**: 37–46.

4 Moth I, Andreasson B, Jensen SB, Bock JE. Sexual function and somatophyschic reactions after vulvectomy. *Dan Med Bull* 1983; **30**: 27.

5 Andersen BL, Cyranowski JC. Women's sexual self schema. *J Pers Soc Psychol* 1994; **67**: 1079–100.

6 McDonald TW, Neutens JJ, Fischer LM, Jessee D. Impact of cervical intraepithelial neoplasia diagnosis and treatment on self-esteem and body image. *Gynecol Oncol* 1989; **34**: 345–9.

7 Corney RH, Crowther ME, Everett H, Howells A, Shepherd JH. Psychosexual dysfunction in women with gynaecological cancer following radical pelvic surgery. *Br J Obstet Gynaecol* 1993; **100**: 73–8.

8 Andersen BL, Woods XA, Copeland LJ. Sexual self schema and sexual morbidity among gynecologic cancer survivors. *J Consult Clin Psychol* 1997; **65**: 221–9.

9 Andersen BL. Surviving cancer. *Cancer* 1994; **74**: 1484–95.

10 Andersen BL, Broffitt B. Is there a reliable and valid measure of sexual behavior? *Arch Sexual Behav* 1988; **17**: 509–25.

11 Andersen BL, Hacker NF. Psychosexual adjustment after vulvar surgery. *Obstet Gynecol* 1983; **62**: 457.

12 Stellman RE, Goodwin JM, Robinson J, Dansak D,

Hilgers RD. Psychological effects of vulvectomy. *Psychosomatics* 1984; **25**: 779–83.

13 Andreasson B, Moth I, Jensen SB, Bock JE. Sexual function and somatopsychic reactions in vulvectomy-operated women and their partners. *Acta Obstet Gynecol Scand* 1986; **65**: 7–10.

14 Weijmar Schultz WCM, Wimja K, Van de Wiel HBM, Bouma J, Janssens J. Sexual rehabilitation of radical vulvectomy patients: A pilot study. *J Psychosom Obstet Gynaecol* 1986; **5**: 119.

15 Tamburini M, Filiberti A, Ventafridda V, DePalo G. Quality of life and psychological state after radical vulvectomy. *J Psychosom Obstet Gynaecol* 1986; **5**: 263.

16 DiSaia PJ, Creasman WT, Rich WM. An alternate approach to early cancer of the vulva. *Am J Obstet Gynecol* 1979; **33**: 825.

17 Rodriquez M, Sevin B-U, Averette HE et al. Conservative trends in the surgical management of vulvar cancer: A University of Miami patient care evaluation study. *Int J Gynecol Cancer* 1997; **7**: 151–7.

18 Weijmar Schultz WCM, Van de Wiel HBM, Bouma J, Janssens J, Littlewood J. Psychosexual functioning after treatment for cancer of the vulva: A longitudinal study. *Cancer* 1991; **66**: 402–7.

19 Cella DF, Tross S. Psychological adjustment to survival from Hodgkin's disease. *J Consult Clin Psychol* 1986; **54**: 616–22.

20 Bloom JR. Psychological response to mastectomy. *Cancer* 1987; **59**: 189–96.

21 Bloom JR, Hoppe RT, Fobair P, Cox RS, Varghese A, Spiegel D. Effects of treatment on the work experiences of long-term survivors of Hodgkin's disease. *J Psychosoc Oncol* 1988; **6**: 65–80.

22 Andersen BL. Sexual functioning morbidity among cancer survivors: Present status and future research directions. *Cancer* 1985; **55**: 1835.

23 Houts PS, Kahn SB, Yasco JM et al. The incidence and causes of job-related problems among employed people with cancer in Pennsylvania. *J Psychosoc Oncol* 1989; **7**: 19–30.

24 Wheatley G, Cunnick W, Wright B, VanKeuren D. The employment of persons with a history of cancer. *Cancer* 1974; **36**: 287–9.

25 Andersen BL, Anderson B, deProsse C. Controlled prospective longitudinal study of women with cancer: I. Sexual functioning outcomes. *J Consult Clin Psychol* 1989; **57**: 683–91.

26 Andersen BL. Predicting sexual and psychological morbidity and improving quality of life for women with gynecologic cancer. *Cancer* 1993; **71**: 1678–90.

27 Roberts CS, Rossetti K, Cone D, Cavanagh D. Psychosocial impact of gynecologic cancer: A descriptive study. *J Psychosoc Oncol* 1992; **10**: 99–109.

Index

Abbreviations used in the index are: HPV = human papillomavirus; VaIN = vaginal intraepithelial neoplasia; VIN = vulvar intraepithelial neoplasia.